Understanding Environmental Health
How We Live in the World

Nancy Irwin Maxwell, DSc
Associate Professor
Department of Environmental Health
Boston University School of Public Health

JONES AND BARTLETT PUBLISHERS
Sudbury, Massachusetts
BOSTON   TORONTO   LONDON   SINGAPORE

World Headquarters

Jones and Bartlett Publishers
40 Tall Pine Drive
Sudbury, MA 01776
978-443-5000
info@jbpub.com
www.jbpub.com

Jones and Bartlett
    Publishers Canada
6339 Ormindale Way
Mississauga, Ontario L5V 1J2
Canada

Jones and Bartlett Publishers
    International
Barb House, Barb Mews
London W6 7PA
United Kingdom

Jones and Bartlett's books and products are available through most bookstores and online booksellers. To contact Jones and Bartlett Publishers directly, call 800-832-0034, fax 978-443-8000, or visit our Web site, www.jbpub.com.

Substantial discounts on bulk quantities of Jones and Bartlett's publications are available to corporations, professional associations, and other qualified organizations. For details and specific discount information, contact the special sales department at Jones and Bartlett via the above contact information or send an e-mail to specialsales@jbpub.com.

This publication is designed to provide accurate and authoritative information in regard to the Subject Matter covered. It is sold with the understanding that the publisher is not engaged in rendering legal, accounting, or other professional service. If legal advice or other expert assistance is required, the service of a competent professional person should be sought.

Library of Congress Cataloging-in-Publication Data
Maxwell, Nancy Irwin
  Understanding environmental health : how we live in the world / Nancy Irwin Maxwell.
    p. ; cm.
  ISBN-13: 978-0-7637-3318-6
  ISBN-10: 0-7637-3318-0
  1. Environmental health. I. Title.
  [DNLM: 1. Environmental Health. 2. Environmental Pollutants—adverse effects. 3. Environmental Pollution—adverse effects. 4. Environmental Pollution—prevention & control. WA 30.5 M465u 2009]
  RA565.M383 2009
  613'.1—dc22

                                                                          2008011316

6048

Production Credits
Publisher: Michael Brown
Production Director: Amy Rose
Associate Editor: Katey Birtcher
Associate Production Editor: Sarah Bayle
Marketing Manager: Sophie Fleck
Manufacturing and Inventory Control Supervisor:
  Amy Bacus

Composition: Cape Cod Compositors, Inc.
Cover Design: Kate Ternullo
Cover Image: © TebNad/Shutterstock, Inc.
Printing and Binding: Malloy, Inc.
Cover Printing: Malloy, Inc.

Printed in the United States of America
12 11 10 09 08   10 9 8 7 6 5 4 3 2 1

In memory of

Benjamin L. Maxwell, Scott R. Maxwell,
and Edward J. Murphy,
whose experiences brought home
the human cost of environmental illness

Contents

Preface

An introductory text like this one, which frames environmental health for a broad group of public health students, should leave its readers with a permanent awareness of environmental influences on health, as well as an appreciation of the societal roots of those influences. Further, it should prepare students who are not focusing in environmental health to engage the environmental health issues that will cross into their professional lives in other domains of public health.

Like many other schools of public health, the Boston University School of Public Health offers two introductory courses in environmental health. One is required of Master of Public Health (MPH) students who are concentrating in environmental health, and also of doctoral students in environmental health. A different course, which I have taught many times, introduces environmental health to MPH students concentrating in other areas—from social and behavioral sciences to biostatistics to health policy and management. These students are a mix of recent college graduates and experienced professionals. And, although the course is designed for MPH students, some undergraduates also seek it out. Thus students bring a wide range of professional and educational experiences to this beginning environmental health course. In particular—and this creates a challenge for both student and teacher—some students have done graduate work in science or medicine, while others have only modest backgrounds in college-level science.

Here are the distinctive features of this textbook. First, it is *briefer* than most introductory environmental health texts. It provides all essential information about environmental health for the MPH student and is designed to stand alone in an introductory course for students in concentrations other than environmental health. At the same time, the brevity of the book gives instructors flexibility to customize their course content by assigning additional readings if they wish to do so. Thus, with supplemental readings this book is appropriate for a unified introductory course in environmental health for MPH students in all concentrations, as offered in some schools and programs in public health. This brief book is also suitable as the environmental health text in a survey course in public health—and in a variety of interdisciplinary courses spanning other fields.

In light of the varied science backgrounds of public health students, this text's *treatment of science content* is designed for readers who have different starting points yet need to end up with the same understanding of the subject matter. An early chapter presents the fundamental science and methods of environmental health, much of which may be unfamiliar even to students with strong science backgrounds. In the rest of the text, sidebars present small bites of general science information at the point where it is first needed to understand an environmental health issue. This format directly addresses the challenge of the varied science preparation of the students, allowing each reader to fill in along the way whatever gaps in background knowledge he or she may have.

The book's *organization* also reflects its intended readership. Environmental health is a sprawling and diverse field, embracing many topics. Traditional topics in the field reflect professional specializations or regulatory domains; as a result, these topics are a mix of hazards (such as toxic chemicals or ionizing radiation), settings (such as occupational health), and environmental media (such as air or water pollution). For those outside the field—a core audience for this textbook—these categories do not easily add up to a coherent whole.

To provide that coherence, this text, more than most, tells a connected narrative, with chapters on the various things people do, as individuals or societies, that create environmental health hazards. After a brief introductory chapter and a substantial chapter on the science and methods of environmental health, there are chapters on the hazards of living with other species, including infectious disease; producing energy from fossil fuels, nuclear fuels, and alternative sources; producing manufactured goods, with the associated pollution; producing food through an industrialized agricultural system; and living in communities, from local to global. Traditional environmental health topics fit easily in this larger framework; as an aid to instructors, a table in the Appendix locates traditional topics within this book's chapter structure. The book's organization gives instructors considerable flexibility in allocating class time to chapters or chapter sections over the course of a semester.

Finally, this text offers a number of pedagogical features that serve both instructor and student. The *writing style* is direct and free of jargon, weaving together narration, explanation, and science. With the nontechnical reader in mind, the text makes explicit many assumptions and connections that are often left implicit, thus guiding the student through unfamiliar territory. *Key terms* serve as stepping-stones for the reader and appear in an extensive glossary of more than 500 items. *Learning objectives* and *study questions* are provided for each chapter, and *supplemental materials* for both instructor and student are available online. The text is enriched by photographs and supported by diagrams, graphs, and tables that summarize or explain important concepts and processes. One series of tables, building chapter by chapter, sets out the complex U.S. regulatory framework for environmental health.

I hope this book will leave students not only with a basic understanding of environmental influences on health, but also with an appreciation of the ways in which we all make the environment we live in.

Nancy Irwin Maxwell
Boston

Acknowledgments

In writing this text, I have benefited greatly from the wisdom and generosity of my colleagues at the Boston University School of Public Health who reviewed draft chapters: Richard Clapp, ever my first reader and formerly a teacher of the introductory environmental health course; Wendy Heiger-Bernays, teacher of the more intensive survey course for students focusing in environmental health; Michael McClean, a committed teacher and insightful critic; and Roberta White, my department chair, who supported this endeavor in ways large and small. As graduate teaching assistants in the introductory environmental health course, Gregory Howard, Patricia Janulewicz, Jessica Nelson, and Megan Romano gave helpful feedback as we used this text in manuscript form. More recently, my colleague Madeleine Scammell has generously used the full manuscript in teaching the same course. Needless to say, any errors that remain are my own.

I thank the many students to whom I have taught environmental health, because they in turn taught me what this textbook should be like. And thanks are also due to Mike Brown, publisher for Jones & Bartlett, who had a long wait for my manuscript but didn't give up; to the anonymous reviewers who provided feedback on the manuscript; and to the editorial staff who turned the manuscript into a book.

Finally, I thank my husband, Keith Maxwell, who has been a sounding board, critical reader, and voice of encouragement throughout the writing of this book. I would not have reached the end of this long road without his support.

A Preview of Environmental Health

Learning Objectives

After studying this chapter, the reader will be able to:

- Define or explain the key terms throughout the chapter
- Describe the scope of environmental health as a field of research and practice
- Articulate key aspects of Western-style development and its impacts

The traditional concept of the "environment" is human-centered, with everything that surrounds us defined as the environment. Science, however, tell us that the **environment** is a complex system of living things and natural processes, and the human species just one player in this web—albeit a player with disproportionate impacts. The field of environmental health is firmly rooted in this scientific understanding of the world, recognizing that the human species creates hazards to the health of the environment. Still, as a branch of public health, the field's core concern is the health of human populations, and its researchers and practitioners think in terms of environmental hazards to human health.

As shown schematically in **Figure 1.1**, **hazards** that are chemical, biological, or physical in nature are at the core of environmental health as a field of study and practice. At the margins of the diagram are genetic traits and social or behavioral hazards. **Chemical hazards**—perhaps the most familiar environmental health threats—include industrial pollutants, pesticides, lead paint, components of cigarette smoke, and a long list of other agents. **Biological hazards** (or biohazards) encompass the agents of infectious disease, but the category is much broader, ranging from molds that trigger allergic reactions all the way to genetically modified food plants. **Physical hazards** stem from contact with some form of energy. Radiation, noise, airborne dust particles, mechanical injury hazards, and extremes of heat and cold are all physical hazards. Thus, environmental health embraces much more than just industrial **pollution**.

However, as shown, the field does not extend to hazards associated with **genetic traits** per se. For example, the health hazards of the chromosomal defect that causes Down syndrome are not environmental health hazards. Still, interactions between genetic traits and environmental hazards—such as the effect of a woman's genetic makeup on her breast cancer **risk** from exposure to man-made chemicals—fall firmly within the scope of environmental health. And many environmental hazards *cause* chromosomal damage, with a wide range of health effects.

At the other end of the continuum, the boundary is fuzzier, but purely **social or behavioral hazards** to health, such as poverty or drug use, are generally seen as outside the field of environmental health. Again, however, environmental health embraces the boundary zone. For example, an interaction between the physiological effects of a social stressor and the asthma risk of air pollution is well within the scope of environmental health. And some hazards that are fundamentally social have effects that fall firmly within environmental health: for example, wars have exposed soldiers and civilians to pesticides and chemical weapons, to radiation from nuclear weapons, and to a host of infectious diseases.

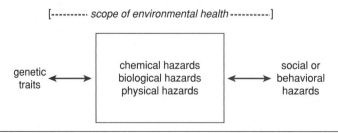

FIGURE 1.1 The scope of environmental health.

Finally, the field of environmental health tends to focus more on man-made (**anthropogenic**) hazards than it does on natural hazards. For example, the science base for understanding natural disasters such as floods, windstorms, earthquakes, landslides, or tsunamis is generally seen as outside environmental health. On the other hand, natural disasters often create environmental health hazards, such as the soup of industrial wastes that Hurricane Katrina left behind in low-lying New Orleans. Moreover, human beings' modifications to the natural environment have produced a **built environment** which, though it provides many benefits, also creates hazards to health.

This textbook, as an overview of environmental health hazards, is fundamentally about how we live in the world. After Chapter 2, "The Science and Methods of Environmental Health," which ensures that readers from different backgrounds share some key concepts, this book is organized around the things we do, as individuals or societies, that create environmental health hazards or expose us to them. Chapter 3, "Living with Other Species," presents a set of natural biological hazards—most prominently, infectious disease—that spring from the fact that human beings are only one species living among many. The burden of infectious disease is especially heavy in the world's lower-income countries.

In Chapters 4 through 7, the focus shifts from the natural setting to modern Western-style development. By the standards of any earlier era, the residents of today's industrialized countries are simply awash in *stuff*—from buildings and cars and home furnishings to clothing, chemicals, and food products. The biologist and early environmentalist Barry Commoner once noted that in an **ecosystem** nothing ever goes away,[1] and so society's stuff, along with its by-products, may move around or be transformed in the environment but will not simply disappear. Thus, modern development, wherever it occurs around the world, brings burdens along with its benefits.

Chapters 4 through 7 address these questions: Where does stuff come from? Where does stuff go? How do we make, use, and dispose of all our stuff? And how do all these activities affect human health? For example, when we consume oil and uranium, they don't disappear, but rather are transformed into energy and wastes. Chapter 4, "Producing Energy," describes the environmental health consequences of using fossil and nuclear fuels, as well as some alternatives to these energy sources. When we produce material goods and food products, we use energy to transform raw materials into products and more wastes, and Chapter 5, "Producing Manufactured Goods," and Chapter 6, "Producing Food," provide this environmental health context for our durable goods, consumer products, and food products. Chapter 7, "Living in the World We've Made," considers the environmental health concerns of sharing the world we have created. This chapter ranges from the hazards of living in local communities—where people consume food and water, use consumer goods, and produce wastes in the form of sewage and trash—to sharing the world's resources and looking toward a global future.

In the 21st century, the underlying reality of environmental health—that our stuff and its by-products may be transformed or moved around, but don't disappear—is playing out in a changed context. We have begun to see clearly the effects of a general failure to exercise foresight at the societal level: that is, a tendency to make decisions about new products and technologies without much regard for the longer term or the bigger picture. At the same time, globalization is now a fact of life. The natural environment, of course, has always been globally connected, but our appreciation of the global scale of pollution and its impacts is more recent. Global trade and travel have become rapid and extensive, with profound implications for environmental health. And with this global perspective, it has become clear that Western-style development is not **sustainable**—that is, the earth simply cannot support the world's entire population in the lifestyle to which the industrialized nations have become accustomed. And this reality in turn is reflected in the enormous disparities in environmental health burdens between the world's industrialized and lower-income countries.

Study Question

As you begin your study of environmental health, note any environmental health problems that have been important in your own life or in areas where you have lived.

Reference

1. Commoner B. *Making Peace with the Planet*. New York, NY: Pantheon Press; 1990.

The Science and Methods of Environmental Health

Learning Objectives

After studying this chapter, the reader will be able to:

- Define or explain the key terms throughout the chapter

- Define and distinguish among the key scientific and methodologic domains of environmental health, and explain how they relate to one another

- Explain how natural environmental processes and the characteristics of individual chemicals together affect the fate and transport of chemicals in the environment

- Describe routes of exposure and excretion, distinguish between exposure and dose and among different measures of dose, and interpret the key features of a dose–response curve based on a rodent bioassay

- Present a conceptual model of exposure, identifying key events or processes as well as estimates of a toxicant or its effects; distinguish between routes and pathways of exposure; and explain the standard units of absorbed dose

- Explain the distinction between descriptive and analytic epidemiologic study designs, compare and contrast the key measures used in surveillance, and discuss criteria for concluding that a statistical association represents a causal connection

- Describe the major steps in a risk assessment for the noncancer and carcinogenic effects of a chemical, explaining the outcome or product of each step, and contrast procedures for the risk assessment of a chemical with those for the risk assessment of a site

- Define risk management, distinguishing it from risk assessment, and give examples of risk management decisions or strategies, noting the relationship between risk management and environmental justice in policy and practice

- Summarize the range of activities that fall under the rubric of risk communication, including public participation in epidemiologic research and in policymaking

- Articulate the key elements of the precautionary principle as it is invoked in environmental health

As a branch of public health, the field of environmental health takes a population perspective. That is, our fundamental concern is not only with the health of individuals, but also with the health of populations—specifically, with environmental factors that pose a risk to the health of populations. As described in Chapter 1, this definition encompasses a wide range of hazards, from chemical and physical toxicants, including radiation and noise, to the biological agents of infectious disease and even interactions with genetic or social factors.

Yet many people, when they think of environmental health, think of pollution—and when they think of pollution, they think of chemicals. In fact, chemical contamination has been at the heart of environmental health concerns in the industrialized nations since the advent of synthetic organic chemicals in the mid-20th century. For this reason, much of this chapter is devoted to describing the science and methods related to chemical exposures and their effects. These approaches are also relevant to other toxicants such as particulates and radiation, as well as to plant and animal toxins.

The first four sections of this chapter describe the science base and research methods that inform our understanding of environmental hazards and their health effects in people.

- From environmental science, we learn about the behavior of contaminants in the environment—their chemical or physical transformations, and their movements with or between environmental media, such as air and water. Taken together, these events are commonly referred to as the **fate and transport** of contaminants in the environment (Section 2.1).
- **Toxicology** is the science of the effects of toxic substances—chemicals including natural toxins, as well as physical hazards such as asbestos fibers and radiation—in humans and other living things (Section 2.2). In a sense, toxicology continues the story of the fate and

transport of environmental contaminants into the interior realm, studying their movements, transformations, and ultimate effects in the body.

- The applied science of **exposure assessment** provides methods to measure or estimate human contact with environmental contaminants (Section 2.3). Exposure can be assessed both outside and inside the body, and so exposure assessment draws not only on an understanding of the processes of environmental fate and transport but also on insights from toxicology.

- Despite the enormous breadth and diversity of environmental health hazards, there is one research method that spans them all. **Epidemiology** (Section 2.4) is a quantitative research method for the study of the distribution and determinants of health outcomes in human populations. By bringing together biological understanding and specialized quantitative methods, epidemiology becomes a tool for documenting connections between environmental hazards and health effects. Specialized epidemiologic methods have been developed to study hazards ranging from chemicals to infectious disease to social factors.

The final four sections of this chapter describe the principles and methods that underlie our actions in addressing environmental health hazards.

- Operating at the interface between science and regulation is **risk assessment** (Section 2.5), an applied science. This process rests on a set of formal procedures for evaluating and integrating scientific information on exposure and toxicity to estimate the real-world public health risk of a hazard. As such, risk assessment is broadly integrative, bringing together information from environmental science, exposure assessment, toxicology, and epidemiology. In environmental health, the formal risk assessment approach is applied mostly to toxicants such as chemicals, particulates, and radiation; however, its influence can be seen in the evaluation of other hazards.

- **Risk management** (Section 2.6) encompasses the very broad range of actions taken to prevent or mitigate environmental health hazards. Risk management decisions are often informed by the results of a formal risk assessment, but of course many decisions must be made in the absence of such an assessment. Unlike risk assessment, risk management must balance risks, benefits, and costs, and also consider the social context of decisions.

- The term **risk communication** (Section 2.7) often refers to the sharing of information about an environmental health risk, such as a hazardous waste site, between experts and the public—a complex process because of differences in the way these two groups tend to conceptualize risk. However, the concept of risk communication also embraces informed consent by research subjects taking part in a study and, more broadly, community participation in epidemiologic research and even in policymaking.

- In contrast to risk assessment and risk management, which are methods for addressing environmental health hazards after the fact, the **precautionary principle** (Section 2.8) calls for the exercise of foresight in deciding whether or how to use new substances or implement new technologies in the first place. This commonsense look-before-you-leap approach to environmental health decision making offers an alternative to the casual adoption of new chemicals and technologies.

The assessment and regulation of environmental health hazards in the United States is complex, involving several major laws and numerous agencies. Moreover, many environmental health issues have international aspects. The federal agencies and other national and international bodies listed in **Table 2.1** play key roles in learning about and addressing environmental risks to health, and will be mentioned at various points throughout this text.

Table 2.1   US and International Agencies and Organizations Most Pertinent to Research and Practice in Environmental Health

---

Agencies within departments of the executive branch of the US government

---

US Department of Health and Human Services
  Public Health Service*—comprises the Department's health-related agencies (as opposed to its health care and human service agencies)
    National Institutes of Health—the primary federal agency for conducting and supporting health research
      National Cancer Institute—conducts and supports research on, and disseminates information on, the causes, diagnosis, prevention, and treatment of cancer
      National Institute for Environmental Health Sciences—works to reduce the burden of human illness from environmental causes, by defining how environmental exposures, genetic susceptibility, and age interact to affect health
        National Toxicology Program—an inter-agency program within the executive branch that evaluates agents of public health concern by developing and applying tools of toxicology and molecular biology; located administratively at the NIEHS
      National Library of Medicine—collects and organizes biomedical science information and makes it available to scientists, health professionals, and the public
    Centers for Disease Control and Prevention—provides a health surveillance system to monitor and prevent disease outbreaks (including bioterrorism), implement disease prevention strategies, and maintain national health statistics
      National Institute for Occupational Safety and Health—conducts research and makes recommendations for the prevention of work-related injury and illness
    Agency for Toxic Substances and Disease Registry—helps prevent exposure to hazardous substances from waste sites on the US Environmental Protection Agency's National Priorities List, and develops toxicological profiles of chemicals at these sites
    Food and Drug Administration—works to ensure the safety of foods and cosmetics (and also the safety and efficacy of pharmaceuticals, biological products, and medical devices)

US Department of Labor
  Occupational Safety and Health Administration—works to ensure the safety and health of US workers by setting and enforcing standards, and by providing training, outreach, and education
  Mine Safety and Health Administration—enforces compliance with mandatory mine safety and health standards to reduce accidents and minimize health hazards

---

US Department of Energy
  Energy Information Administration—provides data, forecasts, and analyses to promote sound policy making, efficient markets, and public understanding regarding energy
  Office of Civilian Radioactive Waste Management—manages and disposes of high-level radioactive wastes and spent nuclear fuel in a manner that protects public health and the environment, as well as national security

---

*The Commissioned Corps of the Public Health Service, a uniformed service of the United States, assigns individuals to assist many federal, state, local, or international organizations.

Table 2.1 *(Continued)*

US Department of Agriculture
   Agricultural Marketing Service—develops quality-grade standards for agricultural commodities and administers programs that regulate marketing
   Animal and Plant Health Inspection Service—protects and promotes US agricultural health, including animal welfare
   Economic Research Service—provides economic research and information to inform decision making on issues related to agriculture, food, natural resources, and rural America
   Food Safety and Inspection Service—responsible for ensuring that the nation's commercial supply of meat, poultry, and egg products is safe, wholesome, and correctly labeled and packaged
   National Agricultural Statistics Service—conducts monthly and annual surveys and prepares official USDA data and estimates of production, supply, prices, and other information

Independent agencies of the executive branch of the US government

US Environmental Protection Agency—responsible for protecting human health and the environment
US Nuclear Regulatory Commission—regulates commercial nuclear power plants and other civilian uses of nuclear materials through licensing, inspection, and enforcement
US Consumer Product Safety Commission—responsible for protecting the public from unreasonable risks of serious injury or death from consumer products

Private, non-profit institutions in the United States

The National Academies—advise the federal government on matters of science and technology
   Institute of Medicine—an honor society of scholars who provide independent advice on matters of biomedical science, medicine, and health
   National Academy of Sciences—an honor society of scholars who provide independent advice in various areas of science
   National Research Council—the operating arm of the National Academies, which conducts most of the National Academies' science policy and technical work

Agencies of the United Nations

World Health Organization—the directing and coordinating authority for health within the United Nations system
   International Agency for Research on Cancer—coordinates and conducts research on the causes of human cancer and the mechanisms of carcinogenesis
United Nations Environment Programme—promotes partnerships to care for the environment, with the goal of improving today's quality of life without compromising that of future generations
   Intergovernmental Panel on Climate Change—a scientific intergovernmental body set up by the United Nations Environment Programme and the World Meteorological Organization (also a UN agency)
UN Scientific Committee on the Effects of Atomic Radiation—scientific advisory group that assesses and reports levels and effects of exposure to ionizing radiation

Descriptions are derived directly from information on these websites. See reference section at end of chapter.

2.1 The Fate and Transport of Environmental Contaminants

The story of human exposure to environmental contaminants begins with the fate and transport of these chemicals—that is, their transformation and movement in the environment. Chemical contaminants in the ambient environment (that is, the general surrounding environment) can be found in air, water, or soil, including soil that is dry and fine enough to become airborne (dust) and soil in bodies of water (sediment). Before describing the movements of air and water in the ambient environment, this section notes some key characteristics of chemicals—for although chemicals are mere passengers in environmental media, they are, in a sense, passengers with preferences.

Physical–Chemical Properties of Chemicals

Chemicals have characteristics, known as physical-chemical properties, that affect their behavior in the environment (**Figure 2.1**). For example, the fate of a liquid chemical spilled on the ground depends partly on its **volatility** *(a)*—the tendency to change into gaseous form (that is, to volatilize). In the environment, a highly volatile liquid chemical that is spilled will move rapidly into a gaseous form that cannot easily be cleaned up. Similarly, **aqueous solubility** *(b)* is the tendency of a chemical to dissolve in water; a highly water-soluble chemical spilled into a lake is likely to become widely dispersed in the water. (Aqueous solubility is often referred to simply as solubility.)

A third property—a chemical's affinity for air versus water *(c)*—reflects whether the chemical is more volatile than soluble, or vice versa. In conceptual terms, such an affinity represents the division, or partitioning, of the chemical between air and water that would occur if the process reached a state of equilibrium. In practice, the shift toward such an equilibrium state in the environment may be rapid or slow.

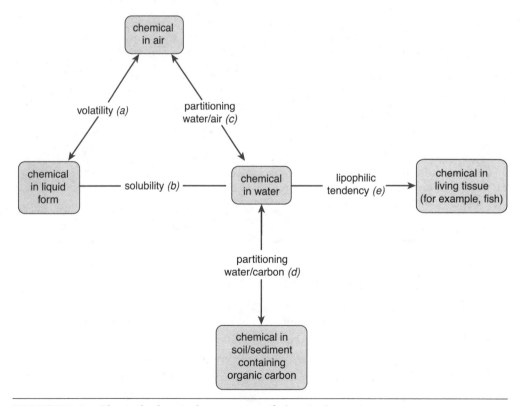

FIGURE 2.1 Physical–chemical properties of chemicals.

Chemicals also show an affinity for soil or sediment—actually, the organic carbon in soil or sediment *(d)*—versus water. Chemicals with a high affinity for organic carbon tend to cling to the sediments of a stream, for example, rather than being found in the water. Finally, chemicals vary in their tendency to move from water to an oily medium *(e)*. Chemicals having such a tendency are called **lipophilic** (fat-loving) or fat-soluble. Lipophilic chemicals in lakes or streams tend to move into the fatty tissues of aquatic organisms, or bioconcentrate; **bioconcentration** is a biological consequence of these chemicals' lipophilic tendency.*

A chemical that tends to bioconcentrate poses a potential threat to organisms through two processes. **Bioaccumulation** is the building up of a chemical in an individual organism's tissues over its lifetime as the organism continues to take in more than it excretes. **Biomagnification** is the process by which a chemical becomes more concentrated in the tissues of organisms at each higher level of the food chain—for example, in big fish that eat smaller fish, and in eagles (or people) that eat the big fish. Thus, bioaccumulation and biomagnification are not properties of individual chemicals but rather processes that take place in organisms and ecosystems.

In practical terms, groups of chemicals with similar properties show similar environmental tendencies. For example, low-molecular-weight solvents such as trichloroethylene and benzene are highly volatile and moderately soluble; they are very likely to become air contaminants, but unlikely to cling to soil. At the other extreme, very heavy chemicals such as polychlorinated biphenyls (PCBs) and dioxins have very low solubility and volatility; they are unlikely to be air or water contaminants, but rather are found in soil or sediment and also reside in fat. Chemicals' behavior can also be affected by environmental conditions; for example, a volatile chemical moves from liquid to gaseous state more rapidly in warmer weather.

Finally, a chemical in the environment does not persist indefinitely as the same chemical but rather is transformed into other chemicals. A chemical's **persistence** in the environment is often quantified as its half-life in air, water, or soil. The **environmental half-life** of a chemical in a given medium is the period of time after which one-half of the original quantity is expected to have been chemically or biologically transformed. The term *half-life* is borrowed from radioactive decay (see Chapter 4); however, unlike radioactive half-life, the environmental half-life of a chemical is only approximate because it is greatly affected by environmental conditions, such as the presence of light or oxygen. The half-life of the pesticide DDT in soil, for example, ranges from about 8 to 15 years. In general, chemicals of higher molecular weight tend to be more persistent. The environmental persistence in soil or sediment of high-molecular-weight, lipophilic contaminants such as DDT or dioxin presents the opportunity for long-term exposures and thus greater potential for bioaccumulation and biomagnification. Even persistent chemicals, however, do not persist indefinitely in the environment, but gradually break down.

---

*Some chemicals, including methylmercury, are not highly lipophilic but do concentrate in the muscle tissue of animals.

The Atmosphere

The earth's atmosphere, though it may seem formless, has a clear structure and regular patterns of movement.

Layers of the Atmosphere

The innermost layer of the earth's atmosphere, called the **troposphere**, extends to an altitude of approximately 8 miles (13 kilometers); within the troposphere, temperature declines with increasing altitude. Most of what we know as weather takes place in the troposphere.

Air in the troposphere is made up mostly of two colorless, odorless gases: by volume, about 78% nitrogen (N_2) and 21% oxygen (O_2). Of the remaining components, known as trace gases, the most abundant by volume is argon, which is chemically inert (that is, under ordinary conditions it does not react with other substances). Other trace gases are more important to life on earth, and to public health: in particular, water vapor (H_2O), carbon dioxide (CO_2), methane (CH_4), nitrous oxide (N_2O), and ozone (O_3) all function as **greenhouse gases**. As the earth radiates heat energy that it has absorbed from sunlight, greenhouse gases in the troposphere absorb some of that heat and reradiate it back toward the earth's surface. This return of energy—a natural greenhouse effect—keeps the earth's climate warm enough to support life.

Above the troposphere lies the **stratosphere**, reaching to an altitude of about 30 miles (48 kilometers). Within the stratosphere, temperature rises with increasing altitude. Roughly in the middle of the stratosphere is a layer in which the concentration of ozone is much higher than at other altitudes within the stratosphere. This **stratospheric ozone layer** absorbs much of the incoming ultraviolet radiation from the sun; without this protection, human beings could not live on the earth. (Ozone formed in the troposphere from anthropogenic pollutants, on the other hand, has negative effects on respiratory health, as described in Section 4.1.)

Beyond the stratosphere lie the two outer layers of the atmosphere: the mesosphere and the thermosphere. The atmosphere does not have a sharply defined boundary at its outer edge, but rather gradually becomes thinner and disappears.

Global and Local Patterns of Air Circulation

On a global scale, prevailing winds at the earth's surface are easterly in the equatorial region (**Figure 2.2**)—these are the trade winds, so named because they carried sailing ships on trade routes from Europe to the Americas. In the mid-latitudes, both north and south, westerly winds prevail; in the polar regions, easterly winds again prevail. These patterns result from the combined effects of two processes—the earth's rotation and vertical air circulation driven by temperature gradients—and can carry air pollutants over long distances, spreading them both horizontally and vertically.

Regular wind patterns also operate at smaller scales. For example, many coastal locations, where the land heats and cools more rapidly than the adjacent water each day, experience onshore winds during the daytime as well as nighttime winds that blow out to sea.

More generally, local and regional weather conditions affect the degree of horizontal and vertical mixing of air, and therefore the dispersion of pollutants in the air. Such dispersion may be

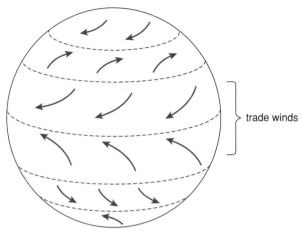

FIGURE 2.2   Global air circulation patterns.

visible near a source—for example, in the form of a **plume** of smoke trailing from a smokestack, becoming broader and less concentrated with increasing distance from the source.

It has been said that "dilution is the solution to pollution"—a view that is both provincial and shortsighted. Yet the reverse is certainly true: Local weather that *prevents* the dilution of air pollution can turn that pollution into an immediate public health threat. The extreme case of such conditions is a **temperature inversion**, in which a mass of cooler, heavier air becomes trapped at ground level—often in a valley—beneath a layer of warmer, less dense air. In such a situation, little mixing occurs, and emissions from local sources can accumulate under this "ceiling," causing pollutants to reach dangerously high concentrations.

Water in the Ambient Environment

Like the atmosphere, the earth's water can transport pollutants at global and local scales, in ways both visible and invisible.

The Global Hydrologic Cycle

The earth's water is connected via a complex web of processes, presented in simplified form in **Figure 2.3**. Not all aspects of this **hydrologic cycle** are readily apparent; though oceans, lakes, and rivers are prominent features of the surface environment, underground water is largely invisible.

As shown, evaporation and precipitation create a continuous exchange of water between the atmosphere and the earth's surface. The great majority of this exchange occurs between the atmosphere and the ocean. Further, the balance of precipitation and evaporation is different on land and sea: The oceans experience a net loss of water through these processes, while land areas experience a net gain. Most of the excess water from precipitation onto land returns to the oceans via rivers; a much smaller volume returns via groundwater.

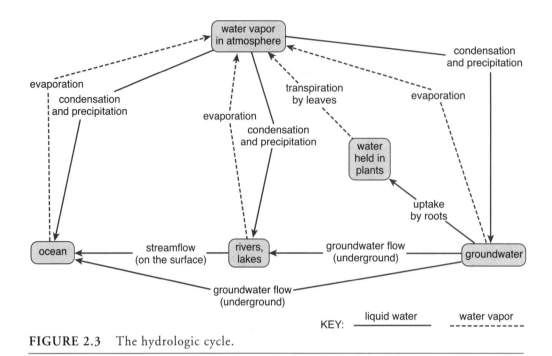

FIGURE 2.3 The hydrologic cycle.

Ocean Currents

Ocean currents play an integral role in moderating the earth's climate, and they also create underwater "climates" supporting populations of fish on which humans depend for food. And, like prevailing winds, ocean currents can carry pollutants long distances. In January 1992, a ship en route from Hong Kong to Tacoma, Washington, lost overboard during a storm several containers of plastic bath toys, including 7200 yellow plastic ducks.[1] The incident occurred near the International Date Line in the northern Pacific Ocean, south of the Aleutian Islands that extend westward from Alaska. Over the next few years, plastic ducks were recovered at Shemya Island, near the western tip of the Aleutians, at several points along the coast of the Alaska panhandle, and on the Washington and Oregon coasts. In 2003, one well-weathered duck turned up near Kennebunkport, Maine, probably having spun off westward in the Pacific and traveled around the globe.[1]

The major surface currents are driven by friction between air and water, and so they mimic the global prevailing winds: easterly near the equator and westerly in the mid-latitudes. But unlike the winds, ocean currents are deflected by the continents so that they form large rotating cells—flowing clockwise north of the equator and counterclockwise south of the equator (**Figure 2.4**). Waters leaving the equatorial region form warm currents; waters returning from the polar regions form cold currents.

Deeper ocean waters also circulate along predictable paths, moving more slowly than surface waters and looping through all the world's oceans like a continuous conveyor belt. This process is largely independent of the surface currents, being driven mainly by differences in the density

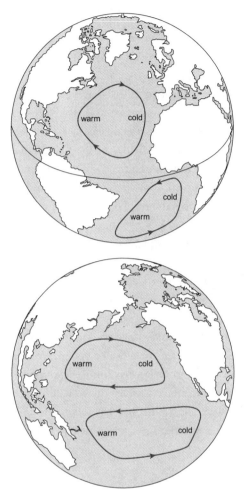

FIGURE 2.4   Major surface currents of the Atlantic and Pacific Oceans.

of the water related to temperature and salinity—and therefore known as the **thermohaline circulation**.

The global thermohaline circulation is propelled by events in the North Atlantic. Here deeper seawater is northbound along the European coast. The northbound water quickly becomes both colder and saltier (because salt is excluded from ice that is being formed). Both these changes make the seawater denser, and as a result it drops suddenly to the ocean floor. This event drives the beginning of a new global circuit by the deep ocean waters.

The Earth's Fresh Water

Lakes and rivers are perhaps the earth's most familiar water features. Typically, rivers begin as small streams that converge in stepwise fashion, ultimately uniting as a river. The area drained by a river and the streams that feed it is referred to as the river's **drainage basin**. Some surface water systems span very large geographic regions—for example, the drainage basin of the Amazon River, with all its tributaries, extends throughout Brazil. Pollutants can travel long distances in rivers and in the sediments they carry.

Confusingly, the term **watershed** is used in two ways: as a synonym for drainage basin (that is, an area); and to refer to the divide between two drainage basins (that is, a line). For example, in the Boston area, a community organization works to protect the Charles River watershed (drainage basin). A three-way watershed (divide) in the Canadian Rockies sends glacial meltwater from the Columbia Icefield to the Atlantic, Pacific, and Arctic Oceans. The Continental Divide in the US Rocky Mountains is another watershed on a grand scale. In environmental health, the term most often refers to a drainage basin, within which sources of pollution might be a concern.

Less visible than rivers, and far less familiar to most people, is the water located underground (see the conceptual model in Figure 2.3 and a more concrete diagram in **Figure 2.5**). Underground water resides in **aquifers**—geologic material that is porous enough to hold and transmit water. Aquifers are most often sand or gravel but can be porous rock such as sandstone, or even fractured rock, and they are typically covered by surface soil.

As precipitation soaks into the ground above an aquifer, water trickles downward through pore spaces. In the topmost subsurface zone, water also moves upward and into the atmosphere. This can occur either via **evaporation** (within the top foot or so) or by a process called **transpiration**, through which water taken up by the roots of plants is released to the atmosphere through their leaves. Whenever more water enters the topmost zone from precipitation than leaves through evaporation and transpiration, water trickles further downward.

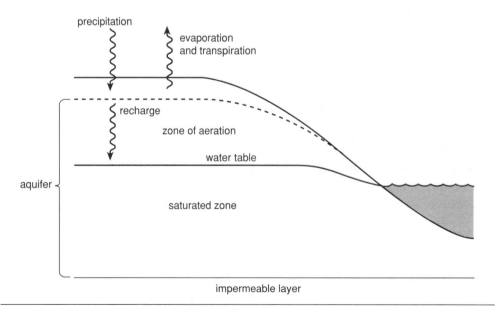

FIGURE 2.5   A water table aquifer.

Below this surface zone of two-way movement of water is a region known as the **zone of aeration**. In this zone, the pore spaces are partly filled by water. Here water moves only downward, and it moves downward only when water from above disturbs it. Water that trickles downward through the zone of aeration **recharges** the aquifer—that is, feeds or replenishes it.

Below the zone of aeration is the **saturated zone**, in which all pore spaces are filled with water. In the saturated zone, water—now called **groundwater**—can move in any direction. Usually, it seeps slowly in response to gradients of elevation and pressure toward a location where water is discharged continuously—for example, via a spring. In most locations, groundwater flows at a rate of only centimeters or inches per day.* In speaking of groundwater flow, the terms **upgradient** and **downgradient** are used in place of *upstream* and *downstream*.

The boundary between the zone of aeration and the saturated zone is called the **water table**. If more water is entering the aquifer (recharge) than is leaving it (discharge), the level of the water table rises; but if recharge is not enough to offset discharge, the water table falls. Typically, there is an annual cycle in the level of the water table related to patterns of precipitation and temperature, evaporation and transpiration.

The area on the ground surface through which rainfall feeds an aquifer is called the aquifer's **recharge area**. The lower limit of the aquifer—the floor—is an underlying layer of rock or clay that is impermeable, or nearly so. In a simple geologic setting like the one just described, the recharge area is directly above the aquifer, with no intervening impermeable layer. This is called an **unconfined aquifer** or **water table aquifer**. The surface of the water table often follows, in muted fashion, the contours of the land surface above. (In fact, contour lines are used to represent the water table surface in maps, much as they are used to represent differences in surface elevation.) If a well is drilled into a water table aquifer—leaving a cylinder made of a fine mesh so that water flows into the borehole—the water level in the well will be the same as that in the surrounding aquifer.

Wastes or other products placed in the ground or on the earth's surface within a water table aquifer's recharge area can contaminate the aquifer. For example, if a chemical such as trichloroethylene is spilled on the ground surface, or dumped into a pit, it can trickle down to the water table. The contamination will then take the form of a plume as the chemical is carried along slowly with the groundwater, gradually dispersing horizontally and vertically—not unlike an airborne plume of smoke. A well that draws water from within such a plume will produce contaminated water.

Similarly, rainwater percolating downward through wastes placed on the ground surface or in a pit can dissolve out or suspend contaminants and carry them along—much as water poured through ground coffee beans dissolves out the substances that turn the water into coffee. Water that has been contaminated by such **leaching** of contaminants is known as **leachate**.

---

*In formations of limestone, mildly acidic groundwater can dissolve the rock, carving out pipelike channels for groundwater, but such "underground rivers" are unusual.

An aquifer that is sandwiched between layers of impermeable (or nearly impermeable) rock is known as a **confined aquifer**. In a confined aquifer, the surface of the groundwater does not rise and fall in response to rainfall as in an unconfined aquifer. Rather, it is largely isolated from local precipitation—although some confined aquifers are replenished by rainfall in a distant location. The water stored in a confined aquifer is under pressure. As a result, if a well is drilled into a confined aquifer, the water level in the well rises above the top of the aquifer. The water pressure may even be great enough that the water rises above the ground's surface, so that no pumping is needed. This type of well is called an **artesian well**.

Where the ground's surface intersects the water table, groundwater is connected to surface water. A spring may be visible on a hillside, for example, as the origin of a small stream. Less obviously, groundwater and surface water connect beneath lakes and streams. In humid regions, the local water table is often higher than a streambed so that groundwater moves into the stream. In arid locations, the local water table is sometimes lower than a streambed; under these conditions, water drains from the stream into the ground.

Today's aquifers were formed long ago and bear the imprint of their geologic histories. In many geologic settings, layers of water-bearing rock alternate with impermeable layers so that aquifers are stacked beneath the earth's surface. Aquifers vary widely in geographic scale. For example, some 25 aquifers are recognized in Massachusetts; in contrast, the extensive Ogallala Aquifer underlies parts of eight US states from South Dakota to Texas.

2.2 Toxicology: The Science of Poisons

The term *environment* suggests something that merely surrounds us, but we are more permeable than we like to think. People contact—and absorb—environmental contaminants mainly by three major **routes of exposure**: **inhalation** (through ordinary continuous breathing), **ingestion** (by eating and drinking), and **dermal contact** (via the skin). Toxicology is the study of how the body processes the toxicants to which it is exposed and, in turn, the ultimate effects of these toxicants in the body.

In toxicology, the term **toxin** is reserved for a naturally produced toxic substance, especially one produced by a plant or animal. The term **toxicant** usually refers to toxic substances that result from human activities, although this definition is stretched to include such naturally occurring agents as toxic metals (for example, arsenic) or radiation that are not produced by a plant or animal. In this text, the term *toxicant* is used except when specifically referring to natural plant or animal toxins.

The Disposition of Chemicals in the Body

Whatever the route of exposure, a chemical is absorbed into the body by passing through cell membranes. From the exposure perspective, the linings of the lungs and digestive tract may be thought of as part of the boundary between the external and internal environments—in effect, as extensions of the skin. In fact, absorption via inhalation and ingestion is much more rapid and complete than dermal absorption because the lungs and digestive tract are designed to absorb oxygen and nutrients, whereas the skin is fundamentally a protective barrier. **Exposure to** environmental toxicants is often defined as *contact with the human envelope*, and the **human envelope** is defined in turn as the boundary that separates the interior of the human body from the exterior environment, as just described. Exposure is quantified as a **dose**, and the term **absorbed dose** refers specifically to the amount of some toxicant that passes through the human envelope, entering the body.

After being absorbed, chemicals are distributed around the body via the bloodstream or the lymph system, and may be metabolized (that is, chemically transformed by enzymes) during the course of this journey. Much, though not all, metabolism of chemicals takes place in the liver. These processes interact: a chemical's path through the circulatory system affects how it is metabolized; and how and where it is metabolized determines its chemical form, which in turn affects whether and how it is stored or excreted. These processes are shown in simplified form in **Figure 2.6**. The term **metabolite** refers to a product of the body's metabolism of a toxicant or toxin.

Lipophilic contaminants, including some pesticides, are stored in fat cells, and lead is deposited in bone (where it substitutes for calcium). Toxicants in such storage depots have been taken out of circulation and are not available to interact with a vulnerable tissue. However, excretion, by removing some quantity of a toxicant from circulation, can allow some of the same toxicant to be released from storage. Chemicals are excreted from the body mostly in exhaled air, urine, and feces, but also in sweat and semen, and by deposition in hair and nails, which in this context are seen as being outside the human envelope. Breast milk may also be a route of excretion; from the perspective of the infant, of course, breast milk becomes a source of ingestion exposure.

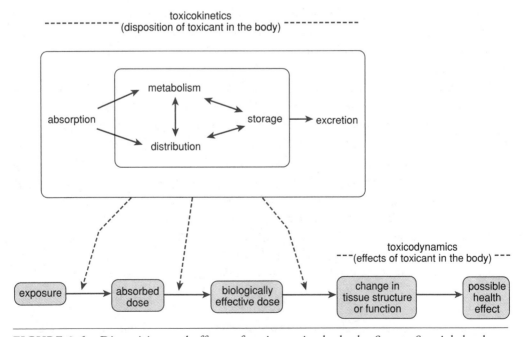

FIGURE 2.6 Disposition and effects of toxicants in the body. *Source*: Special thanks to Wendy Heiger-Bernays and Michael McClean.

The combined processes of **absorption**, **distribution**, **metabolism**, **storage**, and **excretion** of toxicants are referred to as **toxicokinetics** and determine the disposition of a chemical in the body. The net effect of these processes is reflected in the total burden of the chemical or of some breakdown product present in the body at some point in time (the **body burden**). Of more interest in toxicology, however, is the **biologically effective dose**: the quantity of a toxicant or its breakdown product that is available to interact with some vulnerable tissue in the body. Such interactions may result in changes in tissue structure or function, which in turn may have an adverse effect on health; the term **toxicodynamics** refers to these latter processes, which constitute the toxicant's actual effects in the body. Thus, toxicokinetics and toxicodynamics together describe the behavior and effects of toxicants in the body.

Many factors influence the processes of disposition. The characteristics of the exposure itself—for example, a brief exposure (**acute exposure**) versus a long-lasting, low-level exposure (**chronic exposure**)—may influence disposition. Exposures to another toxicant may enhance a toxic effect (**synergism**) or interfere with it (**antagonism**). And finally, many individual characteristics—from age and sex to genetic makeup to health and nutritional status—can affect the fate of a toxicant in the body and make an individual more or less susceptible to its effects. In particular, children's capacity to detoxify chemicals is different from that of adults, and their bodily systems are vulnerable because they are still developing.

Carcinogenesis

The core scientific endeavor of toxicology is to elucidate how biochemical mechanisms of toxicity actually lead to toxic effects in the body—at the level of molecule, cell, organ, or organ system. This discussion focuses on one toxic mechanism, carcinogenicity, because it is pertinent to all cancers, and because the US regulatory framework handles carcinogenicity differently from all noncancer health effects. The mechanisms of noncancer toxicity are many and diverse, and largely outside the scope of this text.

Cancer begins with a change to the genetic code. An organism's genetic code is found in molecules of **deoxyribonucleic acid** (**DNA**) present in the nucleus of each cell. This same type of genetic material, with different information encoded, is found in organisms from animals to plants to bacteria and viruses. In higher animals, including humans, chromosomes are matched up in twos: Human genetic material occurs as 46 chromosomes in 23 pairs. The now-familiar double helix structure of the DNA molecule (see the following sidebar titled "About DNA and the Genetic Code") was first described by British scientists James Watson and Francis Crick in a landmark 1953 article in the journal *Nature*;[2] Crick's working sketch of the molecule appears in **Figure 2.7**.

Mutation is a change to the DNA of a cell.* A mutation that causes local damage within a gene—a small part of the DNA molecule gets changed—is called a **point mutation**. Some point mutations occur spontaneously; others occur when some agent (a **mutagen**) binds chemically to

---

*Prenatal chemical exposures can also have an **epigenetic effect**; that is, a heritable change in how a gene is expressed, without any change to the DNA itself. The study of epigenetic effects is a new and rapidly growing area in environmental health research.

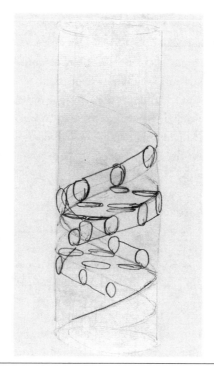

FIGURE 2.7 Francis Crick's early sketch of the DNA molecule still serves as a good representation of DNA's double helix structure: two spiral backbones linked by pairs of bases whose sequence encodes genetic information. *Source*: Courtesy of Wellcome Images.

the DNA, causing a change in its structure. Cells have mechanisms to repair DNA damage, but not all damage gets repaired. Mutations that cause broader structural damage to chromosomes—for example, the loss of large sections or reversing parts of a chromosome—are usually fatal to cells.

Mutations in the cells of the body have varied effects. As just noted, some mutations are repaired by cellular mechanisms; others have effects so severe that they lead to the death of the cell. Still others become the first step on the path to cancer.

Cancer is a disease of cells: A cancerous cell, dividing without restraint, operates outside of the body's normal controls. A malignant tumor, made up of such cells, first *invades* the tissue where it originated, and then *metastasizes* into other tissues, eventually disrupting the functioning of the body. Both genetic and environmental factors can affect an individual's risk of cancer.

Most cancers are believed to result from an accumulation of mutations in genes that direct cell division. Some of these genes (called oncogenes) instruct the cell to divide; others (called tumor suppressor genes) instruct the cell to stop dividing. The mutations that are important for carcinogenesis do one of two things: They either *increase the activity* of genes that instruct the cell to *divide*, or they *inhibit* genes that instruct the cell to *stop dividing*. If enough such mutations accumulate, the result is the runaway proliferation of cells—cancer. Overall, however, the probability of getting enough of the right type of mutations in any given cell is low, making cancer a relatively rare event in the cells of the body.

About DNA and the Genetic Code

The structure of the DNA molecule is the well-known "double helix," a sort of spiraling ladder in which the long strands are composed of sugars and phosphate groups. Each rung is made up of a pair of bases, and it is the sequence of bases that encodes genetic information. A large molecule of DNA is known as a *chromosome*; sections of chromosomes, each encoding a specific heritable trait, are defined as *genes*, each made up of a set of base pairs. In the rungs of the DNA ladder, the same two bases always pair with one another: adenine with thymine, and guanine with cytosine. When a cell replicates, each chromosome unzips, splitting each of its rungs in two; in this way, each half of the chromosome becomes a template to replicate the other half.

For some years, the process of **carcinogenesis** has been described as occurring in stages:

- *Initiation*. A mutation occurs that either enhances instructions to the cell to divide or dampens instructions to stop dividing. This event makes the initiated cell more prone to becoming cancerous. If the mutation is not repaired before the initiated cell divides, the mutation becomes permanent, appearing in all subsequent generations.
- *Promotion*. Various substances, including natural hormones and cigarette smoke, can stimulate cells to divide; in this way, an initiated cell can become a population of cells. Such promotion of the initiated cell does not involve further damage to its DNA. Instead, through repeated cell division, the initiated cell develops into a large group of identical cells—a benign tumor. Promotion has two effects: It increases the number of initiated cells, and, by making cells divide more often, it narrows the window of opportunity for repair of new mutations.
- *Progression*. Critical mutations (those that either enhance instructions to the cell to divide or dampen instructions to stop dividing) continue to occur in the initiated cells of the benign tumor. If enough of these mutations accumulate, the result is cascading cell division—a malignant tumor.

Environmental agents can play a role at each stage of carcinogenesis: as the cause of the critical mutation that initiates carcinogenesis; as promoters of the initiated cell; and as the cause of the critical mutations that constitute progression, leading to the runaway cell division that is cancer. The term **carcinogen** refers to any agent that increases cancer risk.

In more recent thinking,* initiation, promotion, and progression are still the key elements of carcinogenesis, but the process is no longer conceptualized as a neat time sequence, like a three-act play. Instead, in the modern staging of carcinogenesis, in a given performance (that is, tu-

---

*See, for example, Douglas Hanahan and Robert Weinberg. The hallmarks of cancer. *Cell*. January 7, 2000;100:57-70 .

mor) one act may be staged in several scenes, while in another performance two acts may be compressed into one. And in any given performance, each act is staged on its own schedule, with the result that acts may overlap.

Gene–Environment Interaction

As noted in Chapter 1, purely genetic hazards do not fall within the scope of environmental health. However, genetic makeup sometimes affects risk through interaction with an environmental exposure, and such gene–environment interactions are currently of great scientific interest in environmental health.

There are at least three models of gene–environment interaction. First, genetic makeup (that is, genotype) can increase a person's exposure to an environmental **risk factor**—for example, a genetic predisposition to nicotine addiction tends to increase exposure to cigarette smoke. Second, genetic makeup can increase a person's susceptibility to an environmental risk factor. For example, different genotypes might result in the production of larger or smaller quantities of enzymes that determine the capacity of cells to repair DNA damage—damage that is the first step on the road to cancer. And finally, genotype and environmental factors can be independent risk factors for a disease, with a combined effect that is additive or more than additive. For example, both a specific genetic trait and cigarette smoking are known to be independent risk factors for Crohn's disease, a chronic inflammatory bowel disease.[3]

The Dose–Response Relationship

Whatever the mechanism of toxicity, it is useful to establish the quantitative relationship between dose and a toxic effect (response). Such a **dose–response relationship** is typically summarized in a graph plotting dose on the *x*-axis against response on the *y*-axis. In toxicology, the **slope** of the line in such a graph is typically positive—rising from left to right—reflecting increasing toxicity with increasing dose, as shown schematically in **Figure 2.8a**. A steeper slope indicates a more potent toxic effect—that is, a greater increase in toxicity for a given increase in dose.

A second important characteristic of a dose-response relationship is the **threshold** (see **Figure 2.8b**). Again in schematic terms, the threshold dose is the highest dose at which no toxic effect occurs. The practical importance of a threshold (for example, *(a)* in Figure 2.8b) is that doses lower than the threshold dose are without toxic effect. If the threshold dose is zero *(b)*, then as a practical matter there is no threshold and no safe dose.

Now, giving our schematic dose–response relationship a more realistic shape, we show it as a flattened *S*, referred to as a **dose–response curve** (**Figure 2.9a**). In such a curve, the flatter slope in the low-dose region *(c)* reflects the body's ability to partially metabolize, detoxify, or excrete a chemical before it causes a response; as these metabolic processes are overwhelmed at higher doses, the slope of the curve becomes steeper in the middle region *(d)*. At very high doses, the capacity for a toxic response may be overwhelmed, and this effect appears as a plateau at the top of the dose–response curve *(e)*.

Figure 2.9b shows dose–response curves with zero and nonzero thresholds. A wide range of toxicological evidence suggests that nearly all noncancer effects have thresholds; thus a schematic dose–response curve for noncancer effects has the general form of *(f)*. In contrast, the

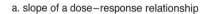

a. slope of a dose–response relationship

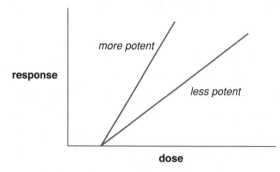

b. threshold of a dose–response relationship

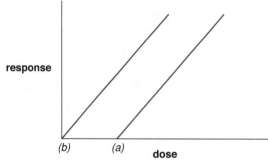

FIGURE 2.8   A schematic representation of the basic dose–response relationship.

mechanistic model of carcinogenesis as a multistage process suggests that any dose, however small, could produce an initiated cell that ultimately results in a malignant tumor. Thus, the schematic dose–response curve for cancer has no threshold (or a zero threshold), taking the general form of *(g)*.

Toxicity Testing

Toxicity testing—the practical work of assessing chemicals' toxicity to living things—complements the core scientific work of understanding the biochemical mechanisms of toxicity. This work, done in support of regulatory decision making, is often referred to as **regulatory toxicology**. In the United States, the National Toxicology Program is the lead agency in conducting regulatory toxicology studies.

In an ideal world, decisions about how to regulate chemicals would be based on studies of health effects in human beings (see Section 2.4 on epidemiology), and in fact such information is used when it is available. But epidemiologic research is limited by ethical standards that rule out deliberately exposing humans to potentially harmful substances. In contrast, toxicity testing in laboratory animals to serve the interests of human health is generally considered to be ethical. As a result, much of the information used to estimate the toxicity of chemicals in humans

a. slope

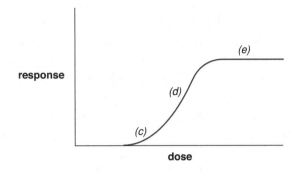

b. threshold/no threshold

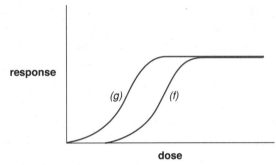

FIGURE 2.9   The dose–response curve.

comes from **bioassays**—toxicity tests in rodents and other laboratory animals. The relatively short lifespan of rodents—about 2 years for mice and rats—also makes such testing practical because even testing for chronic toxicity can be completed in 2 years. Similarly, given that cancer latency—the period between the exposure that initiates a malignant tumor and the recognition of the cancer—is roughly proportional to lifespan, carcinogenicity can be assessed in a 2-year rodent study.

Preliminary Testing for Toxicity

A 2-year chronic rodent study, which gives information on both cancer and noncancer effects, is a costly undertaking (typically, about $1 million to $2 million). For this reason, such studies are done only after preliminary screening for toxicity. Toxicity screening is typically conducted in a tiered process, beginning with tests in microorganisms and cell cultures, proceeding to acute and subchronic studies in rodents, and finally to chronic rodent bioassays. Studies in cells or microorganisms are referred to as *in vitro* studies; those in living animals are referred to as *in vivo* studies.

Screening for mutagenic potential in bacteria reflects the current understanding that mutation is integral to carcinogenesis. The mainstay of mutagenicity testing is the Ames test, an assay in which *Salmonella typhimurium* bacteria are exposed to a chemical. The test compares the rate of occurrence of a specific point mutation at different levels of exposure to the test chemical, with and without the addition of rodent liver enzymes (to metabolize the test chemical), and in multiple strains of the bacterium. Most of the organic chemicals that have been clearly identified as human carcinogens have been shown to be genotoxic in laboratory screens such as the Ames test. A separate laboratory assay for larger-scale chromosomal damage in human or animal cell cultures may also be conducted.

In a study of acute oral toxicity, groups of rodents are administered a dose of the test chemical, usually given all at once; several dose levels are used, including some expected to be lethal. Data from such a study are used to calculate the dose that is acutely lethal to 50% of test animals exposed to it; this 50% lethal dose is abbreviated as the **LD_{50}**. The LD_{50} is expressed in units of milligrams of toxicant per kilogram of body weight (abbreviated as mg/kg). If exposure is by inhalation, an LC_{50} is calculated; this is the concentration of the chemical in air that is acutely lethal to 50% of test animals in a short time, often 4 hours. A more general concept is the ED_{50}, the dose that produces a specific effect (that is, the effective dose) in 50% of test animals.

Further preliminary information about a chemical's toxicity in animals is obtained through the **subchronic rodent bioassay**, a 90-day study. These studies serve at least three purposes. They provide a basis for selecting the doses that will be used in a chronic rodent bioassay. They identify the **target organ**—in the language of toxicity testing, the organ that is affected first as the dose of a test chemical is increased from zero. And they also identify the need for specialized long-term study of particular effects, such as immunotoxicity, neurotoxicity, or effects on reproduction or fetal development. Although rodent bioassays are a standard approach for assessing the toxicity of chemicals, for some chemicals testing in rodents has not proved useful in predicting human risk.

The Chronic Rodent Bioassay

The **chronic rodent bioassay** is about 2 years long, approximately the lifetime of the test animals. Parallel studies are typically conducted in rats and mice; in each study, groups of about 50 animals, male and female, are dosed at three levels, in addition to an unexposed control group. Exposure is most commonly by ingestion (in water or food), less often by inhalation.

Because cancer is a rare disease, very large groups of rodents would be needed to study carcinogenicity at low doses similar to those at which people are typically exposed to environmental chemicals. But such enormous rodent studies are impractical in both logistics and cost; instead, rodents are exposed to very high doses, effectively converting cancer from a rare disease to a common disease and enabling smaller-scale studies. Thus, chronic rodent bioassays are designed to include both a dose high enough to test for cancer without being fatal to the test animals and doses low enough to reveal a no-effect level, if there is one.

Over the course of the study period, the animals are sacrificed, and a complete histopathologic examination is conducted on each animal. This allows the documentation of all cancers as well as a long list of other effects, ranging from gross changes (for example, enlarged liver) to changes at the molecular level. The proportion of rodents showing each effect at each dose is recorded. Specialized testing (for example, for neurotoxicity, immunotoxicity, or reproductive toxicity) is included.

Results of assays in laboratory animals are used to create a dose–response curve for each specific health effect, for example, kidney toxicity. Of course, the results of the assay can document effects only at the doses that were actually administered to the animals in the study, and therefore they give a limited view of the true underlying dose–response curve.

Some of the doses used in a study are given special designations (see **Figure 2.10a**). The *highest* nonzero dose at which *no* effect was observed in a study is called the **no observed adverse effect level** (NOAEL, pronounced "no-ell"), and the *lowest* dose at which an effect *was* observed in a study is called the **lowest observed adverse effect level** (LOAEL, pronounced "low-ell"). Neither the NOAEL nor the LOAEL pinpoints the actual threshold for kidney toxicity, but we can infer that the threshold falls somewhere between the NOAEL and the LOAEL.

However, sometimes all the nonzero doses used in a rodent study show some toxic effect—that is, the study does not identify a NOAEL (see **Figure 2.10b**). In this situation, we can infer only that the threshold is lower than the LOAEL; the study gives no lower bound (other than zero) for the range within which the threshold falls. In this situation, the study does not indicate whether there is, in fact, a threshold.

a. dose–response curve showing NOAEL and LOAEL

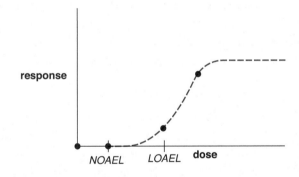

b. dose–response curve showing only LOAEL

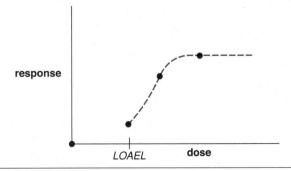

FIGURE 2.10   NOAEL and LOAEL in a dose–response curve.

For a given toxicant of concern, dose–response curves like these are developed for each cancer and noncancer effect documented in the chronic toxicity study, including the effects documented in specialized studies (for example, of immunotoxicity, or reproductive or developmental toxicity). These data help toxicologists learn about mechanisms of action and the behavior of toxicants in living systems.

In the language of toxicology, **reproductive toxicity** is the occurrence of an adverse effect on the reproductive system or reproductive capacity of an organism; **developmental toxicity** is the occurrence of an adverse effect on the developing organism—that is, in utero or during infancy or childhood. The term **teratogenesis** refers specifically to the occurrence of a structural defect in the developing organism resulting from an exposure that occurs between conception and birth, and a **teratogen** is a substance that produces such defects.

2.3 Exposure Assessment: An Applied Science

The preceding two sections describe important processes by which chemicals are transported and transformed—in the environment and in the body—and may cause biological harm. The applied science of exposure assessment is a set of methods to quantify contact between human beings and environmental toxicants. Assessing exposure is quite distinct from assessing toxicity, and both exposure and toxicity are necessary for a health impact to occur. Exposure assessment is important in studying the human health effects of exposure and also in controlling exposures to prevent harm.

Exposure can be assessed both in the external environment and inside the body, drawing on insights from both environmental science (Section 2.1) and toxicology (Section 2.2). In describing exposure assessment, this section first develops a conceptual model of exposure, and then describes how the model is quantified for the practical work of assessing exposure.

Completing the Conceptual Model of Exposure

As described earlier, toxicology provides a conceptual model that begins with the absorption of a toxicant and ends with its effects in the body (Figure 2.6). To consider exposure fully, the model in Figure 2.6 needs to be extended backward to begin with the environmental source of a toxicant. This has been done in **Figure 2.11**, while omitting the details of toxicokinetics provided in the earlier diagram. In Figure 2.11, *boxes labeled with capital letters* represent quantifiable estimates or indicators of a toxicant or its effects in the body, and *links labeled with numbers* designate events or processes that connect those estimates.

Exposure Pathways

Exposure to an environmental contaminant occurs via an **exposure pathway** that begins with the environmental source of the contaminant *(A)* and ends with exposure *(C)*, defined as contact between a toxicant and the human envelope. In some circumstances, the source *(A)* is an ongoing emission—for example, the release of lead into the air from the smokestack of a lead smelter. In other circumstances, the origin of the contamination is harder to pin down in place and time. For example, the lead present in the soil of most US cities today originates from the exhaust of countless moving sources—vehicles using leaded gasoline for decades in the past—

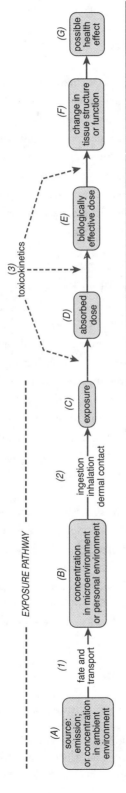

FIGURE 2.11 A conceptual model of exposure and dose. *Source:* Special thanks to Wendy Heiger-Bernays and Michael McClean.

and from the lead paint used on millions of houses, some of which are still shedding lead dust into the environment. It isn't really useful to think about these sources of lead as emissions. Rather, it is more useful to think of the source *(A)* of the lead as its widespread presence in soil, quantified as a concentration.*

From either type of source (A in Figure 2.11), chemicals may be transported in air, water, or soil, sometimes being chemically transformed along the way. These processes, together referred to as the fate and transport *(1)* of environmental contaminants, are described in Section 2.1.

As a result of the processes of fate and transport, a contaminant may be present at some concentration in a person's immediate surroundings *(B)*. Exposure assessors distinguish between **microenvironments** where exposure can occur (for example, a yard whose soil is contaminated by lead, or an office whose air is contaminated by volatile organic compounds) and the **personal environment**, that is, the immediate vicinity of a person's body, wherever that person goes. Thus, a microenvironment is stationary, whereas a personal environment is mobile.

Exposure Routes

Exposure *(C)*—contact between a toxicant and the human envelope—occurs by various routes. Most exposures to environmental toxicants occur via three routes: inhalation, ingestion, and dermal contact *(2)*. These are not the only possible routes of exposure to chemicals—some pharmaceuticals, for example, are delivered by injection into the muscle, and others are sprayed into the nostrils to be absorbed through the nasal lining. But exposure to chemicals present in environmental media is usually by inhalation, ingestion, or dermal contact.

Table 2.2 summarizes the environmental media most associated with these three major routes of exposure. People continuously inhale air, of course, and along with it they inhale dust. Skin, too, may come into contact with soil or dust (for example, while gardening) or water (for example, while swimming or bathing) or with the toxicant itself, particularly in occupational settings. For young children, even dermal contact with food could be substantial in some situations (not shown in table).

People routinely ingest water and food for sustenance. They may also inadvertently swallow small amounts of water (referred to as **incidental ingestion**), perhaps while swimming in a lake or pool. Similarly, if dust is present on the lips, licking the lips leads to incidental ingestion of soil; in the same way, touching the lips with the hands conveys soil to the mouth. Both eating and smoking, for example, result in such **hand-to-mouth exposures**. In certain circumstances, such incidental ingestion can be substantial—for farmers or construction workers, for example, or for toddlers, who spend a lot of time on the ground (and whose hands spend a lot of time in their mouths).

---

*Environmental health practitioners often distinguish between *natural background* concentrations of a substance, such as the lead naturally present in soil as a result of weathering of the earth's surface; *urban background* concentrations of the same substance, such as the lead that is widespread in urban soil from leaded gasoline and lead paint; and the amount of a substance contributed by a specific source of interest, above and beyond these background concentrations, such as the lead from a particular lead smelter.

Table 2.2   Key Environmental Media Associated with the Major Routes of Exposure

Medium of Exposure	Inhalation	Dermal Contact	Ingestion
Air	✓		
Soil	✓(dust)	✓	✓(incidental)
Water		✓	✓
Food			✓

Contact with an environmental contaminant often occurs through multiple exposure routes. For example, a toddler is exposed to lead in the home mainly by ingestion (incidental ingestion of dust via hand-to-mouth activity) and by inhalation (of airborne dust).

Biological Markers of Exposure

The final elements of Figure 2.11, showing the events following exposure, appear previously in Figure 2.6 and are described in the discussion of toxicology in Section 2.2. From the perspective of exposure assessment, the absorbed dose *(D)*, the biologically effective dose *(E)*, and changes in tissue structure or function *(F)* are all quantifiable estimates or indicators of exposure to a toxicant. Such indicators are referred to as biological markers, or **biomarkers**, of exposure.

Quantifying Exposure

It is common wisdom that "the dose makes the poison"—an idea that dates back to Paracelsus, a physician of the late Middle Ages. So, to be of practical use, the conceptual model in Figure 2.11 needs to be filled out with quantitative information. The work of exposure assessment is to translate the event of exposure into an estimate of the dose of a toxicant. This can be done by measuring or modeling the dose, or an estimate can be made on the basis of questionnaires, records, or other data sources.

Measuring or Modeling Dose

In **Figure 2.12**, methods used to quantify exposure have been added across the bottom of the diagram that appeared in Figure 2.11. Specifically, in Figure 2.12, *measurement approaches labeled with lower-case letters* correspond to the quantifiable estimates or indicators labeled with capital letters, and *modeling approaches labeled with lower-case roman numerals* correspond to the events or processes labeled with numbers. Figure 2.12 is complex, and so a detailed explanation is provided here.

Ideally, exposure is quantified inside the body—that is, the absorbed dose *(D)*, the biologically effective dose *(E)*, or a change in tissue structure or function *(F)* is quantified—but often this is not feasible. Instead, external measurements are often made somewhere "upstream" in the exposure model, and mathematical modeling techniques are then used to estimate "downstream" concentrations or doses.

As shown in Figure 2.12, the most basic proxy for dose is simply the concentration of a toxicant in air, water, or soil *(A)*; measurements of these concentrations are made by environmen-

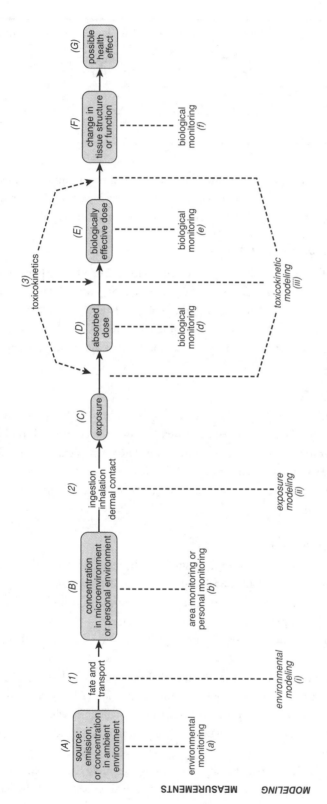

FIGURE 2.12 Measurement and modeling of exposure and dose. *Source:* Special thanks to Wendy Heiger-Bernays and Michael McClean.

tal monitoring *(a)*. A somewhat better proxy is the concentration of the toxicant at or near the location where exposure occurs *(B)*. Measurements may be taken in either the microenvironment or the personal environment.

- Measurements made in the microenvironment where exposure occurs (for example, the concentration of a toxicant in the soil of a yard or the air of a room) are referred to as **area monitoring** *(b)* in Figure 2.12. For example, a modified vacuum cleaner might be used to collect dust samples (**Figure 2.13a**).
- Alternatively, the measurement can be made in the personal environment—that is, the immediate vicinity of the body. For example, a subject in a research study might wear a portable air sampling device (see **Figure 2.13b**), collecting air samples from as close to his or her breathing zone as possible, even as he or she moves through different microenvironments. Measurements of this type are referred to as **personal monitoring** *(b)* in Figure 2.12.

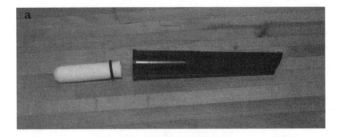

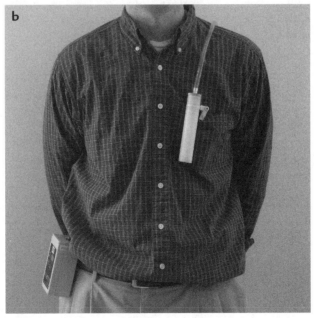

FIGURE 2.13   Area monitoring: a filter inserted into the nozzle of a vacuum cleaner (a) collects dust to be analyzed in a laboratory. Personal monitoring: A portable sampling device (b) incorporates a pump that takes a continuous air sample near the subject's breathing zone; the device also collects a sample of particulate matter over the whole period.

Some sampling devices accumulate a sample throughout an exposure period—for example, a portable air sampling pump might collect a single integrated sample of particulate matter throughout a worker's shift, and the chemical makeup of the sample could be analyzed later in the laboratory. A different device might measure and record second-by-second concentrations of particulate matter throughout the same shift, without collecting any sample. Yet another approach is to collect samples—of soil, for example—from different locations within an area of interest and then mix these samples together to create one composite sample for analysis.

If it is not possible to take a measurement *(b)* of the concentration of a toxicant at or near the location of exposure *(B)*, it may be necessary to derive an estimate of this concentration, using information from farther back along the exposure pathway. Thus, **environmental modeling** *(i)* can be used to estimate the concentration of a contaminant at the location of exposure *(B)*. Such modeling rests on understanding of the processes of environmental fate and transport *(1)* and uses as inputs measurements *(a)* of the concentration of the contaminant in the ambient environment *(A)*. As described in Section 2.1, the environmental fate and transport of chemicals is determined not only by movements of environmental media, such as air or groundwater, but also by the chemicals' own properties.

An estimate of exposure *(C)*, defined as contact with the human envelope, provides a somewhat better proxy of internal dose than do measured or estimated concentrations in environmental media *(B)*. Estimates of exposure rest on two kinds of information: a measurement or estimate *(b)* of the concentration at the location of exposure *(B)*; and **exposure modeling** *(ii)* of contact by ingestion, by inhalation, or via the skin *(2)*. Such modeling rests on assumptions about, for example, the volume of water a person drinks each day, the volume of air he or she inhales (and then exhales); or the area of the skin that is exposed to a contaminant.

All the methods for measuring or modeling exposure described up to this point provide estimates of quantities or processes outside the body. However, for some toxicants, exposure can be quantified *inside* the body. These methods use a measure of one of these indicators:

- The absorbed dose *(D)*, the quantity that passed through the human envelope
- The biologically effective dose *(E)*, the concentration in a specific vulnerable tissue
- Some change in tissue structure or function *(F)* caused by the biologically effective dose

The corresponding biological measurement methods *(d, e, f)* are known collectively as biological monitoring, or **biomonitoring**. As noted previously, the measures themselves are called biomarkers.

For example, the concentration of mercury in hair or fingernails, the concentration of lead in blood (used to screen for childhood lead poisoning), and the concentration of alcohol in exhaled air (the police officer's breathalyzer test for drunk drivers) are all biomarkers offering different windows onto the *absorbed dose*. Similarly, environmental chemicals such as pesticides, heavy metals, and nicotine (or their metabolites) have been measured postnatally in meconium, the fecal matter that accumulates in the fetus during gestation, providing a biomarker of the prenatal absorbed dose. DNA adducts, formed when a chemical binds to a DNA molecule in the nucleus of a cell, are biomarkers of the *biologically effective dose*. And continuous firing of nerve cells is a biomarker of the effect of certain pesticides on these cells—*a change in tissue function*. Biomonitoring techniques are relatively expensive, and all impose some burden on the person whose exposure is being assessed—though providing fingernail clippings, for example, is less invasive than providing a sample of urine or blood. And for many toxicants, no techniques are available to make such measurements in the body.

Finally, biological modeling—specifically, **toxicokinetic modeling** *(iii)*—is sometimes used to predict the ultimate disposition of a chemical from what is known about its toxicokinetics *(3)*—the absorption, distribution, metabolism, storage, and excretion of the chemical. Toxicokinetic modeling is used to estimate the absorbed dose *(D)*, the biologically effective dose *(E)*, or a change in tissue structure or function *(F)* from some upstream measure. Because sophisticated toxicological understanding is required to develop toxicokinetic models, these models are available for a relatively small number of environmental toxicants.

Units of Absorbed Dose

Absorbed dose is usually expressed in units of milligrams of toxicant per kilogram of body weight per day, written as: *mg /(kg*day)*. These units incorporate two important concepts that are probably familiar even if the terminology is not.

First, the mass of contaminant absorbed into the body is **normalized to (averaged over) the body weight** of the person exposed; that is, it is divided by the body weight. This adjustment accounts for the fact that, for example, 10 mg of Chemical X is a greater insult to a 75-kg man than it is to a 100-kg man.

Similarly, the mass absorbed into the body is **averaged over time**—usually, expressed as a daily dose. This adjustment accounts for the fact that, for example, 10 mg of Chemical X absorbed by a 75-kg woman at 5 mg/day over a 2-day period is a different insult from 10 mg of Chemical X absorbed by the same woman at 0.5 mg/day over 20 days.

Thus, to calculate someone's absorbed dose of Chemical X from drinking tap water, these pieces of information are needed:

- The concentration of Chemical X in the water
- The rate at which water is ingested (for example, liters per day)
- The proportion of the Chemical X in the ingested water that is absorbed into the body
- The body weight of the exposed person

For example, the absorbed dose of trichloroethylene to a 70-kg individual who drinks 2 liters per day of water contaminated with trichloroethylene at 5 μg per liter, assuming 100% absorption of the chemical, is calculated as follows:

$$\frac{\dfrac{5 \mu g \text{ chemical}}{\text{liter water}} \times \dfrac{2 \text{ liters water}}{\text{day}} \times 1.0}{70 \text{ kg body weight}}$$

$$= 0.143 \ \mu g/(kg*day)$$

or, in standard dose units, 0.000143 mg/(kg*day)

Similarly, in calculating inhalation exposures, information is needed on the concentration of the chemical in air, the exposed individual's inhalation rate, and the proportion absorbed via the lungs. Calculation of a dermal dose (for example, a gardener's exposure to a chemical in soil) rests on information about the concentration in soil, how much skin is exposed, how much soil clings to the skin, and the rate at which the chemical is absorbed through the skin.

Other Sources of Exposure Information

Approaches other than direct measurement and mathematical modeling are also used to estimate human exposures to environmental hazards. For example, information about contact with environmental media can be obtained using a questionnaire—via in-person interview, telephone interview, or mail survey. Such surveys offer the possibility of direct answers to questions that can't be assessed in the field. For example, how often does the subject apply pesticides in the home? Or, for an exposure via tap water: How much tap water is consumed on a typical day? Does the subject take showers or baths? How often? How long? How hot? Surveys can also be used to gather information on past exposures, from a woman's job history to her history of using hair dye.

In a variation on the questionnaire approach, subjects in an exposure assessment may keep personal records over a period of time—for example, diaries of food consumption or time spent in different activities or locations. Historical exposure information may also come from previously existing documentary sources, such as municipal records of contaminant concentrations in drinking water.

Surrogate measures of occupational exposures—such as a worker's job title or the industry in which he or she is employed—are particularly well developed. This is partly because workplace exposures, which may be high and long-lasting, are of special concern. In addition, the occupational setting, which is more regimented than residential or community settings, lends itself to these approaches.

For example, the classification system used in the US Census Bureau's Economic Census defines thousands of industrial sectors ranging from synthetic rubber manufacturing to silver ore mining to shellfish farming. Similarly, job title might be used as a surrogate for potential exposure to latex gloves in a medical setting—distinguishing among nurses, midwives, physicians, medical technologists, and medical assistants, for example. This approach can be taken a step further by developing a job-exposure matrix—a table that provides an estimate of exposure for each combination of job title (in rows) and hazard (in columns). For example, each job title's exposure to each hazard could be rated on a scale of none–low–medium–high based on measurements or even expert judgment.

In recent years, the **geographic information system (GIS)** has matured into a useful tool for integrating and assessing exposure data. A GIS is a computerized system that combines a database of spatially linked information with application software for spatial analyses and mapping. For example, a GIS might include information used to assess environmental exposures, such as locations where pesticides have been sprayed for mosquito control, or the locations of plumes of solvent contamination in groundwater at different time points, or traffic volumes associated with each quarter-mile segment of a county's roads. In essence, such GIS assessments use location as a surrogate for exposure (see **Figure 2.14**).

Epidemiologic researchers can use geographic information systems to link subjects' addresses with environmental data. For example, in a study of the risk of cancer—a disease with a long latency—associated with contamination of private well water, researchers could link each sub-

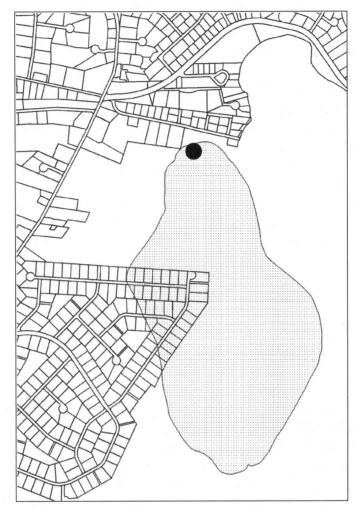

FIGURE 2.14   This GIS map of a chemical plume in groundwater shows that private wells on nearby properties located upgradient of the source are unaffected by the contamination, whereas wells on more distant properties located downgradient are at risk. *Source*: Courtesy of Verónica Vieira.

ject's current home address, as well as past addresses, to environmental data on groundwater contamination for the appropriate time periods. This information can be used to estimate exposures at a series of addresses.

2.4 Epidemiology: A Quantitative Research Method

Epidemiology is a quantitative research method used to document the distribution of health and illness in human populations and also to link health outcomes to risk factors. Simple quantitative methods were first used in the mid-1800s to demonstrate geographic and social differences in the effects of the most pressing health problem of the day, infectious disease. By the mid-1900s, epidemiology had become focused on the chronic illnesses, such as heart disease, which were by then killing more people than were infectious diseases in industrialized countries. In the era of computerized data processing, epidemiologic methods have become heavily analytical and statistical, and epidemiology also continually incorporates new understanding of the mechanisms and genetics of health risks. Infectious disease epidemiology has returned to the foreground in the age of the human immunodeficiency virus and acquired immune deficiency syndrome (HIV/AIDS) and other emerging infectious threats.

The scope of epidemiology today is as broad as public health itself. **Environmental epidemiology** is one of the major sources of information about human disease risk from environmental hazards. In environmental health, epidemiology is used mainly to study risks from chemicals and other toxicants, but also to study risks of noise, injuries, infectious disease, and even social factors. In the study of environmental toxicants, today's epidemiology often incorporates scientific insights from toxicology and practical tools from exposure assessment. In particular, biomarkers of exposure and disease are useful in epidemiology. But even when toxicological understanding is lacking, strong epidemiologic data can form the basis for public health action because it provides information about human beings. Further, actual human exposures are, by definition, within the range of concern, and the health effects studied, although they may be gross endpoints, are meaningful outcomes.

Perhaps the most famous epidemiologic study in the history of public health was conducted by John Snow, a physician, during an 1854 cholera epidemic in London. Hypothesizing that the illness was caused by contaminated drinking water, Snow compared the death rates from cholera according to the water company that supplied individual houses. He documented a more than eight-fold increased mortality among people living in houses served by the Southwark and Vauxhall Company, which drew its water from a heavily polluted region of the Thames River, compared to those served by the Lambeth Company, which drew its water from a part of the Thames not contaminated by London's sewage.[4] The design of Snow's study is fundamentally similar to those in use today.

This section first defines the key measures used to quantify health status in populations, and then outlines descriptive epidemiologic approaches as well as the study designs used to link exposures to health outcomes. The focus is on epidemiologic methods used to study chronic disease, but two specialized branches of epidemiologic research, infectious disease epidemiology and animal epidemiology, are also described.

Key Measures of the Health Status of Populations

Two fundamental concepts—incidence and prevalence—underlie all epidemiology. **Incidence** is the occurrence of *new (incident) cases* of a disease in a given population *during a given period of time*. Because only newly diagnosed cases are counted, measures of incidence are useful in identifying factors that might be associated with the onset of disease.

Mortality can be thought of as the incidence of death: It is the total number of deaths in a given population during a given period of time. Cause-specific mortality can be reported in the same way. Mortality data have certain limitations from a research perspective because mortality from a particular disease can be affected by various factors that operate between diagnosis and death (for example, treatment). Cause-specific mortality is also affected by deaths from other causes—some people who have colon cancer, for example, die in automobile accidents. However, mortality data offer a practical advantage: Because death is the easiest health outcome to ascertain, mortality data are sometimes available where disease data are not. Historically, the earliest surveillance data collected were mortality statistics, and mortality is still an important indicator of the overall health of populations—witness the stark differences in mortality between industrialized countries and lower-income countries.*

In contrast to incidence, **prevalence** quantifies *existing cases* of a disease, specifically, the proportion of a population that has a disease *at a given point in time*. Thus, the prevalence of a disease in a population reflects the incidence of the disease, which contributes to the pool of cases, and also the mortality rate for the disease, which removes cases from the pool. The prevalence of HIV/AIDS in Massachusetts on January 1, 2008, for example, reflects not only factors that affect the onset of the illness but also factors that affect how long people survive with the illness, such as treatment options and the availability of medical care. For this reason, although prevalence figures are useful in assessing the burden of disease or in planning for health services, they are not generally useful in assessing potential risk factors for disease, including environmental risk factors.

The term **morbidity** refers to a diseased (morbid) state, and this can be quantified in a population as prevalence. For example, some sub-Saharan African countries bear a heavy burden of morbidity caused by malaria, as reflected in a high prevalence of malaria infection reported by the WHO.[5]

Various definitions of **disability** have been used in the public health literature and in the movement to protect the rights of people with disabilities, but a core element of the definition is a limitation on a major life activity.[6] Typically, the term *disability* is used to refer to a substantial and/or long-term limitation in a major age-appropriate life activity related to work, school, or caring for oneself. This limitation might be physical or mental. Thus, for example, an inability to walk, or to bathe oneself, or to prepare food, or to make change, or remember one's address could all be considered disabilities. The Americans with Disabilities Act defines disability to include not only such an impairment but also "a record of such an impairment" or "being regarded as having such an impairment."[6] A disability can make an individual more susceptible to the effects of environmental hazards. For example, those with impaired mobility were especially susceptible to injury and death in the wake of Hurricane Katrina, and individuals with chronic lung disease, such as asthma or emphysema, are more susceptible to the respiratory effects of common air pollutants.

---

*As used in this text, the term *industrialized countries* refers to countries in the regions designated by the World Health Organization as *more developed regions* (Europe, North America, Australia/New Zealand, and Japan); and the term *lower-income countries* refers to countries in other areas, designated by the UN as *less developed regions* (World Health Organization. *Definition of Major Areas and Regions.* Available at: http://esa.un.org/unpp/index.asp?panel=5. Accessed July 31, 2006).

Descriptive Epidemiology

Descriptive epidemiology, as the name suggests, simply describes patterns of disease in populations—that is, in existing groups rather than in groups assembled for the purpose of a research study. Further, descriptive epidemiology does not seek to link disease risk statistically to specific factors. Descriptive epidemiologic methods—in particular, disease surveillance—are the everyday tools of environmental health practitioners in city, county, and state health departments. For this reason, this text gives greater emphasis to these descriptive approaches than to the research study designs that are the focus of most courses in epidemiology.

Surveillance

To conduct environmental health **surveillance** is to survey the landscape of illness. Surveillance is fundamentally a comparative exercise. The objective of surveillance is to track and compare disease rates in populations across places, across diseases, or over time. In environmental health, surveillance data often highlight unusual patterns that may provide clues to an environmental risk factor for disease. In public health more broadly, surveillance data are used for policy and planning purposes.

In the United States, state departments of public health typically gather and report disease data. Nearly every state, for example, has a cancer registry—an agency that receives a report of each cancer diagnosis in the state (including the residential address of the patient) and uses this information to track the incidence of various types of cancer and to document geographic patterns. Other health outcomes, from HIV/AIDS to birth defects to gunshot injuries, may also be tracked by state or federal agencies. At the federal level, the US Centers for Disease Control and Prevention (CDC) conducts surveillance, including infectious disease surveillance (see **Figure 2.15**). The CDC also helps states develop their capacity for surveillance, also called *environmental public health tracking*.

The concept of surveillance can be extended to include biomonitoring at the population level. Such **surveillance biomonitoring** often documents exposure rather than illness—for example, monitoring of blood lead concentrations in young children. The concept of surveillance can be further extended to include tracking of health hazards, such as releases of toxic chemicals.

The measure of incidence most commonly used in disease surveillance is the **crude incidence rate**. The crude incidence rate is not an abstraction but rather is tied to a given population and time period. The numerator is simply the number of new cases that arose in the given population during the given time period. The denominator represents both the size of the population at risk and the time period of interest, and thus is quantified as person-years. A denominator of 2000 person-years, for example, might represent a population of 2000 over a 1-year period or a population of 200 over a 10-year period. A crude incidence rate is calculated by simply dividing the numerator by the denominator. For example, 300 new cases of a disease in a population of 100,000 over a 10-year period yields a crude incidence of 0.0003 per year.

The incidence of many diseases is different in males and females; similarly, incidence often varies by age group. Thus, if the crude incidence of lung cancer is different in two towns, the difference may be caused partly or entirely by differences in the age and sex makeup of the towns' populations. Similarly, if the crude incidence of lung cancer is the same in two towns,

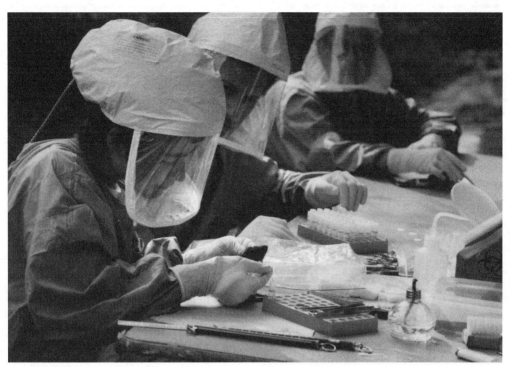

FIGURE 2.15   CDC workers inspect specimens that may be connected to an outbreak of hantavirus, an emerging infectious threat. *Source*: Reprinted courtesy of CDC Public Health Image Library. ID# 7271. Content provider: CDC. Available at: http://phil.cdc.gov/phil/details.asp. Accessed October 3, 2007.

this statistic may obscure a genuine difference in risk. In the example shown in **Table 2.3**, the annual incidence of female breast cancer is 60% higher in Location A than it is in Location B. However, the table also shows that the female population of Location A is somewhat older than that of Location B. Since it is well known that breast cancer is more common in older women, Location A's age makeup may explain, or partly explain, the higher incidence there.

Because comparing incidence across locations and time periods is a fundamental task of surveillance, issues like this one must be addressed. The effects of sex on incidence are usually resolved by reporting separately for males and females. The effects of age on incidence, on the

Table 2.3   Annual Incidence of Female Breast Cancer and Age Distribution of the Female Population in Two Locations for a Given Time Period

Location	Crude Annual Incidence	Proportion of Population in Each Age Group		
		Premenopausal	Perimenopausal	Postmenopausal
Location A	0.0021	0.55	0.09	0.36
Location B	0.0013	0.65	0.10	0.25

other hand, are usually handled through reporting methods that adjust for differences in age distribution. (It is also possible to adjust for both age and sex differences.)

Any method of age adjustment must take account of the separate effects of two factors:

- A population's age distribution (that is, the proportion of the population that falls into each age category)
- The age-specific incidence of disease in each age category

Two basic approaches are used to adjust crude incidence rates so that data for different populations can legitimately be compared. Both approaches use yet another population as a reference—a sort of intermediary for comparison.

One approach is to apply the actual age-specific rates of disease in Location A and those in Location B in their respective populations but substitute the age distribution of a third population used as a reference population (**Figure 2.16**). This yields a hypothetical total number of cases, and thus a hypothetical overall rate of disease, for Location A and Location B. These rates are called **standardized rates** because they have been *adjusted to a standard age structure.* For example, the standardized rate for Location A is the overall rate that *would occur* in Location A if its actual age-specific rates were operating but its population had the age distribution of the reference population. In the United States, the US population as reported in a decennial census is often used as a reference population.

Because the standardized rates for Locations A and B rest on the same age distribution, they can be compared directly (see Figure 2.16). This is typically done in a ratio, called a **standardized rate ratio**, or **SRR** (standardized rate in Location A/standardized rate in Location B). For example, if the standardized rate in Location A is 0.0005 per year, and the standardized rate in Location B is 0.00025 per year, the standardized rate ratio is 2.0, which means that the rate of illness in Location A is twice that in Location B. A standardized rate for just one location is not particularly useful given that it is a hypothetical rate; the point of this approach is to be able to compare standardized rates for different populations by using the ratio.

The inverse approach is taken in calculating a **standardized incidence ratio** (SIR): The age-specific rates of a reference population are applied to the populations of Locations A and B, using their actual age distributions (**Figure 2.17**). This yields the total number of cases that would be expected in Locations A and B if the reference age-specific rates were operating in the local populations. For Location A and Location B, this expected number of cases is then compared to the actual (or observed) total number in a ratio called the standardized incidence ratio (observed cases/expected cases). By convention, the ratio is multiplied by 100. For example, an SIR of 125 for Location A means that the observed number of cases there is 25% higher than the expected number. Here, the term *standardized* refers to the fact that the expected numbers are *adjusted to a standard set of age-specific rates.* In contrast to the SR, an SIR for a single location is useful, because it incorporates the comparison to a reference population. A ratio of observed deaths to expected deaths is a **standardized mortality ratio** (SMR).

Unlike standardized rates, SIRs (and SMRs) for different locations rest on their local age distributions; as a result, the comparability of SIRs depends on how similar or different the local age distributions are. In practice, the effects of differences in local age distributions might be

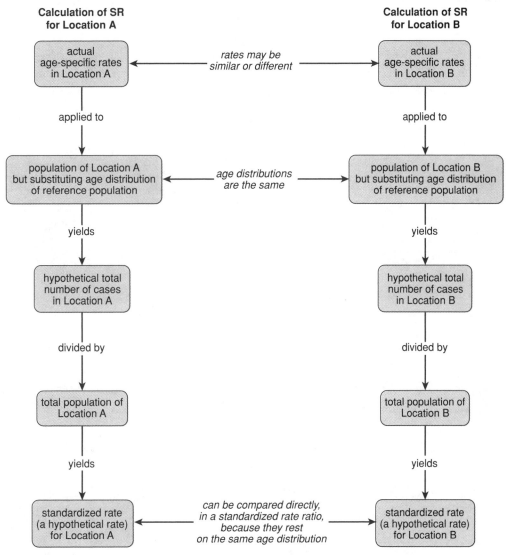

FIGURE 2.16   Standardized rate (SR) and standardized rate ratio (SRR).

substantial or might be so small as to have no practical significance. This effect can and should be assessed in deciding whether it is appropriate to use the SIR in a given situation.

The key methodological drawback of the standardized rate, on the other hand, is its reliance on local age-specific rates. In small populations, age-specific rates are statistically unstable—that is, a change of just a few cases causes a dramatic change in the age-specific rate—and this effect is passed through to the standardized rate. This is why the Massachusetts Department of Public Health, for example, publishes SIRs for cancer, rather than SRs, for the 351 cities and towns of the state, many of which have small populations.

In addition, as time goes by, the reference population used to calculate a standardized rate becomes increasingly remote. Many health departments used the 1940 US Census for decades,

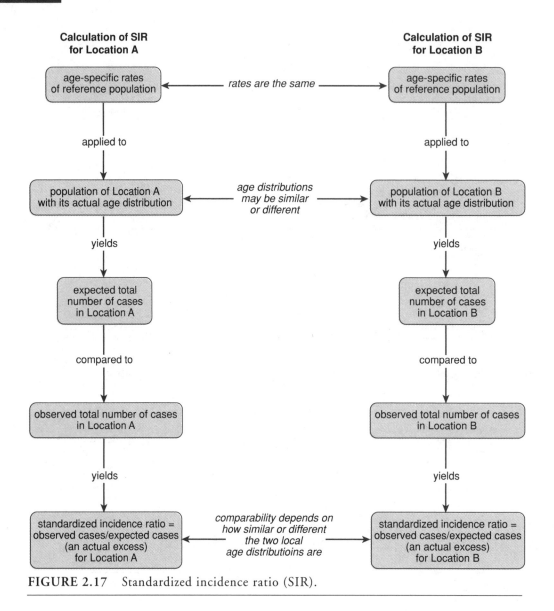

FIGURE 2.17 Standardized incidence ratio (SIR).

and then changed to the 1970 Census, and more recently changed to the 2000 Census. Of course, standardized rates calculated using these different reference populations are not comparable, but most health departments do not have the resources to recalculate SRs and SRRs calculated earlier using a different reference population.

From the community perspective, ordinary citizens are more likely to be able to obtain the total number of cases needed to calculate an SIR than the age-specific case data needed to calculate a standardized rate. This is because health departments, protecting the confidentiality of health data, do not release numbers so small that individuals might be identified. As a result, the SIR is often the statistic of choice for health activists who are concerned about disease in their communities.

When presenting an SR, SRR, or SIR, it is accepted practice to indicate the statistical stability of the rate or ratio by presenting a confidence interval around it. For an example, an SIR of 121 (95% confidence interval 110–133) indicates that the best estimate of the SIR is 121 and there is a 95% probability that the true value lies between 110 and 133.

The Case Series

As described earlier, disease surveillance is conducted on a systematic, ongoing basis in populations. In contrast, the **case series** is simply a set of cases of some disease or condition, often noticed by a clinician, that have some noteworthy characteristic in common. Taken together, the cases might simply be a medical mystery, or they might be seen as an early clue to a risk factor for an illness. For example, a case series of a rare cancer in homosexual men, published in 1982, was an early report on the condition that eventually came to be known as AIDS.[7] Similarly, a series of cases of a rare vaginal cancer in young women provided an early clue to the effects of prenatal exposure to the synthetic hormone diethylstilbestrol (DES),[8] prescribed for more than 20 years in the mid-20th century in the belief that it would prevent miscarriage.

Observational and Experimental Study Designs in Epidemiology

In contrast to descriptive epidemiology, observational and experimental study designs explicitly evaluate associations between risk factors and health outcomes. In an **observational study**, as the name suggests, the investigator does not manipulate exposures but merely observes—and gathers information on—exposures and outcomes. In contrast, in an **experimental study**, the investigator assigns study subjects to different exposure or treatment groups, and then gathers information on outcomes.

Observational studies that use information on exposures and health outcomes ascertained at the community level are called **ecologic studies**. That is, these studies use available community-level data on exposures of interest and previously collected surveillance data on health outcomes. All ecological studies are observational.

In contrast, studies that use individual-level data on exposures and health outcomes compare the experience of two sets of individuals assembled by the investigator for the purpose of the study—people with and without a disease, or people exposed and not exposed to a risk factor. Unlike ecologic studies, an individual-level study design can be either observational or experimental.

Research on environmental health hazards, like other branches of public health research, relies heavily on epidemiologic research. However, only a thumbnail sketch of study designs is provided here, partly because their methodological complexities are beyond the scope of this text, but also because most students of public health will take at least one course in epidemiology.

Group-Level Observational Studies (Ecologic Studies)

As just described, community surveillance documents patterns in rates of disease or death in populations, mostly without attempting explain these patterns or even identify factors that might be associated with these health outcomes. An ecologic study, on the other hand, documents associations between characteristics of communities. In the public health context, the association of interest is often between a health outcome and some other factor. For example, across all the towns of a state, is the mortality rate associated with the presence of manufacturing? With lower average educational attainment? Is the incidence of childhood lead poisoning associated with the presence of an older housing stock? With the percentage of the population in poverty? Analyses such as these, by providing a rich portrait of the public's health, can enhance our understanding of bare surveillance figures.

However, all ecologic studies, because they use data on populations rather than individuals, have limitations. Most important, they cannot link exposure to disease in the same person. Lead poisoning may be more common in towns with old housing, for example, but are the children living in old houses the ones who are being poisoned? Using only data at the population level, it is impossible to know. Further, for methodological reasons too complex to discuss here, analysis of an association using data at the population level can give an incorrect (biased) estimate of the same association at the individual level; this effect is called the *ecologic fallacy*. For these reasons, the ecologic study design is considered useful to *generate* a hypothesis about an association but not to *test* such a hypothesis. Because the work of surveillance is to describe patterns of disease, and because surveillance focuses on patterns across communities, the ecologic study is a natural enhancement to the standardized incidence ratio, as well as a source of new hypotheses for study.

Interestingly, despite the focus in contemporary epidemiology on individual-level study designs (see the following subsection), there is also a growing interest in the effect of truly community-level factors on individual health. For example, a feature of the built environment, or a social stressor such as racial segregation, can be defined only at the community level, though of course any health effects of these factors occur via physiologic mechanisms in individual people. The study of the social determinants of health is known as **social epidemiology**, and analytic methods for **multi-level studies**—that is, studies that include both individual-level and community-level variables—are beginning to emerge in epidemiology.

Individual-Level Observational and Experimental Studies

Unlike ecologic studies, individual-level epidemiologic study designs are used to test a hypothesized association between exposure and outcome. (The term **analytic epidemiology** refers to epidemiologic studies designed to test such a hypothesis.) The three major types of individual-level observational studies are cross-sectional studies, cohort studies, and case-control studies. The simplest of these is the **cross-sectional study**. In this study design, the subjects (for example, a group of workers at a particular facility or in a given industry) are classified on a specific exposure (for example, exposed or not exposed to a chemical in the workplace) and on a health outcome (for example, a neurological deficit). The analysis tests the hypothesis that there is a statistical association between exposure and outcome. A key limitation of the cross-sectional design is that it may not always be clear that the exposure preceded the outcome.

In a **cohort study**, for example, a study of smoking as a risk factor for lung cancer, subjects are selected according to their exposure status (smoker, nonsmoker), and are then compared on disease status (lung cancer, no lung cancer). The key question in a cohort study is: Other things being equal, are the smokers more likely than the nonsmokers to be diagnosed with lung cancer? Cohort studies can be done either prospectively or retrospectively. That is, the subject can be enrolled in a cohort study *before* the health outcome of concern has occurred (a prospective design), and the investigator follows up to determine the health outcomes. Alternatively, the subjects can be enrolled in a cohort study *after* the health outcome of concern has occurred, though the health outcome is unknown to the investigator at the time of enrollment (a retrospective design); again, the investigator follows up to determine the health outcomes.

In a **case-control study**, subjects are selected according to their disease status (for example, lung cancer [cases], no lung cancer [controls*]), and their past exposures are then compared (for example, smoker, nonsmoker). The key question in a case-control study is: Other things being equal, are the lung cancer cases more likely than the controls to have smoked? The case-control design is often used to study rare diseases, such as cancer, because it is impractical to select and follow a cohort of the size needed to generate cancer cases.

In any epidemiologic study, careful assessment of both the risk factor of concern and the health outcome of interest is essential. If subjects are misclassified on either risk factor or outcome, this misclassification will cloud any association that might actually exist, making it difficult or even impossible to discern. The assessment of exposure to environmental risk factors poses unique challenges and uses a distinct set of methods, as described earlier in Section 2.3. Long latency periods, cross-generational effects, and modest relative risks for specific exposures pose methodological challenges in environmental epidemiology.

The epidemiologic study designs just described are considered observational; that is, the investigator sets up a framework for assessing exposures and outcomes, and then observes how the data play out. Other studies have experimental designs, in which the investigator controls the exposure and then follows up on outcome; these designs are variations on the cohort study. One type of experimental study is familiar to the general public: the randomized clinical trial, for example, a trial of a new drug. This is a variation on the prospective cohort study in which subjects are randomly assigned to an exposure group (drug, placebo; or new drug, standard drug) and the health outcome of interest is followed up. In the context of environmental health, it would of course be unethical to expose subjects deliberately to some hazard. Instead, this type of design is used in **intervention studies**: for example, subjects who have asthma and live in public housing are randomly assigned to one of two approaches to improve pest control in their residences, and the impacts on asthma rates of the two approaches are compared.

Evaluating Individual-Level Epidemiologic Studies

In evaluating the results of an individual-level epidemiologic study, the researcher must first assess the statistical significance of the association—that is, assess whether the finding might be due simply to chance. To be considered **statistically significant**, the probability that a finding is due simply to chance must be acceptably low. Often, a less than 5% probability (expressed as $P < .05$) is considered acceptable.

In addition, for a study finding to be considered valid, it must not be attributable to bias or confounding. **Bias** is a systematic error in the way subjects were selected or information was gathered. **Confounding** (from the Latin, to pour together) occurs when a factor that is associated with the

---

*In fact, in modern epidemiology, the definition of a control has become more complex than simply "not diseased," but the simple definition is adequate to the purposes of this overview.

risk factor of interest is itself a risk factor for the health outcome of concern. For example, in a study of body mass index (BMI) and risk of heart attack, if people with a higher BMI are also likely to be older (and if older age is itself a risk factor for heart attack), then part of the apparent effect of higher BMI is actually a result of older age. To see beyond this "pouring together" of the two effects and avoid mistakenly attributing the effect of age to BMI, information on age must be collected and the separate effects of the two risk factors must be teased out by statistical analysis. The phrase "other things being equal" is a colloquial expression of the notion of controlling for confounding.

The term **effect modification** is used in epidemiology when the joint effect of two risk factors is either greater than or less than the effect expected to result from adding their individual effects. Effect modification is analogous to the toxicologic concepts of synergism (the enhancement of a toxic effect) and antagonism (interference with a toxic effect), discussed earlier in this chapter. For example, epidemiologic studies of the lung cancer risk of asbestos exposure have shown that cigarette smoking multiplies the risk of asbestos exposure—a synergistic effect. Unlike bias and confounding, which are nuisance effects to be controlled, effect modification is informative.

Finally, in judging whether a causal connection has been shown, as opposed to merely a valid and statistically significant association, researchers generally consider several factors, including these put forward by the British epidemiologist Sir Austin Bradford Hill in a seminal 1965 article[9]:

- The strength of the association documented (a finding of a 5-fold risk is more convincing than a finding of a 1.5-fold risk)
- The consistency of findings across epidemiologic studies
- An appropriate temporal relationship—that is, exposure to the putative risk factor precedes the development of the disease
- The finding of a dose-response relationship (that is, increasing risk with increasing exposure)
- The biological plausibility of the finding in light of current scientific understanding

Infectious Disease Epidemiology

The distinctive feature of infectious disease, of course, is that it can be transmitted from one individual to another. (Modes of transmission of infectious disease are described in Chapter 3.) This feature makes the methods of infectious disease epidemiology very different from those of chronic disease epidemiology. The core of infectious disease epidemiology is the mathematical modeling of transmission, which is affected by the characteristics of the pathogen (for example, its virulence), of the vector (for example, mosquito or bird), of individual people (for example, their immune status), and of the physical and social environment (for example, the nature and frequency of people's contact with one another).

An infectious disease that is typically present at a low to moderate level in a population or location is considered to be **endemic** there. For example, malaria is endemic in parts of sub-Saharan Africa, but not in Canada. An **epidemic** is the occurrence of disease at an unusually high rate in a population. For example, three deadly epidemics of cholera swept through the United States in 1832, 1849, and 1866.[10] Although the term *epidemic* originally referred only to infectious disease, its use has now been extended to chronic diseases. For example, the increased incidence of childhood asthma is sometimes referred to as an epidemic. The term **pandemic** is reserved for an infectious disease epidemic of global proportions. The influenza pandemic of 1918-1919 infected about one third of the world's population and cost about 50 million lives worldwide.[11] Today's infectious disease specialists are concerned that a small shift in the genetic makeup of the current avian influenza virus (designated the H5N1 variant) could produce another pandemic.

Animal Epidemiology

Epidemiologic methods are sometimes used in animal populations, an endeavor known as **animal epidemiology**, and this research can be useful not only to veterinary science and practice, but also in the service of human health. For example, farm animals or wild animal populations can be used as sentinels in infectious disease surveillance, with the goal of anticipating or preventing an epidemic outbreak in human populations.[12] During the outbreak of bovine spongiform encephalopathy ("mad cow disease") in Great Britain, epidemiologic methods were critical to understanding the nature of the disease, its transmission from cow to cow, and the risk to humans.

Analytic epidemiologic methods have been used to study risk factors for cancer in pet dogs, who get many of the same cancers that humans do and can serve as sentinels for human risk.[13,14] Dogs share with their owners many exposures of the residential environment, indoors and out. In fact, dogs may be more highly exposed to some environmental contaminants—environmental tobacco smoke, for example, because they spend more time breathing indoor air; or pesticides, because they have more contact with household dust indoors or grass and soil outdoors. Dogs offer certain advantages as a study population: They generally eat a consistent diet and have fewer other lifestyle confounders than people do (for example, alcohol consumption), and they have shorter lifespans than humans, which simplifies the study of cancer.[13] Further, participation rates by dog owners in epidemiologic studies of their pets tend to be very high.[14] In recent years, pet cats have come to be seen as potential sentinels for human exposure to flame-retardant chemicals (see Section 5.1) in the home, and especially in household dust;[15] cats' exposure to household dust is enhanced by frequent licking of their paws.

2.5 Risk Assessment: A Regulatory Science

Research in epidemiology and toxicology tells us much about the health effects of chemicals in humans and laboratory animals. But such scientific knowledge accumulates slowly, and questions about a particular chemical, or gaps in theoretical understanding, may be pending for years or even decades.

Meanwhile, government agencies are charged with regulating hazards—for example, setting a limit for the concentration of a chemical in drinking water or deciding how to manage a hazardous waste site. Such policy actions fall under the general rubric of risk management: actions taken to control, or manage, risks to human health (see Section 2.6). In deciding what action to take, regulators do not have the luxury of waiting for scientific certainty to make their decisions easier. In effect, regulators must answer scientific questions that scientists have not yet answered to their own satisfaction.

The process used to bridge this gap is known as risk assessment. Operating in the boundary zone between science and policy, risk assessment is an agreed set of procedures for integrating and interpreting scientific data for the practical purpose of making a decision. Sometimes re-

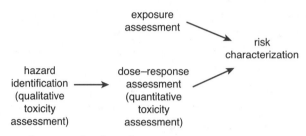

FIGURE 2.18   Basic framework of a risk assessment.

ferred to as a "regulatory science," risk assessment is a formal process for estimating the human health risk of a toxicant or a site by bringing together information on exposure and toxicity. Essentially, risk assessment guidelines establish default procedures for bridging gaps in scientific knowledge in a manner that is both consistent and health protective.

The same basic framework is used whether an individual chemical or a contaminated site is being assessed. The four-step framework shown in **Figure 2.18**, used in most risk assessments conducted by the US Environmental Protection Agency and other government agencies in the United States, was put forward in 1983 in an influential report by the National Academy of Science.* In the exposure assessment step, the risk assessor estimates how much exposure the populations of concern have to the chemical or chemicals of concern. **Hazard identification** is a qualitative evaluation of toxicity with the purpose of establishing the scope of a chemical's health effects (or the presence of multiple chemicals, in the case of a site risk assessment). **Dose–response assessment** quantifies the relationship between dose and effect—that is, it characterizes the dose–response curve for specific toxic effects of the chemical or chemicals of concern. The final **risk characterization** step brings together information on exposure with information on toxicity at different exposures, allowing the risk assessor to estimate the risk to human health. The risk characterization includes an estimate of the uncertainties that are built into it. Each of these concepts plays out somewhat differently in the context of an individual chemical or a contaminated site, as described in the following subsections.

In the real world, the exposure assessment and the toxicity assessment (consisting of the hazard identification and dose–response assessment steps) are not performed in isolation, as it appears in this simplified diagram, but rather inform one another. Perhaps most important, the exposure assessment must consider populations identified in the toxicity assessment as being particularly susceptible to the chemical's effects, while at the same time the toxicity assessment must take account of the exposures estimated for these susceptible populations and also for those identified as most highly exposed.

The basic risk assessment framework—estimating health risk on the basis of exposure and toxicity—can be applied to more than individual chemicals or hazardous waste sites. For example, it can be used to estimate the health risk to workers from an industrial process, or popula-

---

*This 1983 NAS report, *Risk Assessment in the Federal Government: Managing the Process*, is commonly referred to as the Red Book.

tion risks from air pollutants in automobile exhaust. However, this description focuses on risk assessment methods used for individual chemicals and contaminated sites, for which formal procedures have been developed.

Risk Assessment Framework for a Chemical

Somewhat different approaches are typically used to assess the cancer and noncancer effects of chemicals, as described in this subsection. Not all toxic chemicals are carcinogenic, though all carcinogenic chemicals do have some noncarcinogenic toxicity. For this reason, in considering a given chemical, risk assessors integrate what is known about the actual mechanisms that lead to cancer and noncancer effects.

Risk Assessment for Noncancer Effects of a Chemical

In assessing the noncancer health effects of a chemical, the objective of *exposure assessment* is first to identify populations exposed to the chemical of concern, including susceptible or highly exposed subgroups, and then to estimate their exposures. The exposure assessment considers all important sources of exposure, with their associated pathways and routes of exposure, taking account of the physical-chemical properties of the chemical. Exposures are typically quantified using dose units of mg/(kg*day)—that is, the dose is normalized to body weight and averaged over time, as described earlier.

The qualitative step in toxicity assessment—*hazard identification*—establishes the range of noncancer health effects of a chemical. This is accomplished through a review of human case reports, epidemiologic studies of acute and chronic health effects, and short-term and chronic animal bioassays.

The procedures used for the quantitative step in toxicity assessment, *dose–response assessment*, are shaped by the assumption that noncancer effects have a threshold.* Specifically, the existence of a threshold implies that in principle there could be a safe dose. For this reason, dose–response assessment is directed to defining what is called a **reference dose** (RfD), with units mg/(kg*day). The reference dose is a dose that is expected to have no adverse effects in people—specifically, in people who are particularly sensitive to the chemical's effects and who are exposed over a 70-year lifetime.

Unfortunately, the literature on a chemical rarely includes an epidemiologic study of long-term exposure in a sensitive subpopulation. Indeed, the literature might include no dose–response information at all in humans. Therefore, the reference dose for a chemical is usually derived by starting with some other dose that is available in the literature and adjusting it downward to ensure that it is protective of sensitive human beings.

For example, if a reference dose is derived from the NOAEL in a chronic rodent bioassay, the starting value (the rodent NOAEL) is adjusted downward to account for the fact that people may be more sensitive than rodents are, and then adjusted downward again to account for the fact that some people may be more sensitive than most people are. If the starting value is a

---

*Research now indicates that there is at least one exception: The neurotoxicity of lead appears to have no threshold. EPA does not publish a reference dose for lead.

chronic rodent LOAEL rather than a NOAEL, or if the value comes from a short-term rodent study rather than a chronic rodent study, additional downward adjustments are made in deriving the reference dose. An additional downward adjustment may be made to account for gaps in the toxicity data for a chemical.

The actual procedure for making these downward adjustments is to divide the starting value (such as a chronic rodent LOAEL) by one or more **uncertainty factors**, each of which is a hedge against the effects of a specific limitation in the available toxicity data. There are two key decisions in this process. The first is the selection of the dose to be used as the starting value (often the dose for the most sensitive effect in the most sensitive species). The second is the assignment of values of the specific uncertainty factors by which the starting value is reduced in deriving the reference dose. For example, should the starting value be reduced by a factor of 3 to account for a specific limitation in the available data? Or more conservatively, by a factor of 10? These decisions are made by an expert panel, with the opportunity for review by others.

The development of a reference dose is a lengthy process that requires that existing research findings be reviewed and an array of new toxicity studies be undertaken. As a result, the US Environmental Protection Agency (EPA) currently publishes a reference dose for only about 350 chemicals of the many thousands that are produced and used in the United States.

Because the result of dose-response assessment for noncancer effects is a dose, the risk characterization step is a simple comparison of the actual or estimated dose (from the exposure assessment step) to the reference dose:

$$\text{hazard quotient (unitless)} = \frac{\text{actual or estimated dose (mg/kg*day)}}{\text{reference dose (mg/kg*day)}}$$

A **hazard quotient** greater than 1.0 shows that the actual or estimated dose exceeds the reference dose, indicating potential harm to people who are exposed at the actual or estimated dose.

Risk Assessment for the Carcinogenic Effect of a Chemical

The basic procedures of *exposure assessment* in a risk assessment for carcinogenicity are analogous to those in a risk assessment for noncancer effects.

The *hazard identification* step focuses specifically on a chemical's potential to cause cancer in humans. This qualitative evaluation of a chemical's carcinogenicity considers epidemiologic studies as well as chronic animal bioassays, mutagenicity assays, and other short-term tests. The outcome of hazard identification is a designation of the chemical's likely human carcinogenicity, based on expert evaluation of the full body of scientific evidence. Agencies including the US EPA and the International Agency for Research on Cancer (IARC, an arm of the World Health Organization) have defined **weight-of-the-evidence categories** for carcinogenicity (see **Table 2.4**).

In a risk assessment, *dose–response assessment* for carcinogenicity is shaped by the assumption that carcinogenic effect has no threshold. This assumption implies that in principle any dose, no matter how low, carries some risk of cancer. In this context, the concept of a reference dose, or safe dose, is not useful. Rather, the objective of dose–response assessment is to quantify the **cancer slope factor** (CSF): the slope of the dose–response curve, for humans, in the low-dose

Table 2.4 Weight-of-the-Evidence Categories for Carcinogenicity, as Defined by the International Agency for Research on Cancer and the US Environmental Protection Agency

International Agency for Research on Cancer	US Environmental Protection Agency
Group 1: Carcinogenic to humans	Carcinogenic to humans
Group 2A: Probably carcinogenic to humans	Likely to be carcinogenic to humans
Group 2B: Possibly carcinogenic to humans	Suggestive evidence of carcinogenic potential
Group 3: Not classifiable as to carcinogenicity to humans	Inadequate information to assess carcinogenic potential
Group 4: Probably not carcinogenic to humans	Not likely to be carcinogenic to humans

range where human exposures actually occur. The cancer slope factor has units of incremental risk (probability of cancer) per unit increase in dose.

The derivation of a cancer slope factor poses substantial methodological challenges. Only occasionally does the epidemiologic literature provide dose–response information, and therefore the cancer slope factor is typically derived from a rodent bioassay. And, as described earlier, for practical reasons rodents in such studies are given very high doses of the test chemical. Thus, the carcinogenicity data yielded by a rodent bioassay must be extrapolated in two ways: from rodents to people, and from very high experimental doses to much lower real-world exposures.

Sophisticated mathematical models are used to estimate the slope of the human dose–response curve in the low-dose range from rodent data at high doses. Ideally, these models take account of differences in species and differences in dose regimen, while incorporating a health-protective stance. Specifically, assumptions that lead to a steeper slope estimate in the low-dose region are protective of public health.

The cancer slope factor for a particular chemical is decided by an expert panel, with opportunity for review by others. At present, the US EPA publishes a cancer slope factor for fewer than 100 chemicals.

Because the result of a dose–response assessment for cancer effects is a slope, with units of risk (probability) per unit dose, *risk characterization* is accomplished by multiplying the actual or estimated dose (from the exposure assessment step) by the cancer slope factor:

$$\text{dose (mg/kg*day)} * \text{cancer slope factor (risk per mg/kg*day)} = \text{risk}$$

This estimated risk is the **incremental lifetime cancer risk**—the additional cancer risk, over a 70-year lifetime, that would result from the exposures that were assessed.

Table 2.5 summarizes the key steps in a risk assessment for the noncancer and cancer effects of a chemical.

Risk Assessment Framework for a Site

Risk assessment is used to estimate not only the human health risks of individual chemicals, but also risks associated with sites—for example, an operating industrial facility or an abandoned industrial site on which hazardous wastes have been found. Hazardous sites vary widely as to the set of chemicals that is present, the concentrations at which chemicals are found, the envi-

Table 2.5 The Four Major Steps in Risk Assessment as Applied to a Chemical

Step	Noncancer Effects	Cancer
Exposure assessment	Estimate doses at which populations of concern are exposed to the chemical	
Hazard identification	Identify noncancer effects	Assign weight-of-the-evidence classification
Dose–response assessment	Derive reference dose (mg/kg*day); assumes noncancer health effect has a threshold	Derive cancer slope factor (incremental risk per unit dose in mg/kg*day); assumes carcinogenic effect has no threshold
Risk characterization	Calculate hazard quotient (unitless)	Calculate incremental lifetime cancer risk (probability)

ronmental and geographic setting, and the availability of reference doses and cancer slope factors for the chemicals of concern. These complexities are not reflected in the procedural sketch given here. In particular, site risk assessors must draw heavily on the scientific literature and on professional judgment in evaluating potential exposures and in characterizing the toxicity of chemicals for which no reference doses or cancer slope factors have been developed.

A site risk assessment is framed in the same four steps as a chemical risk assessment, but the framework plays out somewhat differently in this context, as shown in **Table 2.6**; for this reason, the first two steps in the risk assessment process are discussed here in reverse order.

In a site risk assessment, the work of *hazard identification* is to characterize the chemical contamination on and from the site. Samples of water, soil, sediments, or air are collected and analyzed for the presence of a long list of chemicals. The concentrations at which individual chemicals are found, in different environmental media at different locations, are reported.

In the context of a site assessment, *exposure assessment* comprises two major tasks. First, the risk assessor constructs plausible scenarios for exposure, identifying groups of people who might be exposed to contaminated environmental media on the site (or from the site), and the activities

Table 2.6 The Four Major Steps in Risk Assessment as Applied to a Site

Step	Noncancer Effects	Cancer Effects
Hazard identification	Through environmental sampling, identify the chemicals present on the site; characterize locations and concentrations of the chemicals in various environmental media	
Exposure assessment	Develop scenarios by which specific populations might be exposed to chemicals on the site; estimate corresponding doses	
Dose–response assessment	For each chemical, obtain published reference dose or develop new one as needed	For each chemical, obtain published cancer slope factor or develop new one as needed
Risk characterization	For each exposure scenario and population, calculate hazard quotient for each chemical and sum across chemicals	For each exposure scenario and population, calculate incremental lifetime cancer risk for each chemical and sum across chemicals

that could bring them into contact with these media. Assumptions made about exposure are intended to include the great majority of the population that is exposed to the site. The exposure scenarios often cover not only current uses of the site but reasonably foreseeable future uses.

In defining exposure scenarios, the risk assessor identifies likely exposure pathways leading to ingestion, inhalation, or dermal exposures to chemicals in various environmental media. For example, the exposure assessment component of a risk assessment for an industrial site abutting a residential neighborhood might include some of these potential exposures to nearby residents:

- Ingestion, inhalation, and dermal exposures to contaminated well water used as tap water
- Dermal and incidental ingestion exposures to contaminated surface water and dermal contact with sediment in a neighborhood pond used for swimming
- Exposures to dust carried from the site by air movements
- Incidental ingestion of soil, dermal contact with soil, or inhalation of vapors on the site itself—for example, by children cutting through the site on their way to and from school
- Consumption of homegrown produce or of fish caught in contaminated waters
- Ingestion of breast milk by infants

The second major task of exposure assessment is to translate each relevant pathway into a concrete dose estimate. Such calculations require a number of inputs, which can be measured, estimated or modeled, or assumed. For example, the risk assessor must quantify the following factors:

- Concentrations of chemicals in various media on the site
- The fate and transport of chemicals or environmental media (for example, the movement of airborne dust from the site into a residential area, or the bioconcentration of a chemical from pond water into fish tissue)
- People's contact with environmental media resulting from various activities
- The likely frequency and duration of people's exposures caused by various activities

Research data provide some basic information—for example, on how much water people typically drink each day, as well as typical inhalation rates and skin areas—and the US EPA has established default values for these factors. However, a site risk assessment often requires many other assumptions to be made. Some are concrete: How often do residents eat locally caught fish, and how much do they eat? How often and for how long do children swim in a contaminated pond? Others require the use of environmental data and scientific understanding, perhaps in the form of mathematical models. For example, given the measured concentration of a chemical in groundwater on the industrial site, what is the expected concentration in water from a private well located downgradient of the site?

As part of a site risk assessment, the core work of *dose–response assessment* is to gather the available toxicity values (reference dose, weight-of-the-evidence classification, and cancer slope factor) for chemicals found on the site—and to derive missing toxicity values for chemicals that are important on the site. Thus, the dose–response step may be relatively straightforward or may require sophisticated scientific work.

In the *risk characterization* step of a site risk assessment, the risk assessor summarizes the cancer risk and noncancer hazard associated with exposure to chemicals on the site, under the exposure scenarios considered. This characterization includes a discussion of the uncertainties embedded in the risk assessment. The risk characterization guides decisions about how best to remediate the site in a manner that will protect public health.

2.6 Risk Management: From Assessment to Action

The term *risk management* refers to the very broad range of actions taken, often by government agencies, to control or reduce environmental risks to human health. The risk management process sometimes begins with the risk characterization derived as the final step in a risk assessment—that is, with a quantitative estimate of the magnitude of a health hazard. However, as risk managers decide whether and how to reduce a given risk, they must consider not only this quantitative estimate of risk but also the regulatory framework, the range of technical options available for controlling the hazard at hand, cost, and social context.[16] This is not a simple matter. Historically, *acceptable risk* has been defined at different times and in different contexts as a specific numerical risk, the lowest risk that is reasonably achievable, the lowest risk that can be achieved using the best available technology, a negligible risk (too small to be of concern), a risk that is comparable to similar existing risks, and a risk that takes account of costs or balancing benefits.

The federal decision-making process also incorporates broader concerns, including the goal of **environmental justice**, which the US EPA defines as equal protection from environmental health hazards and equal access to the agency's decision-making process for people of all incomes and racial or ethnic groups.[17] The agency has named several areas in which it has made environmental justice a priority, including reducing the incidence of elevated blood lead levels and asthma attacks, reducing exposure to toxic air pollutants, ensuring that water is safe to drink and that fish and shellfish are safe to eat, and restoring contaminated sites so that they can be put to use.[18] Thus, environmental justice and the concerns of disenfranchised groups are an explicit factor in some risk management decisions.

The remaining chapters of this text describe many US regulatory provisions or international agreements related to various environmental health hazards. Nearly all of these are efforts at risk management, though this term is not always used. The current section gives a brief preview of the range of activities that fall within the scope of risk management.

Risk Management for Individual Chemicals and Sites

Some risk management decisions are based closely on the results of a risk assessment; for example, US EPA's standards for concentrations of individual chemicals in drinking water are derived from the results of chemical risk assessments.[19] Thus, if a risk assessment has shown that Chemical X is a carcinogen, any exposure to the chemical is assumed to carry some cancer risk, and the goal for the concentration of Chemical X in drinking water is set at zero. The enforceable standard is then set at a concentration that is considered feasible to achieve. Both policy decisions—the choice of a goal and of a feasible standard—are risk management decisions.

Similarly, if a risk assessment has shown Chemical Z to be noncarcinogenic, and a reference dose has been derived, a drinking water standard can be derived from the reference dose. This is done by back-calculating the concentration in drinking water that corresponds to the reference dose, given certain assumptions about body weight and daily consumption of drinking water.

For example, suppose that the reference dose for Chemical Z is 0.000143 mg/(kg*day), or 0.143 μg/(kg*day). Then, a backward calculation would look like this*:

$$\frac{0.143 \ \mu g \ \text{Chemical Z/(kg*day)} * 70 \ \text{kg body weight}}{2 \ \text{liters water/day}} = \frac{5 \ \mu g \ \text{Chemical Z}}{\text{liter water}}$$

The enforceable standard for the concentration of Chemical Z in drinking water might then be set at a concentration somewhat lower than 5 μg/L to account for the fact that people will be exposed from sources other than drinking water.

Risk management decisions about cleaning up contaminated sites are often very complex for several reasons: Numerous chemicals are usually present in more than one environmental medium (for example, in both water and soil); contamination is not evenly distributed across the site; and there may sometimes be several approaches to cleaning up the site using different technologies with different effects and different price tags. Thus, in the context of a contaminated site, risk management is not simply a matter of deriving acceptable target concentrations for individual chemicals. Rather, in making complex decisions about how to remediate contamination, risk managers must incorporate not only information about the toxicity of all the chemicals (including cancer slope factors and reference doses) but also anticipated future uses of the site, the effectiveness of available cleanup options, and costs.

Other Examples of Risk Management

Various approaches can be used to reduce ambient environmental pollution from industrial processes. For example, regulations can require that specific technologies be used to treat wastes before they are released, or industries might be granted allowances to release specified quantities of pollutants. Changes to industrial processes might enable a manufacturer to produce less waste or to substitute less toxic chemicals for those currently being used. Within the occupational setting, federal regulations set limits for the concentrations of some chemicals in workplace air. In some work settings, a hazardous process can be isolated from the rest of the workplace, or individual workers can wear protective gear. All of these approaches to controlling pollution are strategies for risk management.

Not all risk management provisions involve the direct control of pollution. Some regulations set incentives for compliance with standards—or set penalties for noncompliance. Other regulations require information to be gathered and released. For example, federal law requires employers to provide workers with certain information about the chemicals to which they are exposed on the job. Similarly, industrial facilities are required to provide local communities with certain information about chemical releases. Such information can create a powerful incentive to reduce pollution. Other kinds of information are also important in anticipating and managing environmental health risks. For example, various government agencies gather surveillance data on infectious diseases, lead poisoning in children, and other health outcomes.

Finally, much of the work done by local health departments involves the management of environmental health risks. Many city and town governments are responsible for providing water

---

*The corresponding forward calculation appeared in Section 2.3 as an example of calculating a dose of trichloroethylene in drinking water.

supply and sewer service, trash removal, and recycling services. Local governments inspect and regulate food service establishments, manage episodes of foodborne illness, and respond to outbreaks of other infectious diseases. Local health departments also work to manage various environmental hazards related to housing conditions, from controlling rodents to preventing lead poisoning and asthma. Noise is also regulated through local ordinances.

Whatever the hazard, sharing information about a specific risk is usually an important part of risk management. Such activities are referred to as *risk communication*. However, this term includes a much broader range of activities, as described in the following section.

2.7 Risk Communication: Sharing Knowledge

Given that environmental epidemiology, risk assessment, and risk management are all undertaken in the service of public health, what is the role of the public in these endeavors? In recent decades, there has been a gradual shift in the United States away from a purely expert-driven, top-down model of communication with the public on environmental health matters to a more participatory model.

In environmental health, the term *risk communication* usually refers to the exchange or transmission of information about an environmental health hazard between experts and those affected by the hazard. The affected group might be people living near a hazardous waste site, for example, or those affected by a policy decision. Along with risk assessment and risk management, this type of risk communication forms a trio of activities related to understanding and dealing with environmental health hazards. Construed more broadly, risk communication also includes a role for the public in epidemiologic research on environmental hazards and even a role in shaping public policy, as described in the following subsections.

Risk Communication About Environmental Health Hazards

Communication about environmental health hazards between members of the public and scientists or other experts is often complicated by differences in the way these groups perceive risks. Technical experts tend to think of risks in strictly quantitative terms, whereas the public's perception of risks is more affected by other factors. Indeed, the public perception of risk has been formulated as "hazard plus outrage"[20]—that is, the quantitative estimate of risk is modified by a sense of outrage, which is elicited by certain characteristics of the risk.

Research during the 1970s and 1980s identified a number of characteristics of hazards that tend to contribute to public outrage. During this period, research by engineers sought to understand the public's tendency to under- or overestimate risks relative to engineering estimates, while research by psychologists sought to uncover how nonexperts conceptualize risk. Taken together, these two lines of research identified features of hazards that, for members of the public, tend to make the associated risk seem numerically higher and also somehow less bearable.[21-25] That is, these features of hazards tend to generate outrage:

- The consequences of the hazard are serious or irreversible (for example, death or permanent disability).

- The hazard kills large numbers of people at one blow (for example, the risk of a single plane crash that causes 300 deaths, as opposed to the risk of 150 car accidents that cause 300 deaths).
- The hazard simply evokes a gut dread in most people (for example, radiation).
- The hazard is new or unfamiliar, or its consequences are unknown (for example, genetic engineering as opposed to car accidents).
- The consequences of the hazard are unexpected (for example, when a flood of molasses killed 21 people after the rupture of a large storage tank in Boston in 1919).
- The consequences of the hazard are delayed (for example, cancer, with its long latency period) rather than immediate.
- The hazard is perceived as not being within an individual's personal control (for example, a commercial aviation accident as opposed to a car accident while driving).
- The hazard is taken on involuntarily or without knowledge of the risk (for example, the risk of exposure to secondhand smoke as opposed to the risk of smoking).
- The hazard is not natural, but rather manmade (for example, toxic synthetic chemicals).
- The hazard is seen as avoidable or unnecessary—as opposed to, for example, occupational hazards or chemotherapy to treat cancer.
- The victims are nearby (although faraway victims can be brought close by media coverage, especially coverage of identifiable individuals, such as coal miners trapped by a cave-in).

Many environmental health hazards have one or more of these outrage-generating characteristics. In addition, risks that affect people in their homes, such as chemical contamination of drinking water, elicit a powerful emotional response because they strike at the heart of family, security, and even personal identity.[26] Further, the public's outrage tends to be magnified if there are no benefits clearly associated with a risk, if the risk receives a lot of media attention, if the risk results from unethical activities or an unfair process, or if the risk was created by people or institutions they don't trust.[27] Outrage may also be particularly acute in those with past experience of injustice, including residents of lower-income neighborhoods or members of historically disadvantaged racial or ethnic groups.

Thus, professionals who communicate about environmental health risks must understand and acknowledge the roots of outrage in a given situation, and they must be committed to genuine two-way communication with diverse stakeholders—those who are affected by the problem at hand, and who will be affected by the chosen solution. As a general rule, effective risk communication about environmental health issues requires careful planning, genuine collaboration with stakeholders, careful listening and clear speaking, honesty, and compassion, as well as skill in working with the media.[27]

Risk Communication in Environmental Epidemiology

Traditionally, the role of the public in epidemiology has been limited to that of research subject. At a minimum, today's research standards require that subjects give informed consent for their participation after having received information about the potential risks and benefits of taking part in a study.

Without informed consent, research subjects may be exposed to risks that are not apparent to them; historically, members of disenfranchised groups have been particularly at risk of such treatment. In one infamous episode, US Public Health Service researchers at Tuskegee Institute in Alabama studied the progression of syphilis in African American men over many years, without offering them treatment with penicillin when it became available. These events led to reforms at the US Public Health Service and ultimately to current requirements for the informed consent of participants in research.

Still, as important as informed consent is, it reflects a one-way, top-down model of public participation in research. In the 1970s and 1980s, social activism in response to industrial pollution led to more fundamental changes in the paradigm of research and the communication of scientific information. In Niagara Falls, New York, a buried industrial dumpsite known as Love Canal was discovered under a working-class neighborhood (see **Figure 2.19**). In the manufacturing city of Woburn, Massachusetts, industrial solvents dumped near a wetland contaminated the local water supply. In both cities, it was angry local residents who first hypothesized connections between pollution and local health problems, who pressed for health studies and helped shape those studies to be useful to local residents—a new form of activism that has been called "popular epidemiology."[28]

Today, community participation in health research is not unusual. People who have a stake in the outcome of a study—women with breast cancer, for example, or residents of a location being studied—may have some role in planning or conducting the research. This participation

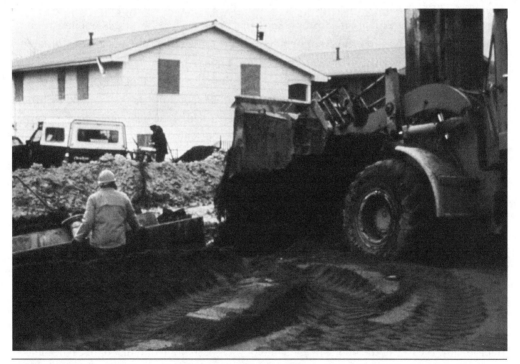

FIGURE 2.19   The Love Canal neighborhood, built over a chemical waste dump, became the scene of bulldozers and boarded-up houses. *Source*: Reprinted courtesy of CDC Public Health Image Library. ID# 5534. Content provider: CDC. Available at: http://phil.cdc.gov/phil/details.asp. Accessed September 26, 2007.

can be as simple as an advisory role grafted onto a traditional top-down research paradigm. At the other extreme is a model known as community-based participatory research. This approach to research rests on three core principles: that those who will be affected by the outcome of a research project should participate in it, from defining the research question to interpreting the results; that there is an equitable sharing of power between researchers and community members; and that the effort emphasizes practical solutions over abstract analysis.[29]

Risk Communication in the Policy Context: The Consensus Conference

Finally, a sophisticated and highly participatory form of risk communication, and one that is very unusual in the United States, is the Danish-style consensus conference. A consensus conference brings together a diverse group of citizens to deliberate a complex issue and offer its collective judgment to government and scientists. In this 3-day process, the panel of citizens is briefed on the issue at hand, given the opportunity to question a panel of experts, allowed to deliberate as a group, and then asked to prepare a report on the issue.

In Denmark, the Danish Board of Technology arranges occasional consensus conferences, whose reports are passed on to the Parliament. More than 20 consensus conferences have been held in Denmark since 1987, on such topics as the use of gene technology in industry and agriculture, the future of fishing, and the use of electronic identity cards. As a general rule, topics are chosen for a Danish-style consensus conference because they are controversial and scientifically complex, and are the subject of current policymaking. Participating in a consensus conference is seen as a civic obligation in Denmark, much like jury duty in the United States.

In 2006, a consensus conference on the subject of biomonitoring—measuring environmental chemicals in people's bodies—was held in Boston by university researchers. The panel's consensus statement[30] was made publicly available and was sent to US policymakers and scientists in the public health arena, although consensus conferences have no formal place in US policymaking at present. Like community-based participatory research, the consensus conference process engages members of the public in the development of scientific knowledge, combining the unique perspectives and expertise of technical experts and lay persons to grapple with an environmental health hazard.

2.8 The Precautionary Principle in Environmental Health

We can learn a great deal about individual toxicants and their health risks from environmental science, from the science of toxicology, from the applied science of exposure assessment, and from the research method of epidemiology, as described earlier in Sections 2.1 through 2.4. In the United States today, such knowledge informs formal decisions and actions mainly through two activities: risk assessment (Section 2.5), an applied science that offers a structured approach for estimating health effects; and risk management (Section 2.6), the amalgam of decisions and actions that are taken to reduce or control the risks of a chemical or a site or an activity. And both risk assessment and risk management now involve formal opportunities for risk communication (Section 2.7)—an exchange of information and viewpoints between technical experts and members of the public.

But for the most part, the activities of risk assessment, risk management, and risk communication occur after the fact—after an industrial process has been put into use, after a toxicant has been released into the environment, after the opportunity to prevent or minimize a hazard has been lost. The historical tendency in the United States has been to introduce new chemicals or processes freely and only later consider their ramifications. In contrast, a strictly precautionary approach would require those introducing a new chemical or activity to show that it is *safe* before it is put into use—but this is, of course, an impossible task.

In countries where a precautionary approach is in place as policy, it is usually articulated in a more nuanced way. In the European Union, for example, the precautionary principle has been stated this way: When there are early warnings of harm from a substance or activity, and the potential harm is serious, it is necessary to take precautionary measures before there is clear proof of harm.[31] (An alternate translation of the original German term is "foresight principle."[32])

The precautionary principle parallels our commonsense notions of taking precautions ("look before you leap"). It also embodies the long-standing preference in public health for primary prevention over secondary prevention, when this is possible. Efforts toward **primary prevention** aim to head off health impacts before they happen (in the environmental health context, for example, by eliminating an exposure that carries a health risk); **secondary prevention** efforts seek to reduce the impacts of a health problem, for example through early detection of a disease. Of all the risk-related activities described earlier, the consensus conference is the most clearly compatible with a precautionary approach.

In environmental health, the most familiar articulation of the precautionary principle is the 1998 Wingspread Statement on the Precautionary Principle (so named because it was agreed at the Wingspread Conference Center in Racine, Wisconsin). This statement adds three elements to the core description of the precautionary principle[33]:

- The proponent of the activity should bear the burden of proof as to the potential for harm.
- When the precautionary principle is applied, the full range of alternatives to the action under consideration must be examined, including no action.
- The process must be open and democratic.

Thus, the precautionary approach is tied to societal goals, asking whether an activity is needed, to what degree its negative impacts can be prevented while still meeting the societal goals, and whether there are other ways to meet the goals with less risk.[34]

Some US policy initiatives and some international agreements, described in Chapter 5, reflect a precautionary approach. For example, the US Toxic Substances Control Act is precautionary in spirit, despite practical barriers to its full implementation. Two international agreements—the Kyoto Protocol on global climate change and the Montreal Protocol on Substances that Deplete the Ozone Layer—reflect a precautionary approach to problems that are global in scale and will respond only slowly to control measures. And the European Union has recently established a program for the *R*egistration, *E*valuation, *A*uthorisation and *R*estriction of *C*hemicals (REACH), under which new chemicals can be authorized only after toxicity testing (with more testing required for higher-volume chemicals) and a weighing of their potential risks against their potential socioeconomic benefits.[35]

Finally, an approach known as **health impact assessment**—the assessment of the likely health impacts in a population of a proposed policy or action, before it is implemented—has been gaining traction, mostly in the international setting. The World Health Organization, for example, supports the use of health impact assessments for several reasons.[36] First, this approach links decision-making in non-health sectors to the public health sector. In addition, it is a participatory approach that involves communities affected by important decisions before those decisions are made. And finally, because it is anticipatory, and considers positive as well as negative impacts, the health impact assessment is seen as compatible with a sustainable approach to development.

The health impact assessment has no formal place in the US regulatory framework at present, although there is growing interest in this approach.[37] (The US National Environmental Policy Act calls for an evaluation of the *environmental* impacts of proposed federal projects; see Chapter 4.) Instead, the risk assessment/risk management paradigm that remains dominant in US regulation calls for individual existing health risks to be quantified and then managed, one by one. The absence of foresight embodied in this approach has led to numerous missed opportunities for primary prevention of human health impacts from environmental hazards, including many of those discussed in coming chapters.

Study Questions

1. Contrast the typical profiles of higher- and lower-molecular-weight chemicals as to their physical-chemical properties and their behavior in the environment.
2. Assess the advantages and disadvantages of epidemiology and rodent bioassays as sources of information about the human health effects of environmental chemicals.
3. Suppose that a surveillance biomonitoring program has measured concentrations of polybrominated diphenyl ethers (PBDEs) in women's breast milk, with the goal of describing exposure at the population level. Much is still unknown about the toxicity of these common flame-retardant chemicals (described in Chapter 5). Would you recommend that the results of the biomonitoring be reported back to the study participants? Why or why not?
4. Explain why risk assessors use a reference dose to quantify noncarcinogenic toxicity, but use a cancer slope factor to quantify carcinogenic toxicity.
5. Suppose that you work for a state health agency and have been asked to review a site remediation plan for an abandoned industrial facility, which is adjacent to a neighborhood that has long borne an inequitable burden of industrial contamination. How would you incorporate concerns about environmental justice as you consider the plan?
6. As you read the rest of this text, try to identify an environmental health topic that you think would be appropriate for a Danish-style consensus conference.

References

1. Hohn D. Moby-Duck, or the synthetic wilderness of childhood. *Harper's Magazine.* January 2007:39–62.
2. Watson J, Crick F. A structure for deoxyribose nucleic acid. *Nature.* 1953;171(4356): 737–738.

3. Lewis C, Whitwell S, Forbes A, Sanderson J, Mathew C, Marteau T. Estimating risks of common complex diseases across genetic and environmental factors: the example of Crohn disease. *J Med Genet.* 2007;44:689–694.

4. Snow J. *On the Mode of Communication of Cholera.* 2nd ed. London, England: Churchill; 1855. Reprinted as *Snow on Cholera.* New York, NY: Hafner Publishing Co.; 1965.

5. World Health Organization. *Africa Malaria Report 2003.* 2003. Available at: http://www.rbm.who.int/amd2003/amr2003/amr_toc.htm. Accessed January 7, 2008.

6. US Equal Employment Opportunity Commission. *Facts about the Americans with Disabilities Act.* Available at: http://www.eeoc.gov/facts/fs-ada.html. Accessed February 7, 2008.

7. US Centers for Disease Control. A cluster of Kaposi's sarcoma and *Pneumocystis carinii* pneumonia among homosexual male residents of Los Angeles and Orange Counties, California. *MMWR Morb Mortal Wkly Rep.* 1982;31(23):305–307.

8. Herbst A, Ulfelder H, Poskanzer D. Adenocarcinoma of the vagina. Association of maternal stilbestrol therapy with tumor appearance in young women. *N Engl J Med.* 1971;284(15): 878–881.

9. Hill AB. The environment and disease: association or causation? *Proc R Soc Med.* 1965;58: 295–300.

10. Rosenberg CE. *The Cholera Years: The United States in 1832, 1849, and 1866.* Chicago: University of Chicago Press; 1962.

11. Taubenberger JK, Morens DM. 1918 influenza: the mother of all pandemics. *Emerg Infect Dis.* 2006;12(1).

12. Halliday JEB, Meredith AL, Knobel DL, Shaw DJ, Bronsvoort BMd, Cleveland S. A framework for evaluating animals as sentinels for infectious disease surveillance. J R Soc Interface. 2007;4:973–984.

13. Vastag B. Giving new meaning to the word "watchdog"? *J Natl Cancer Inst.* 1999;91(2): 112–114.

14. Bukowski J, Wartenberg D. An alternative approach for investigating the carcinogenicity of indoor air pollution: pets as sentinels of environmental cancer risk. *Environ Health Perspect.* 1997;105(12):1312–1319.

15. Dye J, Venier M, Zhu L, Ward C, Hites R, Birnbaum L. Elevated PBDE levels in pet cats: sentinels for humans? *Environ Sci Technol.* 2007;41(18):6350–6356.

16. US Environmental Protection Agency. *2006–2011 EPA Strategic Plan: Charting Our Course, 2006.* Available at: http://www.epa.gov/ocfo/plan/2006/entire_report.pdf. Accessed March 26, 2008.

17. US Environmental Protection Agency. *Environmental Justice.* Available at: http://www.epa.gov/compliance/environmentaljustice/index.html. Accessed November 10, 2007.

18. Johnson S. *Reaffirming the U.S. Environmental Protection Agency's Commitment to Environmental Justice, 2005.* Available at: http://epa.gov/oswer/ej/pdf/admin-ej-commit-letter-110305.pdf. Accessed March 26, 2008.

19. US Environmental Protection Agency. *Setting Standards for Safe Drinking Water.* Available at: http://www.epa.gov/safewater/standard/setting.html. Accessed November 5, 2007.

20. Sandman P. Risk communication: facing public outrage. *EPA Journal.* November 1987:21–22.

21. Starr C. Social benefit versus technological risk: what is our society willing to pay for safety? *Science.* 1969;165:1232–1238.

22. Lowerance W. *Of Acceptable Risk: Science and the Determination of Safety.* Los Altos, Calif: William Kaufman, Inc.; 1976.

23. Rowe W. *An Anatomy of Risk.* New York, NY: John Wiley and Sons; 1977.

24. Slovic P, Fischhoff B, Lichtenstein S. Rating the risks. *Environment.* 1979;21(3):14–39.

25. Slovic P. Perception of risk. *Science.* April 17, 1987;236: 280–285.

26. Fitchen JM. When toxic chemicals pollute residential environments: the cultural meanings of home and home ownership. *Hum Organisation.* 1989;48:313–324.

27. Covello V. Risk communication. In: Frumkin H, ed. *Environmental Health: From Global to Local*. San Francisco, Calif: Jossey-Bass; 2005:988–1009.

28. Brown P. Popular epidemiology and toxic waste contamination: lay and professional ways of knowing. *J Health Soc Behav*. 1992;33(3):267–281.

29. Scammell M. Roots of community research. *Race, Poverty and the Environment*. 2004;XI(2): 23–26.

30. Lay Panel of the Boston Consensus Conference on Biomonitoring. Consensus statement measuring chemicals in people—what would you say? Boston Consensus Conference on Biomonitoring; December 11, 2006; Boston, Mass.

31. European Environment Agency. *Late Lessons from Early Warnings: The Precautionary Principle 1896–2000*. Luxembourg: Office for Official Publications of the European Communities; 2001.

32. Kriebel D, Tickner J, Epstein P, Lemons J, Levins R, Loechler E, et al. The precautionary principle in environmental science. *Environ Health Perspect*. 2001;109(9):871–876.

33. Wingspread Conference. *Wingspread Statement on the Precautionary Principle*. Available at: http://www.sustainableproduction.org//precaution/stat.wing.html. Accessed February 7, 2008.

34. Kriebel D, Tickner J. Reenergizing public health through precaution. *Am J Public Health*. 2001;91(9):1351–1355.

35. European Commission. *REACH*. Available at: http://ec.europa.eu/environment/chemicals/reach/reach_intro.htm. Accessed January 25, 2008.

36. World Health Organization. *Why Use HIA?* Available at: http://www.who.int/hia/about/why/en/index.html. Accessed May 22, 2008.

37. US Centers for Disease Control and Prevention. *Health Impact Assessment*. Available at: http://www.cdc.gov/healthyplaces/hia.htm. Accessed April 9, 2008.

Websites Used as Sources for Table 2.1

US Department of Health and Human Services

US Department of Health and Human Services. HHS: What We Do. Available at: http://www.hhs.gov/about/whatwedo.html/ Accessed March 21, 2008.

US Public Health Service. US Public Health Service. Available at: http://phs-nurse.org/Overview.htm Accessed March 22, 2008.

National Institutes of Health. About NIH. Available at: http://www.nih.gov/about/index.html Accessed March 22, 2008.

National Institutes of Health. Institutes, Centers & Offices. Available at: http://www.nih.gov/icd/ Accessed March 22, 2008.

National Cancer Institute. NCI Mission Statement. Available at: http://www.cancer.gov/aboutnci/overview/mission Accessed March 22, 2008.

National Toxicology Program. About the NTP. Available at: http://ntp.niehs.nih.gov/index.cfm?objectid=7201637B-BDB7-CEBA-F57E39896A08F1BB Accessed March 22, 2008.

National Institute for Occupational Safety and Health. About NIOSH. Available at: http://www.cdc.gov/niosh/about.html Accessed March 22, 2008.

US Department of Labor

Occupational Safety & Health Administration. OSHA's Mission. Available at: http://www.osha.gov/oshinfo/mission.html Accessed March 22, 2008.

Mine Safety and Health Administration. MSHA's Mission. Available at: http://www.msha.gov/MSHAINFO/MISSION.HTM Accessed March 22, 2008.

US Department of Energy

US Department of Energy. Energy Information Administration. Available at: http://www.doe.gov/organization/energyinformationadmin.htm Accessed March 21, 2008.

US Department of Energy. Program Offices. Available at: http://www.doe.gov/organization/program_offices.htm Accessed March 21, 2008.

US Department of Agriculture

US Department of Agriculture. Agencies and Offices: Agricultural Marketing Service (AMS) Overview. Available at: http://www.usda.gov/wps/portal/!ut/p/_s.7_0_A/7_0_1OB?contentidonly= true&contentid=AMS_Agency_Splash.xml&x=14&y=10 Accessed March 21, 2008.

US Department of Agriculture. Agencies and Offices: Agricultural Research Service (ARS) Overview. Available at: http://www.usda.gov/wps/portal/!ut/p/_s.7_0_A/7_0_1OB?contentidonly=true& contentid=ARS_Agency_Splash.xml&x=17&y=13 Accessed March 21, 2008.

US Department of Agriculture. Agencies and Offices: Animal and Plant Health Inspection Service (APHIS) Overview. Available at: http://www.usda.gov/wps/portal/!ut/p/_s.7_0_A/7_0_1OB? contentidonly=true&contentid=APHIS_Agency_Splash.xml&x=10&y=6 Accessed March 21, 2008.

US Department of Agriculture. Agencies and Offices: Economic Research Service (ERS) Overview. Available at: http://www.usda.gov/wps/portal/!ut/p/_s.7_0_A/7_0_1OB?contentidonly=true& contentid=ERS_Agency_Splash.xml&x=9&y=5 Accessed March 21, 2008.

US Department of Agriculture. Agencies and Offices: Food Safety and Inspection Service (FSIS) Overview. Available at: http://www.usda.gov/wps/portal/!ut/p/_s.7_0_A/7_0_1OB?contentidonly= true&contentid=FSIS_Agency_Splash.xml&x=15&y=10 Accessed March 21, 2008.

US Department of Agriculture. Agencies and Offices: National Agricultural Statistics Service (NASS) Overview. Available at: http://www.usda.gov/wps/portal/!ut/p/_s.7_0_A/7_0_1OB? contentidonly=true&contentid=NASS_Agency_Splash.xml&x=7&y=11 Accessed March 21, 2008.

Independent executive agencies

US Environmental Protection Agency. About EPA. Available at: http://www.epa.gov/epahome/ aboutepa.htm Accessed March 22, 2008.

US NRC. About NRC. Available at: http://www.nrc.gov/about-nrc.html Accessed March 22, 2008.

US Consumer Product Safety Commission. About CPSC. Available at: http://www.cpsc.gov/ about/about.html Accessed March 22, 2008.

Private nonprofit institutions

The National Academies. About the National Academies. Available at: http://www.nationalacademies .org/about/ Accessed March 25, 2008.

National Academy of Sciences. About the NAS. Available at: http://www.nasonline.org/site/PageServer? pagename=ABOUT_main_page Accessed March 25, 2008.

Institute of Medicine. About the Institute of Medicine. Available at: http://www.iom.edu/CMS/ AboutIOM.aspx Accessed: March 25, 2008.

National Research Council. Welcome to the National Research Council. Available at: http://sites .nationalacademies.org/nrc/index.htm Accessed March 25, 2008.

Agencies of the United Nations

World Health Organization. About WHO. Available at: http://www.who.int/about/en/ Accessed March 25, 2008.

International Agency for Research on Cancer. Home page. Available at: http://www.iarc.fr/ Accessed March 25, 2008.

Intergovernmental Panel on Climate Change. About IPCC. Available at: http://www.ipcc.ch/ about/index.htm Accessed March 25, 2008.

UN Scientific Committee on the Effects of Atomic Radiation. About Us. Available at: http://www .unscear.org/unscear/en/about_us.html Accessed March 25, 2008.

Living with Other Species

Learning Objectives

After studying this chapter, the reader will be able to:

- Define or explain the key terms throughout the chapter

- Distinguish among the major types of pathogens

- Explain the distinct and varied ways in which infectious disease can be transmitted

- Describe key strategies for reducing the transmission of infectious diseases

- Compare the burden of infectious disease and infection-related cancers in industrialized and lower-income countries, noting which mode of disease transmission makes the largest contribution to global mortality

- Describe governmental roles in managing infectious disease risk in the United States

Humans exist within ecosystems, which encompass other animals, plants, and microscopic organisms in a complex web of relationships. This close coexistence, which offers many benefits, is also the source of infectious disease among people (Section 3.1), a leading cause of global mortality and morbidity. In addition, people sometimes fall victim to poisons produced by animals, plants, or fungi (Section 3.2). Finally, living intermingled with other species also causes allergies and asthma (Section 3.3), which occur when humans' necessary defenses against a multitude of threats are misdirected against harmless substances.

3.1 Infectious Disease

All animals are habitats for other organisms—the result of millions of years of co-evolution. The human body is **host** to many small organisms because it offers sheltered conditions and nutrients that enhance the organisms' reproduction. Many of these organisms are harmless, and some are even helpful. For example, large populations of bacteria in the gut and on the skin ordinarily prevent disease-causing bacteria from establishing colonies. Thus, some relationships between microorganisms and their animal hosts are mutually beneficial; the associations we call **infectious diseases** are those that are troublesome to the animal host. An infectious disease that can be transmitted to humans from nonhuman animals, either domestic or wild, is called a **zoonosis**, or a zoonotic disease. Influenza, rabies, and anthrax are all zoonoses.

The term **pathogen** identifies an infectious agent that, when it becomes established in a host organism—that is, when it infects the host—causes a specific infectious disease in the host. Pathogenic bacteria, for example, cause a large number of distinct diseases in people and other animals. Other factors, such as genetic traits or environmental conditions, may contribute to the risk of illness, but the pathogen is the factor without which a specific infectious disease cannot occur.

The great variety of symptoms in infectious diseases results from the wide range of processes that can be triggered as a pathogen makes its home in the human body. To give just two examples: The diarrhea caused by some pathogenic *Escherichia coli* bacteria occurs because the bacteria secrete a toxin that stimulates the production of an enzyme that changes the fluid balance in the intestine;[1] and the chills and fever that characterize malaria occur when, at one point in a complex life cycle, large numbers of parasites are released into the bloodstream by bursting red blood cells.[2]

Death and disability from infectious disease have figured prominently in human experience, and so these diseases have been closely observed for many centuries. Early scientists distinguished among diseases with different symptoms and appreciated that different diseases might have distinct causes. It was well understood by the 16th century, for example, that close contact with a sick person increased the risk of some diseases—including smallpox, leprosy, and syphilis—but not others. For many years, the elusive causal factor for the other diseases was characterized as a sort of atmospheric emanation known as a **miasma** rising from the earth (in the 17th-century belief) or from rotting organic matter (in the 19th-century version).[3] For example, miasmas were thought to cause malaria (the name of the disease is derived from the Italian for *bad air*).

As of the early 19th century, scientists who believed that diseases could be caused by germs were still in the minority. Although microbes had first been observed under the microscope in the 17th century, evidence that they caused disease accumulated only slowly. But in 1876, everything changed: the scientist Robert Koch isolated the anthrax bacterium and demonstrated that it produced the disease in cattle. By the end of the 19th century, scientists had documented the infectious agents of typhoid fever, leprosy, malaria, tuberculosis, cholera, diphtheria, tetanus, plague, and other illnesses.[3]

Present scientific understanding of infectious disease is extensive and sophisticated, yet much is still unknown about the complex and ever-evolving relationships among human beings, pathogens, and the environment. This section treats the following topics:

- The major classes of pathogens and their key characteristics
- Immunity and vaccination against infectious disease
- The transmission of infectious disease, including transmission via closeness or contact, transmission through fecal-oral exposures, and foodborne and vectorborne transmission
- Infectious disease as a cause of cancer
- The burden of infectious disease mortality worldwide
- Approaches to controlling infectious disease
- The US regulatory framework for managing infectious disease risk

Types of Pathogens

Several types of infective agents act as human pathogens. **Worms** are multicellular organisms that can be as small as 1 mm in diameter* but that can range to more than 1 m in length (see **Figure 3.1**). Worms are not microorganisms; even the smallest are visible to the naked eye. Parasitic worms are also known as helminths.

Protozoa are single-celled organisms. These microorganisms are approximately 10 microns in diameter—1/100th the diameter of a small worm—and were some of the first organisms seen under a microscope. A protozoan cell has a true nucleus that contains DNA, and most protozoa can move actively about in the environment. Among the illnesses caused by protozoan parasites are malaria and cryptosporidiosis, a disease that affected more than 400,000 people in a 1993 waterborne disease outbreak in Milwaukee. Pathogenic worms and protozoa are **parasites**: They must spend at least a small part of their life cycle inside an animal host, on which they depend for certain benefits.

Like protozoa, **bacteria** are single-celled organisms. With a typical diameter of about 1 micron, bacteria are smaller than protozoan parasites (see **Figure 3.2**). They lack a true nucleus with a membrane, instead simply containing a mass or ring of DNA. And, unlike parasites, most bacteria can live their full life cycle outside the body of the host organism, living in water or soil, for example. Tuberculosis, cholera, tetanus, and Lyme disease are examples of diseases caused by bacteria, as is infection with pathogenic *E. coli*.

---

*1 millimeter = 0.001 meter; 1 micron = 0.001 millimeter; 1 nanometer = 0.001 micron.

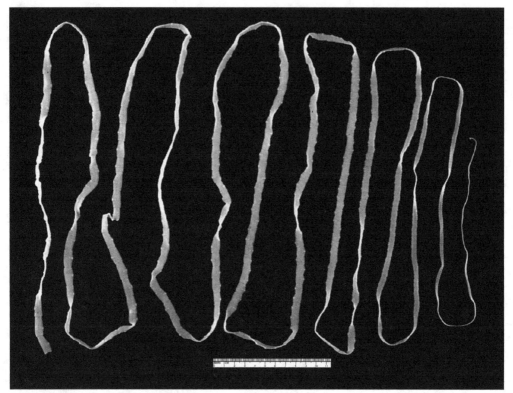

FIGURE 3.1 Usually ingested in an immature form in undercooked meat, the adult *Taenia saginata* tapeworm frequently reaches 15 feet in length and can live for years in the small intestine. *Source*: Reprinted courtesy of CDC Public Health Image Library. ID#5260. Content provider: CDC. Available at: http://phil.cdc.gov/phil/details.asp. Accessed October 3, 2007.

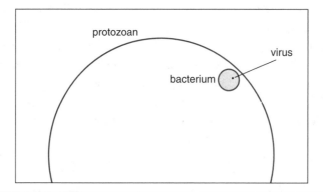

FIGURE 3.2 Approximate relative size of protozoan, bacterium, and virus.

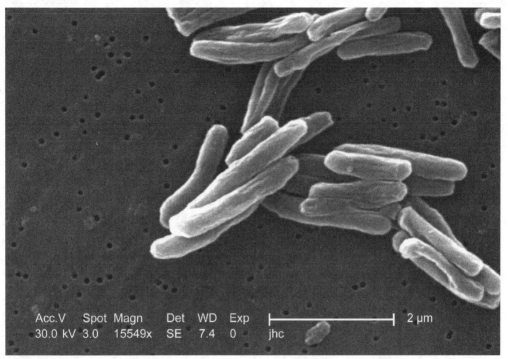

Acc.V   Spot Magn   Det   WD   Exp   2 µm
30.0 kV 3.0   15549x   SE   7.4   0   jhc

FIGURE 3.3 This scanning electron micrograph image shows several *Mycobacterium tuberculosis* bacteria; as the name suggests, this organism causes TB. *Source*: Reprinted courtesy of CDC Public Health Image Library. ID# 8438. Content provider: CDC/Dr. Ray Butler; Janice Carr. Available at: http://phil.cdc.gov/phil/details.asp. Accessed September 21, 2007.

Some bacteria are aerobic, requiring free oxygen to survive; other species can survive only in an anaerobic environment (that is, an environment lacking free oxygen); and still others can tolerate either condition. Some species of bacteria can take on the form of **spores**—dormant cells with a hard coating—to survive inhospitable conditions such as a dry environment, returning to their active, or vegetative, form when they find themselves in better conditions (for example, in the human body). Some bacteria cause injury to cells by invading body tissues and multiplying (infection); others cause injury by secreting a toxin (intoxication). Much of the terminology used to describe bacteria reflects their traditional classification by shape—round (*cocci*), spiral (*spirilli*), or rod-shaped (*bacilli*), like the tuberculosis bacteria in **Figure 3.3**—and their response to laboratory staining techniques. Certain molds and yeasts, single-celled fungi slightly larger than bacteria, can also cause human disease.

Unlike the unicellular protozoan and bacterium, a **virus**, at about 50 nanometers, is simply a strand of genetic material (DNA or RNA*) with a coat of protein. Lacking a cell wall, most viruses do not survive long outside a host organism. A virus cannot reproduce outside the host, but rather

*In some viruses, RNA (ribonucleic acid), rather than DNA, carries the genetic code.

uses the host cell's biochemical machinery to make copies of its own genetic material and assemble new viruses. Functionally, viruses are parasites—they cannot reproduce without the host organism—but the term *parasite* dates from an era when viruses were unknown and is more often used to refer to worms and protozoa. Viral pathogens cause influenza, measles, polio, Ebola hemorrhagic fever, dengue fever, and hantavirus pulmonary syndrome, among other illnesses.

Finally, **prions** are simply proteins found on the surface of normal nerve cells of some mammalian species, including humans. These prion proteins exist in normal and abnormal forms, which have the same chemical makeup but different shapes. As is true of all proteins, a prion's shape is a critical part of its identity and affects its function. The shape of the normal prion gives it a weak and flexible structure; the shape of the abnormal prion makes it rigid and nearly indestructible. The abnormal prion also has the special property of inducing nearby normal prions to convert to the abnormal shape through a mechanism that is not fully understood. When established in the brain, the abnormal prions produce a set of degenerative brain illnesses (encephalopathies). Because abnormal prions form plaques that create holes in the brain, producing a sponge-like appearance at autopsy, these diseases are called **transmissible spongiform encephalopathies** (TSEs). Prion diseases emerged from relative obscurity in the 1990s when it became clear that abnormal prions could be transmitted to people who ate beef from cattle suffering from "mad cow disease."

The Body's Defense Against Pathogens

The body's immune system distinguishes substances that are "self" from those—such as bacteria and viruses—that are foreign. The first time the body is exposed to such a foreign substance (called an **antigen**), the immune system responds by mounting a counterattack. This immune response includes the production of special proteins (**antibodies**) and cells to eliminate the antigen. The person experiences the disease, but if he survives he is protected against the same disease in the future because his immune system is now prepared to respond effectively. Such immunity, produced by one's own immune system, is called **active immunity**, and it is usually permanent.

A **vaccine** is an antigen preparation that is administered to a person—by injection, by mouth, or by nasal spray—to produce an immune response while bypassing illness. The antigen in a vaccine has been modified so that it does not cause illness (for example, bacterial cells in the vaccine may be dead or weakened), although it still evokes the immune response. An individual who has been vaccinated is protected against the disease in the future, without ever having actually been ill. This, too, is active immunity, produced by one's own immune system.

Alternatively, a person may acquire **passive immunity** from a vaccine that contains antibodies—ready-made protection against attack—rather than antigens. Infants in utero acquire passive immunity from antibodies transported across the placenta. Unlike active immunity, passive immunity is temporary.

From a public health perspective, the larger goal in vaccinating an individual is not just to keep that person from getting sick, but to keep him or her from spreading disease to others. **Herd immunity** refers to the practical protection experienced by a community when enough of its members have immunity against a disease that it becomes difficult to maintain a chain of infection. That is, the higher the proportion of those in the group who are immune, the less likely that a sick person will transmit the disease to someone who is vulnerable. The proportion of the group that must be immune to achieve herd immunity depends on how readily the disease is passed from one person to another, as well as on environmental factors such as crowding. By coupling the effects of aggressive vaccination and herd immunity, a disease can actually be eradicated—a goal that has been achieved for smallpox and is now being eyed for polio.

The term **vaccine-preventable diseases** refers to the set of diseases for which a vaccine is presently available. The US Centers for Disease Control and Prevention lists the following vaccine-preventable diseases as illnesses that once killed or disabled many US children and adolescents but that are now uncommon in the United States:

- Diphtheria
- *Haemophilus influenzae* type B
- Hepatitis A
- Hepatitis B
- Measles
- Mumps
- Pertussis (whooping cough)
- Pneumococcal disease
- Polio
- Rubella (German measles)
- Tetanus (lockjaw)
- Varicella (chickenpox).

Vaccines have also been developed for Lyme disease, rabies, typhoid fever, cholera, plague, anthrax, and other diseases.

The Transmission of Infectious Disease

Pathogens are flexible and opportunistic travelers, and so infectious disease is transmitted in many different ways. However, most of those ways are variations on three major modes of transmission: by closeness or contact, by some environmental medium (including food), or by vector. In the context of infectious disease, the term **vector** (from the Latin verb *to carry*) refers to a living transmitter of pathogens.

Transmission Through Closeness or Contact

Microbes can pass from person to person through simple proximity.* For example, coughing and sneezing spray droplets into the air. Droplets from a person with an infectious respiratory disease contain pathogens, which can be passed to a nearby person who inhales the suspended droplets during the brief period before they settle out of the air. Those traveling in commercial

---

*Strictly speaking, the term *contagious disease* refers to infectious disease transmitted person to person through closeness or contact, though in casual usage it sometimes appears synonymous with *infectious disease*. The term *communicable disease* is used with varied meanings and is not used in this text.

airliners are often acutely aware of this kind of transmission. Diseases transmitted by droplet include respiratory illnesses caused by bacteria (for example, diphtheria, tuberculosis, and pertussis [commonly called whooping cough]) or viruses (for example, influenza, measles, mumps, and rubella [commonly called German measles]). Some of these diseases can also be transmitted in finer aerosols that stay suspended in air for a longer period and that can penetrate deeper into the respiratory tract. Other pathogens, including streptococcal bacteria, the herpes simplex-1 virus (HSV-1), and the infectious mononucleosis virus, are transmitted mainly by direct oral contact.

Respiratory secretions or saliva can also be passed from person to person via an object in the environment, such as a shared handkerchief, a utensil, or a computer keyboard. An object that passively transmits pathogens in this way is called a **fomite**. For example, toddlers in day care transmit disease via fomites by mouthing and sharing toys. Pathogens vary in their capacity to survive such a passage through the environment.

Infectious diseases can also be transmitted via sexual contact. Major sexually transmitted diseases (also called venereal diseases) include the bacterial illnesses syphilis and gonorrhea, as well as the herpes simplex-2 virus (HSV-2, also known as genital herpes) and the human papillomavirus (HPV). Some pathogens that are sexually transmitted, such as the hepatitis B and hepatitis C viruses and the human immunodeficiency virus (HIV) that causes acquired immune deficiency syndrome (AIDS), can also be transmitted in blood. This can occur through medical procedures such as blood transfusions or via syringes acting as fomites: Drug users might share syringes, for example, and shortages of new syringes sometimes lead to the reuse of syringes in medical settings.

Transmission of diseases through closeness or contact can be reduced mainly through personal behaviors (for example, covering the nose when sneezing, not sharing utensils, preventing sexual transmission) or by remediating overcrowded conditions. Further, most of the diseases that can now be prevented by vaccination are diseases transmitted through closeness or contact.

As described in the following section, many diarrheal diseases are transmitted by ingestion of water contaminated by fecal waste. But another type of fecal transmission is more akin to transmission by closeness or contact. Recently documented events of transmission of the H5N1 avian influenza (bird flu) virus to humans are believed to have occurred when the victims inhaled bird droppings that had become **aerosolized** (that is, dried and reduced to very fine airborne particles). Hantavirus, which causes severe respiratory illness, can be transmitted to people via aerosolized rodent feces in the same manner. Thus, although the bird flu virus and hantavirus can be transmitted in fecal matter, exposure is via inhalation, and the resulting illness is respiratory.

Fecal–Oral Transmission of Diarrheal Disease

Many diseases transmitted via environmental media are fecal in origin. When a person has an infectious diarrheal disease, his or her feces contain pathogens. If another person somehow ingests even a small amount of this fecal matter, he or she is exposed to the pathogens via the **fecal–oral pathway**. In this way, one person's **infectious diarrheal disease** becomes the next person's **disease of fecal origin**, and these two terms refer to the same set of diseases. The list of diseases of fecal origin includes cholera and typhoid fever (both bacterial), dysentery (which can be caused either by a bacterium or by a protozoan parasite), the protozoan illnesses giardiasis and cryptosporidiosis, and the viral diseases hepatitis A, Norwalk virus, and polio. Both giardiasis and cryptosporidiosis are zoonotic illnesses that affect wild animals and farm animals as well as people.

How does one come to inadvertently ingest fecal pathogens? Much as a fomite can transmit contagious diseases from person to person, usually over short distances, water can act as a passive transmitter of infectious disease organisms through the natural environment, sometimes over long distances (**waterborne transmission**; see *a* and *b* in **Figure 3.4**). For example, a community might release untreated sewage into a river from which a downstream community draws its drinking water. For decades in the 19th and early 20th centuries, the city of Buffalo, New York, dumped its sewage into the Niagara River, with the result that the downstream city of Niagara Falls had high rates of cholera. Similarly, a well that is located downgradient of a privy or a septic system can supply water tainted by fecal waste. In some areas of Cape Cod in Massachusetts, where septic systems and small house lots are combined with heavy reliance on private drinking water wells, groundwater has been carefully monitored by the regional planning agency for decades to detect any evidence of contamination. Finally, water at beaches and in swimming pools can be contaminated so that swimmers are exposed via incidental ingestion of the water.

In the industrialized countries, such **waterborne illness** is largely—though not completely—controlled, through treatment of both sewage and drinking water (see Chapter 7). In many lower-income countries, however, waterborne illness caused by large-scale fecal contamination of rivers, lakes, and wells is a central fact of life. Diarrheal disease, transmitted by ingesting contaminated water, is the major health impact of such contamination and a leading cause of mortality and morbidity in lower-income countries. Dermal contact carries a different risk: If a person with a skin wound swims or bathes in water contaminated by sewage, the wound can become infected. Left untreated, such a wound infection may progress to septicemia (blood poisoning).

Although water is the dominant environmental medium in fecal–oral transmission, as indicated by the heavy lines in Figure 3.4, it is not the only one. Uncontrolled fecal waste can also contaminate the ground *(c)*—a common problem in regions where the latrine (a simple pit in

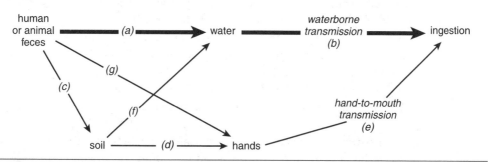

FIGURE 3.4 Fecal–oral transmission of disease via water, soil, and hands in a setting with no treatment of sewage or drinking water.

the ground, used as a toilet) is a common means of waste disposal. In the industrialized world, exposure to human fecal waste on the ground is mostly limited to recreational activities, such as camping or playing at playgrounds. Dried fecal waste quickly becomes mixed with dust, so this exposure might not be obvious. People can also be exposed to feces of farm animals or pets. In any setting, young children are particularly likely to have these exposures because they spend time playing on the ground—getting soil on their hands *(d)* and putting their hands into their mouths, resulting in **hand-to-mouth transmission** of pathogens *(e)*. Particularly in lower-income countries, worm diseases are common among young children. Adults' hands, too, can convey pathogens along the fecal–oral pathway as fingers touch the mouth in eating, smoking, or gesturing. Contaminated soil can also add to the pathogen load of rivers, lakes, or groundwater *(f)*.

To prevent direct contamination of the hands with fecal matter *(g)*, those who live in industrialized countries are routinely taught to wash their hands before preparing or eating food, and after using the toilet, changing a baby's diaper, or aiding a sick or disabled person with toileting. Actual behavior may be less careful, however. For example, a recent study of handwashing among female college students found that only 63% washed or rinsed their hands after using the toilet, and only 38% washed with soap.[4] Other research indicates that men are less likely than women to wash their hands after using the toilet.[5] The goal of handwashing is not to kill microorganisms but rather to remove them, and this is best accomplished through the use of soap and warm running water, vigorous rubbing for at least 20 seconds, and careful drying of the hands.[6] In lower-income countries, facilities for effective handwashing may not be readily available.

Although the terminology used to describe the transmission of infectious diarrheal disease is modern—exposure pathways, fecal–oral transmission—the ideas are not new. An article published in the *Journal of the American Medical Association* in 1898, for example, describes an exposure pathway that today we might label "incidental ingestion of fecal matter":

> An English practitioner refers to the fact that many cases of typhoid fever occur in the autumn, and attributes the cause of the disease to games, such as marbles and peg-top, which are played in the street during this time of the year after the cricket season is over. In playing marbles a boy frequently licks his fingers to prevent the marble slipping, and the whip-cord of a top is wet in the mouth for the same reason. In this way germs are conveyed into the alimentary tract. . . . These games may therefore be a great source of danger to children living a town life. . . . In his own city of Sheffield, he says that he has seen the contents of yard-vaults [cesspools] shoveled out into the streets or roadway in large heaps to be carted away afterward, but leaving behind remainders lodged between the stones of the road, upon and near which the open-air games of boys are daily practiced. . . . Contaminated water in his opinion is not the only source of typhoid and other filth fevers among boys.[7]

Transmission of Nonfecal Organisms Found in Water or Soil

Although many pathogens found in water or soil are of fecal origin, these media are also natural reservoirs for many nonfecal pathogens. Just two nonfecal waterborne pathogens are described here, chosen simply to demonstrate the broad range of ways by which pathogens can be transmitted in water.

Guinea worm disease (dracunculiasis) is a waterborne parasitic illness. When a person drinks water containing Guinea worm larvae, the parasite matures in the body. Ultimately, a worm up to 3 feet long emerges through a skin wound, usually when the skin is immersed in water. The worm immediately spills larvae back into the water, restarting the cycle of disease.[8] Guinea worm disease was once widespread in sub-Saharan Africa but is now uncommon, largely because of the widespread use of simple methods to filter water (see **Figure 3.5**)—a public health success story.

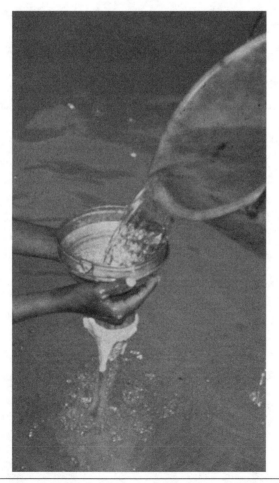

FIGURE 3.5 Use of a simple strainer like the one being demonstrated here—a metal funnel and a piece of filter cloth—can filter out water fleas that carry the larval Guinea worm parasite. *Source*: Reprinted courtesy of CDC Public Health Image Library. ID# 8206. Content provider: CDC. Available at: http://phil.cdc.gov/phil/deatils.asp. Accessed September 26, 2007.

Legionella bacteria are transmitted by very different means—in the water droplets of fine aerosol sprays, which are inhaled. Some shower heads, whirlpool spas, and ultrasonic humidifiers produce such a fine spray. Aerosols can also be created in the cooling towers of large air-conditioning systems (where air is blown through water to cool the water by evaporation) and then carried via ambient air or through air-conditioning ducts.[9] Air-conditioning ducts were the source of the first identified outbreak of the pneumonia-like *Legionella* illness (Legionnaires' disease) at an American Legion convention in 1976.

Soil is also a natural reservoir for several pathogens important to human health. Spores of the bacterium *Clostridium tetani*, which causes tetanus (lockjaw), are widespread in soil and can survive there under dry conditions for many years. People are most commonly exposed to *Clostridium tetani* via a skin wound. For example, a deep puncture wound from stepping on a rusty nail can result in a tetanus infection—not from the nail or the rust, but from bacteria in soil that the nail embeds into the wound. In lower-income countries, newborns and their mothers are at risk of tetanus infection because of unhygienic birthing conditions. The bacterium produces a neurotoxin that causes muscle spasms, beginning in the head and neck. Spores of the anthrax bacterium, *Bacillus anthracis*, are also widespread in soil.

Foodborne Transmission

Any infectious illness transmitted in food is a **foodborne illness**. In a setting without sewage treatment or drinking water treatment, several fecal–oral exposure pathways lead through food (see *l* in **Figure 3.6**; this figure adds **foodborne transmission** of fecal disease to the pathways depicted in Figure 3.4). As shown in Figure 3.6, water tainted by human sewage may be used in the preparation of food *(h)*, or small amounts of contaminated soil may be present on food *(i)*—for example, if vegetables are not adequately washed. Unwashed hands can also compromise the cleanliness of food preparation *(j)*.

Finally, the humble housefly, by landing first on fecal waste and then on food, can transfer bacteria and protozoan parasites that cling to its feet *(k)*. Unlike the inanimate fomite,

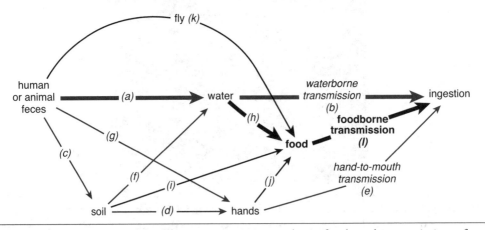

FIGURE 3.6 Addition of foodborne transmission to basic fecal–oral transmission of disease, in a setting with no treatment of sewage or drinking water.

the housefly is a living transmitter of pathogens—a vector. Still, its function is strictly mechanical—it plays no biological role in the life cycle of the pathogen—so it is termed a **mechanical vector**. This type of transmission can be reduced by screening the vents of privies to prevent flies from entering the waste pit, by putting screens in windows and doors, and by covering food.

Thus, in a setting without treatment of sewage or drinking water, human fecal contamination so dominates foodborne illness that it is difficult to separate out other sources of food contamination. In contrast, in industrialized nations, because fecal wastes are generally controlled and tap water is generally clean, both human fecal contamination and other sources of foodborne illness are often readily identifiable. Some foodborne hazards originate far "upstream" in the food supply, long before food products reach consumers; these hazards are described in Chapter 6.

Foodborne Illness in the Industrialized Countries

Despite the routine treatment of both wastewater and tap water, food is sometimes contaminated by human fecal matter. For example, shellfish can be contaminated by sewage waste before being harvested—and might also be eaten raw so that pathogens survive the trip to the table. More often, human fecal contamination of food occurs when someone fails to wash his or her hands thoroughly after using the toilet and before preparing food. Such handwashing is important not only at home but also in food service settings. This is why local health codes require restaurant workers to wash their hands after using the toilet and before returning to work. Noncompliance with these procedures can result in transmission of an illness such as hepatitis A from one worker to a number of customers before the outbreak becomes apparent and is traced to its source.

However, in the industrialized nations, most foodborne illness is not of human fecal origin, but comes from other sources. Pathogens can be present on food when we bring it home from the store. For example, small quantities of fecal matter from animals eaten as food, such as poultry or cattle, may contaminate the carcass during processing (detailed in Chapter 6), and thus animal fecal pathogens can be present on raw meat when it is purchased. Similarly, nonfecal pathogens can be present on food at the time of purchase. Pathogens present on food can contaminate utensils and other kitchen equipment. Careful washing of fruits and vegetables removes soil that might harbor pathogens; this is particularly important if a food is to be eaten raw.

Even human skin is a potential source of pathogens, especially if a person has infected cuts or sores on the hands; thorough handwashing is important even if no infection is present. And control of mechanical vectors, such as houseflies or cockroaches (see **Figure 3.7**), which are attracted to food and can carry pathogens on their feet, is also important.

Basic Levers for the Control of Foodborne Illness

In reality, microbial contamination of food is a fact of life. However, many hazards can be prevented or controlled by following some general practices for safe food handling. As the term *food safety* is typically used in environmental health, it focuses on procedures to prevent food-

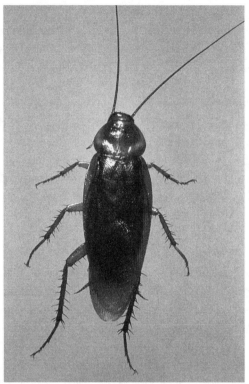

FIGURE 3.7 Cockroaches, which are widespread household pests, can serve as mechanical vectors in the transmission of foodborne pathogens. *Source*: Reprinted courtesy of CDC Public Health Image Library. ID# 6319. Content provider: CDC. Available at http://phil.cdc.gov/phil/details.asp. Accessed September 26, 2007.

borne illness at the point where food is prepared, by controlling the environment in which pathogens find themselves. Toxins found in nature, including some to which people might be exposed via food, are described in Section 3.2.

If pathogenic bacteria are to survive and prosper in food, their basic needs must be met. Most human pathogens (which are adapted to live in the human body and also to survive a passage through the ambient environment) survive and multiply at temperatures from 40°F to 140°F—a temperature range known in food safety as the **danger zone**. Bacteria also require water and nutrients, and individual species have other requirements (such as an aerobic environment, or an anaerobic environment) or tolerances (for a high-salt environment, for example).

In favorable conditions, the growth of a population of bacteria follows a typical pattern (see **Figure 3.8**). During the first 1 to 4 hours in a new environment, bacteria multiply only slowly. This early period is known as the **lag phase**. The lag phase is followed by a period of logarithmic growth (the **log phase**), followed in turn by a plateau as the bacterial population exhausts the resources of its environment.

Thus, two basic levers for the control of bacterial contamination of food are time and temperature, and a general rule of thumb in food safety is "keep it hot, or keep it cold, or don't keep

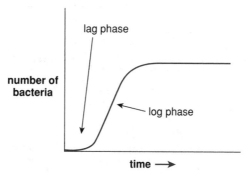

FIGURE 3.8 A schematic bacterial growth curve.

it." That is, although the lag phase offers a sort of grace period, the key to food safety is to limit the time that food spends in the danger zone. Food should be stored cold and cooked to a high enough temperature to kill pathogens. (Instructions for specific foods should be followed; the recommended temperatures for broiled meat and poultry, for example, are higher than 140°F.) Some foodborne pathogens form spores that can survive inhospitable conditions. Of course, cleanliness—of hands, work surfaces, and implements—is also a key to controlling foodborne illness, as detailed in the following subsection.

Some Important Foodborne Pathogens

When we think of foodborne illness, we tend to think of vomiting and diarrhea, and indeed these are common symptoms. But in fact, foodborne pathogens cause a range of symptoms, and do so by a range of mechanisms. Some foodborne pathogens cause symptoms in the host simply through **infection**—for example, by invading tissues or causing inflammation. Other species produce toxins that cause the symptoms of foodborne illness; this type of illness is called **intoxication**. Usually, intoxication occurs when pathogens produce a toxin in food, which is then eaten, but some pathogens produce toxins in the body.

Some important foodborne pathogens in the United States are described briefly here and summarized in **Table 3.1**.

Nontyphoid *Salmonella* species (that is, excluding *Salmonella typhii*, which causes typhoid fever) are common in the feces of poultry and therefore often contaminate raw poultry during processing. When people become sick from *Salmonella*-contaminated poultry, it is usually for one of two reasons: Either the poultry was not cooked to a high enough temperature to kill organisms; or alternatively, the bird was properly cooked but it was contaminated *after cooking* by an implement or a cutting board that had been in contact with the raw bird. This is known as **cross-contamination** of cooked food by raw food. If the recontaminated cooked bird is then allowed to sit for long enough at room temperature, the bacterial population will increase dramatically. Illness from nontyphoid *Salmonella*, which causes vomiting and diarrhea, occurs only after ingesting a very large number of organisms.[10]

Campylobacter species, like *Salmonella*, are common contaminants of raw poultry; *Campylobacter* it is now the leading cause of bacterial diarrheal illness in the United States.[10]

Table 3.1   Key Characteristics of Some Common Foodborne Pathogens

Pathogen	Common Source	Common Food	Aerobic/ Anaerobic	Spore-forming?	Toxin-producing?
Salmonella species	Poultry/fecal	Poultry	Aerobic	No	?*
Campylobacter species	Poultry/fecal	Poultry, raw milk	Aerobic	No	No
Listeria monocytogenes	Widespread in environment	Raw milk, soft cheeses	Aerobic	No (but hardy)	No
E. coli O157:H7	Cattle/fecal	Ground beef, leafy greens	Aerobic	No	Yes (produced in the body)
Staphylococcus aureus	Human skin	Ham salad, chicken salad	Aerobic	No	Yes (heat-stable)
Clostridium botulinum	Soil	Home-canned food	Anaerobic	Yes	Yes (heat-sensitive)

*Salmonella has traditionally been considered not to produce a toxin, but recent evidence suggests that it may do so.

Data from: US Food and Drug Administration. *Foodborne Pathogenic Microorganisms and Natural Toxins Handbook, 2005.* Available at: http://vm.cfsan.fda.gov/~mow/intro.html.

Analyses of poultry products purchased in stores show that *Campylobacter* and *Salmonella* are widespread in both conventionally and organically grown poultry, but the strains present in the conventionally grown poultry are much more likely to be resistant to common antibiotics.[11,12]

Although nontyphoid *Salmonella* and *Campylobacter* are the two most common foodborne illnesses in the United States, they are rarely fatal to those who are made ill (see **Table 3.2**). In contrast, **Listeria monocytogenes** is the least common of the six illnesses described here, but also the most fatal. *Listeria* organisms are widespread in mammals and birds and also in soil. Among

Table 3.2   Estimated Annual Illnesses and Deaths in the United States from Six Foodborne Pathogens During the 1990s

Agent	Cases of Illness	Deaths
Salmonella (nontyphoid)	1,341,873	553
Campylobacter species	1,963,141	99
Listeria monocytogenes	2493	499
E. coli O157:H7	62,458	52
Staphylococcus species	185,060	2
Clostridium perfringens	248,520	7

Adapted from: Mead P, Slutsker L, Dietz V, McCraig L, Bresee J, Shapiro C, et al. Food-related illness and death in the United States. *Emerg Infect Dis.* 1999;5(5): 607–625:Table 3.

non-spore-forming organisms, *Listeria* is unusually resistant to heat, cold (it can multiply in refrigerated foods), and drying.[10] *Listeria* has been documented in many types of foods but is
most associated with raw milk and soft ripened cheeses. This foodborne pathogen causes serious
illness, with symptoms including septicemia (blood poisoning) and meningitis; pregnant
women can suffer spontaneous abortion or stillbirth.[10]

One pathogen of particular concern in recent years is a strain of the bacterium *Escherichia
coli* (*E. coli*). There are hundreds of strains of *E. coli*, many of which are normally present in the
human gut. The strain known as *E. coli* O157:H7 can be present in the intestines of healthy
cattle and can contaminate meat during processing. In people, *E. coli* O157:H7 produces a
toxin after colonizing the intestines, and the toxin damages the lining of the intestine, causing
bloody diarrhea, sometimes severe. In some people, especially in children under 5 years and the
elderly, the infection also causes destruction of red blood cells and kidney failure; this complication, called hemolytic uremic syndrome, can be fatal.[13] The most common vehicle for illness
from *E. coli* O157:H7 is ground beef: Although adequate cooking does kill this pathogen, the
heat must reach the organisms wherever they have been left by processing, and it is harder to
heat the interior of a hamburger than the surface of a steak. Moreover, ingesting as few as 10 organisms can cause illness.[10] An early outbreak of *E. coli* O157:H7 occurred when cider was
made from apples that had fallen from trees and become contaminated by cow manure.

Staphylococcus aureus (commonly called *staph*) is a normal inhabitant of human skin but is
present in very large numbers in boils and other sores or cuts and is usually passed to food
through poor hygiene* practices on the part of someone preparing food. Ham salad and
chicken salad are common vehicles for staph illness because contamination occurs after cooking, in handling the meat. If the meat then sits at room temperature—for example, on a buf-
fet—the organisms multiply and produce a toxin, which causes illness. Because the toxin is
heat-resistant, reheating food (such as a sliced cooked ham) will not prevent illness. Staph
causes gastrointestinal illness.

Poisoning by *Clostridium botulinum* is commonly known as botulism. *Clostridium* is an
anaerobic, spore-forming organism that produces a toxin that can be denatured by heat.
Clostridium is widespread in the soil in the environment and may therefore be present on vegetables, for example. Historically, the classic vehicle for botulism was home-canned food, although home canning is less common today than in the past. If green beans, for example, are
inadequately heated during canning, spores can survive the canning process and germinate in
the anaerobic environment of the can, producing a toxin. Although the toxin can be denatured
by heat, this requires boiling for some time. Thus, if the food is only quickly reheated, the toxin
causes illness. Botulinum toxin is a potentially fatal neurotoxin; early symptoms include weakness, vertigo, and difficulty swallowing and breathing.[10] *Clostridium botulinum* spores (some-

---

*In this text, the term *hygiene* is used in the sense of cleanliness, mainly as it relates to infectious disease
risks. Historically, this term was used broadly to refer to public health as the science of preventing disease
and maintaining health, and this usage survives in the term *industrial hygiene* as a synonym for *occupational health*.

times present in honey) do not germinate in the adult gut but can germinate in the gut of infants, and infant botulism can be fatal.[10]

Finally, **scombroid poisoning** (not listed in Table 3.2) is caused by a toxin produced by certain types of bacteria, acting on certain amino acids in foods, when conditions of time and temperature are not adequately controlled. Scombroid poisoning is most associated with the spoilage of fish, especially tuna and related fish (for example, mahi mahi, bluefish, sardines, mackerel, amberjack, abalone), but it has also been tied to the production of Swiss cheese.[14] Once the toxin is formed, it is not inactivated by cooking, canning, or freezing; the symptoms, which sometimes require hospitalization, can include a drop in blood pressure, headaches, and vomiting and diarrhea.[14]

Vectorborne Transmission

A host species that transmits an infectious disease to another host species is called a **biological vector** of the disease, and a disease that is transmitted in this way is called a **vectorborne disease**. (Diseases that might be transmitted by a mechanical vector such as a housefly, which is not a host species, are not considered vectorborne diseases.) Many biological vectors are **arthropods**, a group that comprises insects (such as mosquitoes, flies, lice, and fleas) and arachnids (including ticks, mites, and spiders). However, mammalian hosts can also transmit diseases to people.

Many arthropods transmit disease among larger animals by taking blood meals from them (**Figure 3.9**). Such an *arthropod-borne virus* is called an **arbovirus**. For example, the West Nile virus, which can cause encephalitis, infects humans, birds, and certain species of mosquito. When one of these mosquitoes bites an infected bird, it draws blood that contains the virus. In the mosquito, the virus migrates to the saliva glands, and when the mosquito later bites another

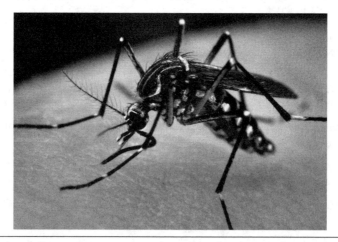

FIGURE 3.9 An *Aedes aegypti* mosquito, the vector for dengue fever, takes a blood meal from a human host. *Source*: Reprinted courtesy of CDC Public Health Image Library. ID# 9252. Content providers: CDC/Prof. Frank Hadley Collins, Dir., Cntr. for Global Health and Infectious Disease, Univ. of Notre Dame. Available at: http://phil.cdc.gov/phil/details.asp. Accessed August 21, 2007.

Table 3.3 Comparison of Fomite, Mechanical Vector, and Biological Vector

Transmitter of Disease	Living Transmitter?	Host Organism?
Fomite	no	no
Mechanical vector	yes	no
Biological vector ("vectorborne" illness)	yes	yes

bird (or a person), the mosquito injects saliva containing viruses into the new host. Thus, a biological vector, such as a mosquito, functions differently from a mechanical vector, such as the housefly passively depositing pathogens that are stuck to its feet (see **Table 3.3**). Some biological vectors are themselves made ill by the pathogens they transmit, but most are not. Dengue fever (also known as breakbone fever for the severe joint pain it causes) is another arbovirus disease, carried by mosquitoes between people and monkeys.

There are many variations on the basic framework of vectorborne transmission by arthropods, reflecting the diverse interconnections that are possible among pathogens and their hosts in ecosystems. For example, a pathogen may require more than one host species to complete its life cycle: The protozoan parasites that cause malaria (*Plasmodium* species) pass through some developmental life stages in humans and others in the mosquito vector (*Anopheles* species). Alternatively, the vector may require multiple hosts to complete its life cycle, with the pathogen merely along for the ride. For example, Lyme disease is caused by a bacterium (*Borrelia burgdorferi*) that is found in the blood of the tick vector (see **Figure 3.10** and **Figure 3.11**). A tick larvum, after taking a blood meal (usually from a bird), molts into a nymph; which, after taking a blood meal (usually from a

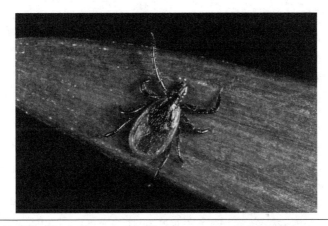

FIGURE 3.10 The black-legged tick (*Ixodes scapularis*), shown here on a blade of grass, transmits Lyme disease among a number of mammalian hosts, including humans. *Source*: Reprinted courtesy of CDC Public Health Image Library. ID# 1669. Content providers: CDC/Michael L. Levin, Ph.D. Available at: http://phil.cdc.gov/phil/details.asp. Accessed September 19, 2007.

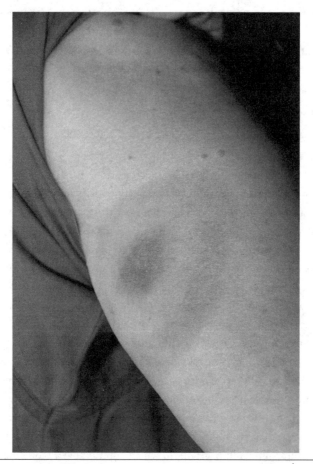

FIGURE 3.11 The "bulls-eye" rash around a tick bite on this woman's arm is characteristic of the infection known as Lyme disease. *Source*: Reprinted courtesy of CDC Public Health Image Library. ID# 9873. Content providers: CDC/James Gathany. Available at: http://phil.cdc.gov/phil/details.asp. Accessed September 13, 2007.

mouse or a person), molts into an adult tick; which, after taking a blood meal (usually from a deer or a person), produces eggs that hatch into larvae. At any stage of the tick's life, the bacterial pathogen can be passed to a new host when the tick takes a blood meal.

In contrast, the insect vector for typhus—the body louse—simply moves from person to person through close proximity (explaining why this disease, which was once common, most often afflicted armies, prisoners, and others living in crowded conditions). The bacterial pathogen (*Rickettsia prowazekii*) is not passed via the bite of the louse but rather is present in the louse's feces. The louse leaves both bites and feces on the skin of its human victim. The bites are itchy, and by scratching, the victim rubs the louse feces into the bites. The rickettsial infection is fatal to the louse.

Arthropod vectors transmit many other illnesses, including two that have historically appeared as large-scale epidemics: plague (a bacterial illness transmitted by rat fleas) and yellow fever (a viral illness transmitted by mosquito). Two parasitic vectorborne diseases that, like malaria, cause much morbidity in warm climates are onchocerciasis (river blindness), caused by a parasitic worm and transmitted by black flies, and African sleeping sickness, caused by a protozoan parasite and transmitted by tsetse flies.

Although most vectorborne transmission is by arthropod vectors, nonarthropod vectors can also transmit disease via bite. For example, a raccoon or squirrel infected with rabies carries the virus in its saliva and can transmit it to a person by biting.

Vectorborne transmission is commonly managed using two basic approaches. One is to reduce the vector population through the use of pesticides or by modifying the environment—for example, draining a swamp to reduce mosquito populations or managing rubbish to reduce rodent populations. The other is to prevent contact between vectors and people—for example, people can choose their clothing to prevent contact with ticks, or use screens or nets to prevent contact with mosquitoes. In some high-malaria regions, the use of bed nets impregnated with pesticide has been successful in reducing transmission of the disease by mosquitoes. Insect repellents, as the name suggests, drive pests away but do not kill them.

A Complex Web of Transmission

For purposes of introducing basic concepts of infectious disease, this text has described transmission by closeness or contact, by environmental medium, and by biological vector as if these were all quite distinct. Yet in functional terms, it is clear that a sneeze, a child's toy, a sexual encounter, aerosolized fecal matter, a polluted river, a housefly, a raw oyster, undercooked meat or poultry, an ultrasonic humidifier, a tick, and a rabid squirrel all play fundamentally similar roles in transmitting disease. In natural settings, infectious agents are transmitted by varied and flexible means, blurring any neat distinctions that might be drawn. Further, there is increasing concern that pathogens might be deliberately transmitted—that is, used as weapons, called **bioweapons**—on a larger scale than has been seen in the past.

The transmission of anthrax illustrates the complexities of disease transmission. This zoonotic disease occurs mostly in large herbivores including cattle, sheep, and goats. Infected animals shed spores in urine and feces, and other animals become infected by ingesting spores in soil while grazing. Anthrax spores can persist in soil for decades and are dispersed in the environment by wind. Spores are also thought to be effectively dispersed in the environment on the feathers of vultures and other scavenging birds who have fed on infected carcasses.[15] Most people are exposed to anthrax spores through close contact with an animal or its hide or wool. Most often, the spores enter via a skin wound; less frequently—but more fatally—spores are inhaled. People can also become ill by eating the meat of an infected animal. Last but not least, if anthrax spores can be effectively aerosolized for greater airborne dispersion, they could be used by terrorists as a weapon—an act of **bioterrorism**. This complex picture of anthrax transmission combines elements of transmission by biological vector (cow or sheep); by closeness or contact (with the animal's hide or wool); by mechanical vector (vulture); by air, soil, feces, or food; and perhaps even by intent.

Finally, the web of infectious disease transmission is always changing. Scientists now recognize a set of **emerging (or reemerging) infectious diseases**—illnesses that have only recently been identified or are making an unexpected comeback. HIV/AIDS, the H5N1 avian influenza, Ebola hemorrhagic fever, severe acute respiratory syndrome (SARS), bovine spongi-form encephalopathy and the associated illness in humans, dengue fever, hantavirus, *E. coli* O157:H7, and drug-resistant malaria are all in this group. Within a few decades, AIDS emerged from obscurity to become a global health threat of enormous proportions. At any time, the constant shuffling of the genome of the avian influenza virus might produce a variant that is readily transmissible between humans—and when this happens, infected travelers are likely to spread it around the world before they know they are sick. These emerging diseases serve as a reminder that pathogens and vectors are resilient and flexible, and that the effects of human activities can ripple through a global ecosystem.

Infectious Disease as a Cause of Cancer

The International Agency for Research on Cancer (IARC), which evaluates the carcinogenicity not only of chemical and physical hazards but also of infectious agents, has designated several pathogens as known or probable human carcinogens. (An infection can increase cancer risk through various mechanisms—for example, through chronic irritation, resulting in cell prolif-eration and increased opportunity for mutation.) Known infectious causes of cancer were esti-mated to account for about 18% of cancers worldwide in 2002.[16] Taken as a group, the lower-income nations have both a higher incidence of infectious disease and a greater popula-tion than the industrialized nations do. Thus 26.3% of cancers in the lower-income nations in 2002 but only 7.7% of cancers in the industrialized nations in the same year are attributable to infectious causes. As shown in **Figure 3.12**, most of these are cancers of the liver, cervix, or stomach.

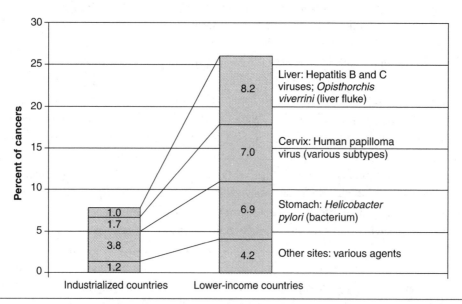

FIGURE 3.12 Percentage of cancers by infectious agents in industrialized and lower-income countries. *Data from*: Parkin DM. The global health burden of infection-associated cancers in the year 2002. *Int J. Cancer* 2006;118;3030–3044: table XI.

Global Patterns of Infectious Disease Mortality

As described earlier, there are a great number of human pathogens. Yet a relatively well defined set of illnesses account for most deaths from infectious disease worldwide—a total of approximately 14.9 million in 2002.[16] Diseases transmitted by closeness or contact predominate—in **Figure 3.13**, all categories except diarrheal diseases and malaria fall into this group. The burden of death from lower respiratory infections (26% of infectious disease deaths) and HIV/AIDS (19%) is particularly heavy. Among deaths from childhood diseases, more than half are from measles, and most others are from pertussis (whooping cough) or tetanus. Malnutrition contributes heavily to infectious disease mortality, both by increasing susceptibility to disease (for example, to pneumonia) and as a complication of illness (for example, measles). Indeed, the World Health Organization estimates that malnutrition is an underlying factor in more than half of childhood deaths worldwide.[17]

Simple mortality statistics, of course, cannot capture the full impact of infectious disease in morbidity and in economic and social costs. Even so, mortality patterns reveal much about the burden of disease and about disparities in that burden. Worldwide, 26% of all deaths were from infectious disease in 2002, the most recent year for which detailed infectious disease mortality statistics are available.[18] Overall, infectious disease is a more prevalent cause of death where overall child and adult mortality are high, as shown in **Table 3.4**, which groups countries by mortality stratum and geographic region, following the World Health Organization's reporting format. As shown, only African countries appear in the highest mortality stratum. Further, the proportion of mortality from infectious diseases is higher in African countries than in countries in other regions, even those with comparable overall mortality. In the low child/low adult mortality stra-

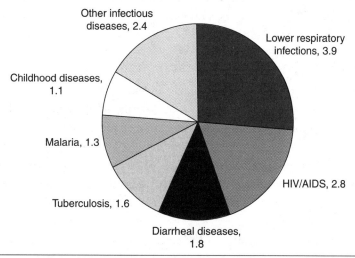

FIGURE 3.13 Estimated deaths worldwide from leading infectious causes, 2002 (millions of deaths). *Data from*: World Health Organization. *Statistical Annexe, World Health Report 2004—Changing History*; Table 2. Available at: http://www.who.int/whr/2004/en. Accessed February 7, 2008.

Table 3.4   Percentage of Worldwide Deaths That Are from Infectious Disease, by Mortality Stratum and Geographic Region

Mortality Stratum	Geographic Region					
	The Americas	Europe	Eastern Mediterranean	Africa	Southeast Asia	Western Pacific
High child/very high adult				66		
High child/high adult	33		36	60	31	
Low child/high adult		4				
Low child/low adult	11	7	8		23	11
Very low child/very low adult	5	6				11

Empty cell indicates no countries in geographic region and mortality stratum.

Data from: World Health Organization. *The World Health Report 2004—Changing History, 2004.* Statistical Annexe, Table 2. Available at: http://www.who.int/whr/2004/en/. Accessed: February 7, 2008.

tum, the countries of Southeast Asia stand out as having a heavy burden of death from infectious disease. The United States falls in the stratum of very low child and very low adult mortality.

By the 1960s and 1970s, experts in the United States and other industrialized nations were riding a wave of optimism, believing that infectious disease was no match for modern medicine. But by the end of the century, that optimism had been deflated by the emergence of new diseases, the reemergence of old ones, and the stubborn hold of infectious disease as a major cause of mortality and morbidity in much of the world.

Strategies for Managing Infectious Disease Risk

Before the microbial causation of disease was widely understood, two main strategies were used to control or prevent infectious disease.[3] One was quarantine—the practice of isolating sick or potentially sick persons so that they could not infect others. Quarantine addressed the fear of person-to-person contagion. The word itself derives from the 14th-century Venetian practice of requiring ships to wait at anchor in port for 40 days before anyone was allowed to disembark. Modern terminology distinguishes between **isolation** (the separation of persons who have an infectious illness) and **quarantine** (the separation of persons who have been exposed to an infectious agent and may become ill).[19]

The second main strategy, beginning in the early 19th century, was **sanitation**—specifically, the removal of decaying organic matter, sometimes even extending to the draining of swamps—to prevent miasmas from rising out of this matter. In the name of sanitary reform, public sewer systems were built and procedures were set up to remove garbage from cities. These measures, though they rested on a misunderstanding of disease causation, provided a substantial benefit to public health by reducing sources of exposure to fecal matter and to insect and rodent vectors of disease.[3] This sanitary reform movement laid the foundation for the field of environmental health.

In the 20th and 21st centuries, isolation/quarantine and environmental interventions including sanitation have been supplemented by other tools of modern infectious disease control. Chemical pesticides are widely used to control vectors of disease. Vaccination and antibiotics (pharmaceuticals that kill or inhibit bacteria), aided by intensive disease surveillance, have become central to the battle to control infectious disease. Surprisingly, though vaccination against smallpox was adopted rapidly after it was introduced in 1796, almost 100 years passed before vaccines for any other diseases were developed. Today vaccines for more than 20 diseases have been developed.

Although antibiotics remain an important weapon in the battle against infectious disease, bacterial resistance to antibiotics is a growing problem. Over time, a population of bacteria can become largely resistant to a specific antibiotic if, at the outset, some of the bacteria have a genetic makeup that confers resistance. This is the familiar phenomenon of "survival of the fittest," as occurs in natural selection—except that in this case, the selection factor is a man-made antibiotic. With the widespread use of antibiotics in both humans and animals, such antibiotic resistance has become a major public health concern.

Of particular concern at present is a virulent antibiotic-resistant strain of *Staphylococcus aureus*. Known as **methicillin-resistant** *Staphylococcus aureus* (MRSA), the strain is also resistant to related antibiotics, including penicillin and amoxicillin. MRSA is widespread in hospitals and commonly found on the hands of health care workers, and most cases of MRSA are associated with invasive procedures in a health care setting, leading to infections of surgical wounds or of the bloodstream, for example.[20] Such infections are referred to as hospital-acquired MRSA or health-care-associated MRSA. A much smaller number of MRSA infections occur outside health care settings, and are referred to as community-acquired, or community-associated MRSA. Drug resistance has also created challenges in the treatment of tuberculosis, HIV/AIDS, and malaria.

US Regulatory Framework for Managing Infectious Disease Risk

In the United States today, the US Centers for Disease Control and Prevention (CDC) develops disease-specific guidelines for the vaccination of children and adults and provides these recommendations to the states. The individual states can then adopt the recommendations, requiring children to have immunizations before entering school in the state. States also set rules for exemptions from the vaccination requirements—for example, for medical or religious reasons. Similarly, each state is responsible for isolation and quarantine within its own borders. At the national level, CDC has the authority under the US Public Health Service Act to use isolation or quarantine to prevent infectious diseases from being brought into the country (see **Table 3.5**). (This table is the first in a series of similar tables that place regulatory provisions within the traditional regulatory domains of environmental health; each subsequent table in the series will fill in additional pieces of the US regulatory picture.) There are limitations on this power, however, and it has rarely been invoked.

Table 3.5   Overview of US Regulatory Framework for Environmental Health Hazards (1)

Environmental Health Domain	Major Laws and Key Provisions for the Control of Environmental Health Hazards
Biological hazards	*Public Health Service Act (PHSA)—development of guidelines for vaccination; use of quarantine or isolation to prevent entry of infectious diseases into the United States; conduct of surveillance and investigation of outbreaks*
Air pollution	
Ionizing radiation	
Alternative energy sources	
Hazardous wastes	
Occupational health	
Industrial water pollution	
Toxic chemicals	
Pesticides	
Food supply	
Sewage wastes and community water supply	
Municipal solid waste	
Consumer products	
Environmental noise	

Note: New information appears in italics.

The CDC also conducts infectious disease surveillance for a list of nationally notifiable diseases, using data collected voluntarily by the states. Finally, the CDC investigates epidemics and foodborne disease outbreaks, and does research and public education on infectious disease. At the international level, the World Health Organization (WHO) conducts infectious disease surveillance and prevention programs and responds to outbreaks.

As described earlier, food handling practices are important in preventing foodborne illness. However, events that occur upstream in the food supply system are also important. The US regulatory framework focuses on these upstream risks (see Chapter 6); requirements for treating sewage and drinking water are also important (see Chapter 7).

3.2 Poisons in Nature

Several types of poisons—produced by animals, plants, algae, or fungi—can cause illness in people. For example, nature arms some animals with poisons, which they use mainly to defend against predators or to subdue their own prey, usually by biting or stinging.[21] Some of the best known among the many species of venomous snakes worldwide are the cobra, viper, copperhead, diamondback rattlesnake, and coral snake. Some scorpions and spiders (for example, the black widow and brown recluse; see **Figure 3.14**) are also venomous, as are some marine creatures including stingrays and scorpionfishes.

Both the medicinal and poisonous properties of plants have long been recognized. Many plants cause gastrointestinal upset or minor skin irritation (for example, poison ivy), and some have more serious health effects. Livestock, because of exposures through foraging, often suffer the effects of plant toxins. Of particular note for human risk is the castor bean plant, whose seeds contain ricin—a toxin so potent that eating a mere five or six seeds can be fatal to a child.[22]

Some organs of **pufferfish** (also called fugu, blowfish, and several other names) contain potent neurotoxins—tetrodotoxin, saxitoxin, or both—that may cause death from respiratory paralysis.[23,24] In Japan, where this fish is considered a delicacy, some fish cutters are specially trained to remove the organs that contain the toxins, without contaminating the rest of the fish. However, depending on the location where pufferfish are caught off the US Atlantic Coast, the entire fish (rather than only certain organs) can be toxic, or the fish can be free of these toxins—and thus the US Food and Drug Administration advises consumers to eat pufferfish only from sources known to be safe.[24]

Both animals and plants, when eaten as food, can serve as the vehicles for toxins produced by smaller organisms—for example, algae or fungi. For example, the tiny marine algae known as dinoflagellates, which are near the base of the oceanic food chain, produce toxins. These toxins

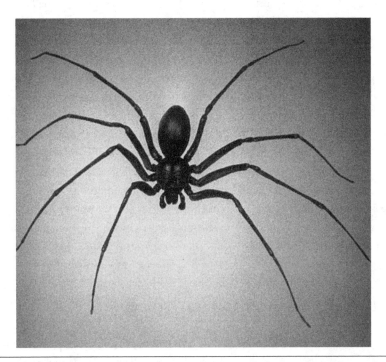

FIGURE 3.14 The venomous brown recluse spider—including legs, about the size of a US quarter—is found in several south-central states in the United States. *Source*: Reprinted courtesy of CDC Public Health Image Library. ID# 6268. Content providers: CDC/Andrew J. Brooks. Available at: http://phil.cdc.gov/phil/details.asp. Accessed August 21, 2007.

accumulate up the levels of the food chain, ultimately reaching concentrations in shellfish or finfish tissues that can poison people who eat these food animals.[21] **Paralytic shellfish poisoning** (also called saxitoxin poisoning), which has symptoms ranging from tingling and numbness to respiratory paralysis,[25] occurs most often in people who have eaten mollusks. **Ciguatera poisoning**, marked by gastrointestinal, neurological, and cardiovascular symptoms,[26] is typically caused by eating warm-water reef fish, such as barracuda, grouper, or snapper. During warm weather, dinoflagellate populations in coastal waters can multiply rapidly, giving the water a reddish color—a phenomenon known as a "red tide."

Plants, especially grain plants used as food, can serve as the vehicle by which people are exposed to toxins produced by molds or other fungi (**mycotoxins**). For example, the mold *Claviceps purpurea*, commonly known as ergot, is a parasite that affects grains of rye and other cereals in the field. Ergot produces a mycotoxin; the symptoms of ergot poisoning (**ergotism**) include vasoconstriction, especially in the extremities, leading to gangrene. Historically, ergotism was a common and much-dreaded condition, known in the Middle Ages as St. Anthony's fire because of the characteristic blackened gangrenous limbs.[22]

Unlike ergot, the mold *Aspergillus flavus* grows mainly on crops in storage,[27] affecting especially peanuts and corn. Under favorable conditions this mold produces **aflatoxins**, which might then be present in food products, including peanut butter. On the whole, storage conditions are much better controlled and less conducive to the growth of mold in industrialized countries. In these countries, foods are rarely contaminated with aflatoxins at concentrations high enough to cause acute toxicity, though such outbreaks occur occasionally in lower-income countries.

More important, aflatoxin exposure is associated with increased risk of hepatocellular carcinoma, the most common form of primary liver cancer. This is one of the most common cancers worldwide (although relatively rare in the United States and western Europe), occurring at especially high rates in sub-Saharan Africa, China, and Southeast Asia. Hepatitis B is also a risk factor for hepatocellular carcinoma—and the risk from combined exposure to hepatitis B and aflatoxin is much greater than the sum of the separate risks.[28] Together, these two risk factors account for the great majority of hepatocellular carcinoma in high-risk regions.[28,29]

Finally, some mushrooms (which, like molds, are a type of fungus) are poisonous to humans. Many species of mushrooms grow wild, and there is no simple way to distinguish harmless species from poisonous ones. Poisonous mushrooms cause a wide range of symptoms, including gastrointestinal and neurological effects, and occasionally death.[30] Worldwide, most deaths from mushroom poisoning are caused by eating *Amanita phalloides*, also called the "death cap."[22]

3.3 Allergy and Asthma

As described earlier, the normal immune response to an antigen—a potentially harmful foreign substance such as a microbe—is to produce antibodies and cells to eliminate the antigen. But sometimes a person's immune system mounts an unnecessary response to a substance that is foreign but harmless; such a substance is called an **allergen**, and the abnormal response is **allergy**, a type of immune disease. Many common substances can act as allergens, including pollens, molds and mold spores, animal dander, dust mites, and cockroach droppings.

On first exposure to a specific allergen, a person who is genetically predisposed to allergy produces allergen-specific antibodies that become concentrated in the respiratory tract. This series of events is called **sensitization**: From this point forward, whenever the body is presented with this allergen, the antibodies will cause the release of chemical mediators (for example, histamine), which in turn produce the symptoms of an allergic reaction. Depending on the mediators and where they act, the reaction can be in either the upper airway (nose and throat) or the lower airway.

In the upper airway, exposure to a specific allergen—in a person who has previously been sensitized to the allergen—triggers an attack of **allergic rhinitis** ("hay fever"), with symptoms of sneezing, runny nose, and watery eyes. These symptoms can persist for some time—for example, during the season when certain pollens or molds are widespread.

Events in the lower airways are more complicated. Here, exposure to a specific allergen—in a person who has previously been sensitized to the allergen and who has asthma as a chronic underlying condition—triggers an asthma attack.* **Asthma** is an immune illness in which the bronchi (the two major airways that serve the two lungs) are chronically inflamed and also hyperreactive. That is, they are prone to sudden muscle constriction that reduces the diameter of the bronchi (an effect known as **bronchoconstriction**), which in turn reduces the flow of air to and from the lungs. An **asthma attack** is an acute flare-up of the chronic condition, with increased inflammation and bronchoconstriction, as well as an overproduction of thick mucus. Together these changes produce symptoms of coughing, wheezing, and shortness of breath. An asthma attack can be extremely debilitating or even fatal. In a person with chronic asthma, acute attacks can be triggered not only by exposure to an allergen but also by exposure to a simple respiratory irritant such as cigarette smoke, chemical fumes, fragrances, irritating air pollutants, or even cold air.

Allergy and asthma, though often expressed in the respiratory system, are fundamentally immune conditions, and noninhalation exposures can be important, as can nonrespiratory reactions. For example, an allergic reaction to eating peanuts (an ingestion exposure) can include asthma symptoms, as well as nausea, abdominal pain, and shock.

Much more is known about allergic sensitization and asthma triggers than is known about the root causes of chronic asthma. Still, the convergence of two lines of evidence indicates that at least some causes of asthma are to be found in the environment.[31] First, research has shown that the prevalence of asthma is higher in industrialized countries than in lower-income countries, and that asthma prevalence in industrialized countries is increasing. Second, there is clear evidence that exposure to secondhand tobacco smoke (that is, from other people's smoking), as well as to certain chemicals used in occupational settings, can cause asthma. Thus, it seems likely that the increase in asthma prevalence is somehow tied to environmental features associated with modern development.

One possibility, known as the "hygiene hypothesis,"[32] suggests that today's children are on the whole less exposed to bacteria and viruses—because they live in cleaner houses, have fewer siblings, and have less contact with animals—and that this makes them more susceptible to

---

*Although most asthma is allergic asthma, occurring through the mechanism described here, there are also other types of asthma.

asthma. The idea is that the immune cells that mount the body's response to pathogens also tend to dampen other immune cells' inappropriate response to allergens. Thus, if a hygienic environment *reduces* the immune response to pathogens, a paradoxical effect is an *increase* in allergy and asthma. The hygiene hypothesis remains a work in progress.[33] Both the immune system and the lungs are immature at birth and continue to develop during childhood, making children more vulnerable than adults to the onset of asthma.

Modern development certainly brings new allergens: latex gloves, medicines, chemicals in the home and workplace. The modern lifestyle can also bring greater exposure to some natural allergens—for example, warmer and more airtight houses can increase exposures to dust mites and molds. And burning coal and oil produces irritant gases that can trigger asthma attacks. Clearly, even though the roots of allergy and asthma are in humans' coexistence with other species, these health conditions are also affected by modern development.

Study Questions

1. Describe three distinct ways in which infectious disease is routinely transmitted via the hands, giving an example of a pathogen for each.
2. Identify a factor you could change to reduce your risk, or your family's risk, of infectious disease, explaining why this change would be effective.
3. Based on your reading of this chapter, design a poster that gives basic tips for food safety at home, written for readers with a high school education.
4. In the event of a human influenza outbreak in a US state, under what conditions do you think it would be appropriate for the state government to use quarantine and/or isolation to control the outbreak?
5. Describe the health connection between hepatitis B infection and exposure to aflatoxin, and explain the global pattern of disease that results.

References

1. Black RE. *Escherichia coli* diarrhea. In: Wallace RB, Doebbeling BN, eds. *Maxcy-Rosenau-Last Public Health and Preventive Medicine.* 14th ed. Stamford, Conn: Appleton & Lange; 1998: 243–245.
2. Kachur SP, Bloland PB. Malaria. In: Wallace RB, Doebbeling BN, eds. *Maxcy-Rosenau-Last Public Health and Preventive Medicine.* 14th ed. Stamford, Conn: Appleton & Lange; 1998:313–326.
3. Rosen G. *A History of Public Health.* Expanded ed. Baltimore, Md: Johns Hopkins University Press; 1993. Originally published in 1958.
4. Drankiewicz D, Dundes L. Handwashing among female college students. *Am J Infect Control.* 2003;31(2):67–71.
5. Johnson HD, Sholcosky D, Gabello K, Ragni R, Ogonosky N. Sex differences in public restroom handwashing behavior associated with visual behavior prompts. *Percept Mot Skills.* 2003;97(3 Pt 1):805–810.
6. US Centers for Disease Control and Prevention. *General Information on Hand Hygiene.* Available at: http://www.cdc.gov/nceh/vsp/cruiselines/hand_hygiene_general.htm. Accessed December 2, 2007.

7. JAMA 100 years ago. *JAMA.* 1998;297(23):1862.

8. Hopkins DR. Dracunculiasis. In: Wallace RB, Doebbeling BN, eds. *Maxcy-Rosenau-Last Public Health and Preventive Medicine.* 14th ed. Stamford, Conn: Appleton & Lange; 1998:254–255.

9. Breiman RF, Butler JC. Legionellosis. In: Wallace RB, Doebbeling BN, eds. *Maxcy-Rosenau-Last Public Health and Preventive Medicine.* 14th ed. Stamford, Conn: Appleton & Lange; 1998: 246–248.

10. US Food and Drug Administration. *Foodborne Pathogenic Microorganisms and Natural Toxins Handbook, 2006.* Available at: http://vm.cfsan.fda.gov/~mow/intro.html. Accessed March 20, 2007.

11. Cui S, Ge B, Zheng J, Meng J. Prevalence and antimicrobial resistance of *Campylobacter* spp. and *Salmonella serovars* in organic chickens from Maryland retail stores. *Appl Environ Microbiol.* 2005;71:4108–4111.

12. Luangtongkum T, Morishita T, Ison A, Huang S, McDermott P, Zhang Q. Effect of conventional and organic production practices on the prevalence and antimicrobial resistance of *Campylobacter* spp. in poultry. *Appl Environ Microbiol.* 2006;72(5):3600–3607.

13. US Centers for Disease Control and Prevention. *Escherichia coli* O157:H7. Available at: http://www.cdc.gov/ncidod/dbmd/diseaseinfo/escherichiacoli_g.htm. Accessed March 24, 2007.

14. US Food and Drug Administration. *Foodborne Pathogenic Microorganisms and Natural Toxins Handbook: Scombrotoxin.* Available at: http://www.cfsan.fda.gov. Accessed May 25, 2006.

15. US Department of Agriculture, Animal and Plant Health Inspection Service. *Epizootiology and Ecology of Anthrax, 2006.* Available at: http://www.aphis.usda.gov/vs/ceah/cei/taf/emerginganimalhealthissues_files/anthrax.pdf. Accessed March 20, 2007.

16. Parkin DM. The global health burden of infection-associated cancers in the year 2002. *Int J Cancer.* 2006;118:3030–3044.

17. World Health Organization. *World Health Organization Report on Infectious Diseases: Removing Obstacles to Health Development.* Available at: http://www.who.int/infectious-disease-report/index-rpt99.html. Accessed February 7, 2008.

18. World Health Organization. *Statistical Annexe, World Health Report 2004—Changing history.* Available at: http://www.who.int/whr/2004/en/. Accessed February 7, 2008.

19. US Centers for Disease Control and Prevention. *Fact Sheet: Isolation and Quarantine, 2004.* Available at: http://www.cdc.gov/NCIDOD/dq/sars_facts/isolationquarantine.pdf. Accessed July 15, 2006.

20. US Centers for Disease Control and Prevention. Overview of healthcare-associated MRSA. Available at: http://www.cdc.gov/ncidod/dhqp/ar_mrsa.html Accessed March 20, 2008.

21. Russell FE. Toxic effects of animal toxins. In: Klaassen CD, ed. *Casarett and Doull's Toxicology: The Basic Science of Poisons.* 5th ed. New York, NY: McGraw-Hill; 1996:801–839.

22. Norton S. Toxic effects of plants. In: Klaassen CD, ed. *Casarett and Doull's Toxicology: The Basic Science of Poisons.* 5th ed. New York, NY: McGraw-Hill; 1996:841–853.

23. US Food and Drug Administration. *Foodborne Pathogenic Microorganisms and Natural Toxins Handbook: Tetrodotoxin.* Available at: http://www.cfsan.fda.gov. Accessed May 25, 2006.

24. US Food and Drug Administration, Center for Food Safety and Applied Nutrition. *Consumer Advisory: Only Eat Puffer Fish from Known Safe Sources.* Available at: http://www.cfsan.fda.gov/~dms/adpuffer.html. Accessed October 17, 2007.

25. US Food and Drug Administration. *Foodborne Pathogenic Microorganisms and Natural Toxins Handbook: Various Shellfish-Associated Toxins.* Available at: http://www.cfsan.fda.gov. Accessed May 25, 2006.

26. US Food and Drug Administration. *Foodborne Pathogenic Microorganisms and Natural Toxins Handbook: Ciguatera.* Available at: http://www.cfsan.fda.gov. Accessed May 25, 2006.

27. Kotsonis FN, Burdock GA, Flamm WG. Food toxicology. In: Klaassen CD, ed. *Casarett and Doull's Toxicology: The Basic Science of Poisons.* 5th ed. New York, NY: McGraw-Hill; 1996:909–949.

28. Yu MC, Yuan J-M. Environmental factors and risk for hepatocellular carcinoma. *Gastroenterology.* 2004;127:S72–S78.

29. Omer RE, Kuijsten A, Kadaru AMY, Kok FJ, Idris MO, El Khidir IM, et al. Population attributable risk of dietary aflatoxins and hepatitis B virus infection with respect to hepatocellular carcinoma. *Nutr Cancer.* 2004;48(1):15–21.

30. US Food and Drug Administration. *Foodborne Pathogenic Microorganisms and Natural Toxins Handbook: Mushroom Toxins.* Available at: http://www.cfsan.fda.gov. Accessed May 25, 2006.

31. Baldi I, Tessier J, Kauffmann F, Jacqmin-Gadda H, Nejjari C, Salamon R. Prevalence of asthma and mean levels of air pollution: results from the French PAARC survey. *Eur Respir J.* 1999;14:132–138.

32. Strachan D. Hay fever, hygiene and household size. *BMJ.* 1989;299:1259–1260.

33. Strachan D. Family size, infection and atopy: the first decade of the "hygiene hypothesis." *Thorax.* 2000;55(suppl 1):S2–10.

Producing Energy

Learning Objectives

After studying this chapter, the reader will be able to:

- Define or explain the key terms throughout the chapter

- Describe the fossil fuel cycle, its environmental impacts, and its occupational risks

- Explain why the fossil fuel cycle produces the major air pollutants that it does, and describe the major health risks associated with particulates and pollutant gases

- Explain the relationship between particulate size and the fate of inhaled particulates in the body

- Explain how exposures to lead and methylmercury are linked to the use of fossil fuels, describe their health effects, and explain why there are social disparities in exposure to these pollutants

- Explain in simple terms how pollutant gases increase the temperature of the troposphere, and describe the anticipated environmental and human health effects of global climate change

- Compare the estimated time frames for using up reserves of fossil and nuclear fuels, in the United States and globally

- Describe key approaches to managing the various public health risks associated with reliance on fossil fuels

- Describe the US regulatory framework for managing the public health risks associated with air pollution from the use of fossil fuels

- Describe radioactive decay, distinguishing between ionizing and non-ionizing radiation and among alpha, beta, and gamma radiation

- Describe the nuclear fuel cycle

- Explain how exposure to ionizing radiation is measured

- Summarize the human health risks of ionizing radiation and of the nuclear fuel cycle

- Describe the key natural and anthropogenic sources of exposure to ionizing radiation

- Describe key approaches to managing the public health risks associated with reliance on nuclear fuels

- Describe the US regulatory framework for managing the public health risks associated with the use of nuclear fuels

- Describe the range of alternatives to traditional fossil and nuclear energy sources, weighing their advantages and disadvantages

Industrialized society requires tremendous inputs of energy—to power manufacturing processes, transport goods and people, heat and cool buildings, and make possible countless activities of the modern lifestyle. Much of this energy comes from fuels—substances that release energy when they are changed, mostly through burning or nuclear fission. This chapter considers the resources that produce most of our power—the fossil fuels that have been the mainstay of modern industrial development (Section 4.1); uranium, the nuclear option that emerged in the later 20th century (Section 4.2); and alternatives to these dominant energy sources (Section 4.3). Each section describes, for a given energy source, how energy is produced, the associated environmental and health impacts, and the US framework for regulating its processes and wastes. In addition, Section 4.1 describes the processes of global climate change and the contribution of fossil fuels to this daunting problem.

4.1 Energy from Fossil Fuels

For thousands of years, humans' most important energy sources (other than their own muscle power) were draft animals, wind, water, wood, and charcoal made from wood. Coal deposits near the earth's surface were mined in Britain in the 12th century, and perhaps even under Roman rule, but it was not until the early 19th century that coal was used on a large scale. By the mid-20th century, oil and natural gas had joined coal as leading energy sources for European and American industry, heating, and transportation. Electricity—a highly transportable *form* of energy that can be generated from a windmill, water power, or the burning of fossil fuels—came into wide use in the industrialized countries in the late 19th century. During the 20th century the world, and especially the industrialized nations, became ever more dependent on fossil fuels for energy. In the United States today, fossil fuels provide about 85% of our energy.[1]

Fossil fuels—coal, petroleum, and natural gas—are formed from decayed plants and animals laid down millions of years ago and then subjected to heat and pressure underground. The term *fossil fuels* is also used to refer to fuels, such as gasoline, that are derived from oil, coal, or natural gas. Fossil fuels contain **hydrocarbons** and are also known as **hydrocarbon fuels** (see the sidebar titled "About Organic Chemicals, Hydrocarbons, and Fuels," which follows). Unlike water and wind power, and even wood fuel, fossil fuels cannot be renewed on the human time scale: They are considered **nonrenewable energy resources**.

As will be described later, the fossil fuel "cycle" is an extension of the natural global carbon cycle. But on the human time scale, the use of these nonrenewable resources is not a cycle but rather a one-way process in which fuels are extracted from the earth and then burned. This section addresses the following series of topics:

- How we extract fossil fuels from the earth and how long we can expect to do so
- The suite of air pollutants produced by burning fossil fuels
- These pollutants' health impacts, at the local or regional scale

About Organic Chemicals, Hydrocarbons, and Fuels

For the most part, *organic chemicals* are those that contain carbon (there are a few exceptions, including carbon dioxide and carbon monoxide, which are classed as inorganic compounds). Carbon is special: It forms many different compounds because it has the unique ability to bond to itself in long chains, rings, and combinations of these. Some organic compounds, known as *hydrocarbons*, are composed only of hydrogen and carbon. Methane (with one carbon atom), propane (with a chain of carbon atoms), and benzene (with a ring of carbon atoms) are examples of hydrocarbons. Most hydrocarbons are combustible, and our most familiar fuels—coal, oil, natural gas—all contain hydrocarbons. These fuels are referred to both as *hydrocarbon fuels* and as *fossil fuels*, a term that alludes to their prehistoric origins.

- The impact on the global climate of burning fossil fuels
- US regulatory approaches to controlling pollution from the burning of fossil fuels

Extraction of Fossil Fuels

Coal, a solid fuel, is mined from the earth. Petroleum, also called crude oil, is a gooey liquid; it is pumped from underground deposits where it often occurs with natural gas (which is indeed a gas at ordinary temperatures). Workers in coal mines and oil and gas fields face an array of occupational hazards, many of them physical in nature.

Environmental and Human Health Effects of Coal Mining

Traditionally, coal was mined underground, and many underground mines are still active. In recent decades, however, **surface mining** (also called **strip mining**) has become more common. In surface mining, enormous trucks are used to remove the earth overlying a seam of coal—a process that generates great quantities of dust. In the most extreme form of surface mining, entire mountaintops are removed and neighboring valleys are filled with the earth. In this way, a landscape is leveled; in addition, the long-term stability of the filled valleys is uncertain. Even underground mines scar the surface landscape: Forests over coal mines have often been cut down for railroad ties and for timbers to shore up the mineshafts.[2] The center of US coal production has shifted in recent decades from Appalachia to the western states, where the coal deposits have lower sulfur content and surface mines can be excavated on a massive scale. The coal is transported by rail in single-cargo, single-destination trains of 100 cars or more.[3] In 2002, more than 1 billion tons of coal were shipped within the United States, almost two thirds by rail.[4]

Because any form of coal mining disturbs the earth's surface and creates waste rock, **acid mine drainage** is a common problem at both active and abandoned coal mines. Acidic drainage from mines develops because pyrite (iron sulfide) is typically present in coal and waste rock piled at mine sites (including metal mines as well as coal mines). When pyrite in coal or waste rock is exposed to water and air, a chemical reaction produces sulfuric acid, often aided by a species of bacterium that thrives in an acid environment. As a result, rainwater percolating through the waste rock, or draining through the mine shafts, is made acidic. Because it is acidic, the water mobilizes metals from soils and rock, and it also dissolves minerals, creating suspended solids in the runoff. Thus, acid mine drainage produces a combination of high acidity, high concentrations of metals, and high concentrations of dissolved solids—as well as a characteristic orange color resulting from the presence of iron oxide—in the streams or groundwater into which it drains. Acid mine drainage typically originates from a large area, because mines are such sprawling operations, and can continue for decades after a mine is closed or abandoned.

A coal mine is an inherently dangerous working environment. The job of a coal miner carries well-known risks to life and limb, as well as to the lungs. An underground mine in particular, with its blasting and digging, is a dusty environment. Miners are exposed not only to coal dust but also to silica (quartz) dust because quartz is widespread in the earth's crust. When particulates lodge in the lungs, tissues react to this physical irritant by forming excessive fibrous tissue (scar tissue). This condition, known as **fibrosis**, makes lung tissues less flexible and thus interferes with breathing. Fibrosis associated with exposure to coal dust is called **pneumoconiosis** (also known as black lung), and fibrosis associated with exposure to silica is called silicosis. Both conditions cause a debilitating loss of lung function. Bands of such scar tissue can form throughout the lung but are often concentrated around the small airways (respiratory bronchioles, described later in this chapter).

In the past, miners worked with little or no respiratory protection (**Figure 4.1**) and were exposed to dust at very high concentrations. In the industrialized nations today, there are controls on dust, and miners wear protective gear that substantially reduces their exposure to coal and silica dust, though it does not eliminate it. In some lower-income countries, miners still work with little protection. Miners are also at risk of poisoning from carbon monoxide, which can be released from pockets in the coal as it is disturbed by mining.

In addition to these inhalation hazards, coal miners are at risk of acute injury and death from accidents involving machinery, cave-ins, and fires or explosions. In the United States, the annual rate of fatal injury among coal miners for 2000–2004 was about 33 per 100,000 workers, making coal mining one of the country's most dangerous jobs.[5]

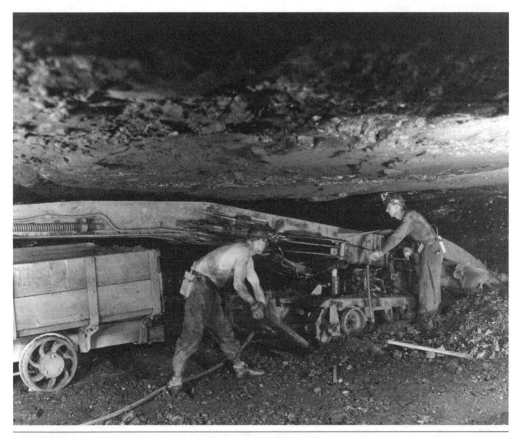

FIGURE 4.1   US coal miners, circa 1930–1960, wear no respiratory protection as they operate a mechanized coal bin loader. *Source*: Reprinted courtesy of CDC Public Health Image Library. ID# 9558. Content providers: CDC/Barbara Jenkins, NIOSH. Available at: http://phil.cdc.gov/phil/details.asp. Accessed August 21, 2007.

The risk of fire or explosion is ever present in a coal mine. The elements of the "fire triangle"—the three components that together are sufficient to cause a fire—are fuel, heat, and oxygen. Of these, fuel (the coal itself) and oxygen are already present in a coal mine so that only a source of heat, such as friction or electrical sparks from tools or heavy machinery, is needed to start a fire.[6] The "explosion pentagon" adds two elements to the fire triangle: a confined space and fuel that is finely dispersed and suspended in air. An underground mine is a confined space. Thus, if fine coal dust is suspended in the air, only heat is needed for an explosion to occur; and, on the other hand, if heat is present, all that is lacking is for coal dust to be suspended in the air.[6]

Environmental and Human Health Effects of Oil and Gas Extraction

Typically, crude oil must be pumped to the surface, though some oil deposits are under pressure so that no pumping is required. Natural gas, which consists mainly of methane, is often extracted along with crude oil from the same geologic formations. Extraction of petroleum produces wastes of oily water and rock fragments, and some liquid wastes are disposed of by injecting them deep underground. Some oilfields are located offshore, which complicates the extraction process.

Taking oil and natural gas from the earth requires powerful drilling equipment and releases high-pressure streams of oil and gas. Workers are at risk of accidental injury, overexposure to noise and vibration, and extremes of cold or heat, depending on location.[7] Hydrogen sulfide (an asphyxiating gas) and radon gas (a source of ionizing radiation; see Section 4.2) may be mixed in with natural gas.[7] And some components of crude petroleum—still in solution as the oil comes from the earth—will be considered hazardous chemicals after they are separated out at the refinery. Like many other workers, oil and gas workers also use some chemicals on the job—for example, solvents to clean drilling gear.

From the oilfield, crude oil is distributed to refineries by ship and via an extensive pipeline infrastructure. In the United States, it is the Trans-Alaskan pipeline that appears most often in the news—because it crosses the pristine Alaskan wilderness—but many more miles of pipeline crisscross the continental United States. Pipelines carry Central Asian oil to ports and Western markets, and pipelines on the floor of the North Sea and the Gulf of Mexico carry oil to shore.

These deliveries, via tanker ship or pipeline, come at some cost to the environment. In 1989, the tanker *Exxon Valdez* ran aground in Prince William Sound, an inlet on Alaska's southern coast; over the next few days, the ship leaked about 11 million gallons of crude oil into the Sound. The spill caused extensive environmental contamination and much harm to wildlife, and its lingering effects are still being evaluated. The oilfield at Prudhoe Bay, on Alaska's north slope near the Alaskan National Wildlife Refuge, has been plagued by spills, with the most recent occurring in 2006.

Refined fuel products (such as gasoline and diesel fuel) are distributed from petroleum refineries by rail and truck. Refineries are industrial facilities that produce not only various fuels but also nonfuel products (such as lubricating oils, petroleum jelly, and asphalt) and organic chemicals to be used as inputs to other industries.

Like petroleum, natural gas is often distributed by a pipeline network; in this case, the branching system reaches individual homes and other buildings. When cooled to a very low temperature (about −260° F), natural gas becomes a liquid; such **liquefied natural gas (LNG)** is transported in tanker ships, in which the low temperature can be maintained. When the tanker reaches its destination, the natural gas is warmed to a gaseous state for distribution by pipeline. Currently, the United States has three LNG terminals on the East Coast, one on the Gulf Coast, and one in the Gulf of Mexico; about 40 more such terminals have been proposed or approved.[8]

The Time Horizon for Fossil Fuels

Global supplies of fossil fuels, though substantial, are finite. It is estimated that the world's recoverable coal reserves could last up to 200 years at the current rate of use.[9] However, this global average disguises coal's uneven distribution around the globe. Further, substantial increases in coal consumption are anticipated as oil reserves dwindle and as the economies of lower-income countries grow—particularly that of China, which holds an estimated 12% of global recoverable coal reserves.[9] The United States alone holds 26% of the world's recoverable reserves; Austria, Germany, Poland, and the countries of the former Soviet Union together account for another 40%.[9]

At the present global average rate of consumption, the world's proved petroleum reserves will last only about 40 years.[10,11] Further, the world's oil reserves, like its coal reserves, are unevenly distributed—and the biggest consumers are not those with the largest reserves. The United States, the largest single consumer of oil, imports more than half of the oil it uses; at the present rate of consumption of its own reserves, the United States could run out of domestic oil in as little as 11 years.[10]

The Middle East, on the other hand, is home to about 60% of the world's proved reserves of petroleum and about 40% of the world's proved reserves of natural gas.[11] Outside of the Middle East, Venezuela and Nigeria have substantial proved reserves of both oil and natural gas. In addition, Russia, Libya, and Kazakhstan have substantial oil reserves; and the United States and Algeria have substantial natural gas reserves.[11] These critical natural resources have been a source of geopolitical tensions for decades, and no doubt this will continue to be true.

On a somewhat more optimistic note, the term *proved reserves* is a conservative estimate of oil and gas resources. It refers to quantities that are nearly certain to exist in known reservoirs, and which could be extracted using current technologies and under current economic conditions.[11] In the future, oil could be discovered in new locations, or extracted from different types of geologic formations (for example, oil shale)—and these more costly approaches are likely to appear more economically attractive as oil becomes scarcer. Still, there can be no doubt that the era of unlimited fossil fuel consumption is drawing to a close, and that global dependence on these fuels is not a sustainable energy option.

Air Pollution from Burning Fossil Fuels

Most combustion products from burning fossil fuels are released into the atmosphere, becoming **air pollution**—a term that has traditionally referred to pollution of the troposphere. All combustion is fundamentally the same basic oxidation process (see the following sidebar titled "About Combustion"). However, this simple picture is complicated by both the conditions of

---

About Combustion

At its most basic, *combustion* is a chemical reaction that requires a hydrocarbon fuel, the presence of oxygen, and an initial source of heat. Heating causes the hydrocarbon fuel to break down and recombine with the oxygen, forming water (H_2O) and carbon dioxide (CO_2). This oxidation reaction also releases heat energy, causing the combustion to continue as long as fuel remains. Extra heat energy, beyond that needed to maintain the combustion, can be put to use for human purposes. When not enough oxygen is immediately present for a hydrocarbon fuel to burn completely, carbon monoxide (CO) is formed instead of CO_2.

---

burning and the characteristics of the fuel. In particular, combustion under real-world conditions is often incomplete, and fossil fuels are more than just hydrocarbons. Further, some air pollutants from the burning of fossil fuels set in motion complex secondary impacts.

This section describes the sources and environmental fates of key air pollutants from burning fossil fuels, beginning with the most basic products of any combustion; then describing other substances that can be released by burning, depending on the makeup of the fuel; and finally noting the distant environmental effects of acidic secondary pollutants. Because this picture is already a complicated one, the pollutants' various direct human health effects—many, but not all, respiratory in nature—are presented in a separate section following this one.

Basic Products of Combustion: Oxides and Particulates

The various combustion processes of an industrial society produce many of the same pollutants, though their profiles vary. As shown in **Table 4.1**, we burn fossil fuels to power vehicles of all types, to generate electricity, and to heat commercial and residential buildings. In addition, some heavy manufacturing facilities, including petroleum refineries, metal smelters, and pulp and paper mills, are powered directly by burning fossil fuels.

Because combustion is oxidation, the combustion of fossil fuels produces several oxides; the most important sources of these pollutants are indicated by check marks in Table 4.1. Carbon dioxide (CO_2), a natural constituent of the atmosphere, is released any time fossil fuels are burned. In contrast, carbon monoxide (CO) is mainly a product of inefficient burning when vehicles idle, and thus carbon monoxide pollution is attributable mainly to cars.

Nitrogen is plentiful in the atmosphere, and thus oxides of nitrogen—the gases nitrous oxide (N_2O), nitrogen dioxide (NO_2), and, if combustion is incomplete, nitric oxide (NO)—are produced by burning. These reactions occur especially at the high temperatures that are typical of processes that convert one form of energy to another; thus, cars and power plants are the major sources of these pollutants. Nitrogen dioxide is a brownish gas that is a visible marker of air pollution. In the world of air pollution, NO_2 and NO are together referred to as NO_x, pronounced "nox."

Table 4.1 Key Sources of Major Air Pollutants from the Burning of Fossil Fuels

| | Sources of Pollutants | | | |
Pollutant	Vehicles (gasoline, diesel)	Electric Power Plants (coal, oil)	Heating Buildings (oil, natural gas)	Manufacturing (coal, oil, natural gas)
Basic products of the combustion process				
Carbon dioxide (CO_2)	✓	✓	✓	✓
Carbon monoxide (CO)	✓			
Nitrous oxide (N_2O)	✓	✓		
Nitrogen dioxide (NO_2), Nitric oxide (NO)	✓	✓		
Sulfur dioxide (SO_2)		✓		(some)
Particulate matter (PM)	✓	✓	✓	✓
Other pollutants liberated by combustion				
Mercury (from coal)		✓		(some)
Lead (from leaded gasoline)	✓			
Volatile organic compounds (from gasoline)	✓			

Sulfur is present in most coal and crude oil; however, it is refined out of most fuels derived from crude oil, and the sulfur content of natural gas is very low. Thus, sulfur dioxide (SO_2) gas is produced mainly when coal or sulfur-containing oil fuel is burned—mostly in power plants, but also in aging boilers still being used in manufacturing. Sulfur oxide (SO) may also be formed but does not persist as a stable compound. SO and SO_2 are known as SO_x ("sox"). Because sulfur is refined out of gasoline and heating fuels, cars and furnaces do not produce SO_x. In the atmosphere, some sulfur dioxide is converted to tiny water-soluble particles known as sulfates.

Finally, burning of fossil fuels adds to the burden of particles in the air. In environmental health, and especially in the regulatory context, the term **particulates** or **particulate matter (PM)** refers to a complex mixture that can include both small solid particles and fine liquid droplets (aerosols).* The actual makeup of airborne particulate matter varies, but often includes not only soil particles (dust), but also sulfates, metals, and organic chemicals. A common organic component of particulates is a group of compounds known as **polycyclic aromatic hydrocarbons (PAHs)**; the name describes their structure of multiple carbon rings fused together).

---

*Long, narrow fibers, such as asbestos fibers (not produced by the burning of fossil fuels), are also considered particulates.

PAHs, which are present in petroleum and are also a product of incomplete combustion, are ubiquitous in the environment.

Concentrations of airborne particulate matter are measured as mass per unit volume of air—milligrams or micrograms per cubic meter (mg/m^3 or $\mu g/m^3$). Per unit of energy output, burning of coal produces a much greater mass of particulates than burning of oil, which in turn produces more than burning of natural gas.

Other Pollutants Liberated by Combustion: Mercury, Lead, VOCs

The burning of fossil fuels releases not only the ordinary products of complete and incomplete combustion but other substances as well, reflecting the composition of the fuel (Table 4.1). For example, **mercury** is naturally present at low concentrations in most coal, as are various other metals. But mercury is an unusual metal—liquid at room temperature and easily volatilized at warmer temperatures. Thus, unlike, for example, iron and aluminum found in coal, which remain in the ash when the coal is burned, elemental mercury vaporizes and moves into the atmosphere. The quantity released per ton of coal burned is small, but we burn many tons of coal, and mercury is strongly neurotoxic, as described later.

In the atmosphere, elemental mercury (also called metallic mercury) can be carried with air currents for some time, but eventually it settles out or is deposited with rain or snow. Once the elemental mercury reaches the earth's surface, certain species of bacteria convert the mercury from its elemental form to a different form: an organic compound called **methylmercury**.* This conversion occurs mostly in the sediments of oceans, lakes, and rivers. Methylmercury is taken up by algae, the first rung on an aquatic food chain that leads through zooplankton, small invertebrates, and fish of increasing size. Although methylmercury is not highly lipophilic, it does become concentrated in the muscle of fish.

Through the processes of bioaccumulation and biomagnification, methylmercury collects at higher concentrations up the food chain. Methylmercury is found at highest concentrations in large predator fish, such as tuna or swordfish (in salt water) and bass or pike (in fresh water). Most human exposure to mercury liberated by the combustion of fossil fuels is exposure to methylmercury through eating fish. Although mercury has been known as a neurotoxicant for more than a century, the importance of the coal-to-fish-to-table exposure pathway has only recently been appreciated. Infants in utero can be exposed to methylmercury consumed by the mother.

Like mercury, **lead** has long been known to be neurotoxic at high doses. However, in contrast to mercury, which occurs naturally in coal, lead was deliberately added to gasoline to improve engine performance. In the early 1920s, General Motors and E. I. DuPont formed a new corporation to produce gasoline to which an organic lead compound, tetraethyl lead, had been added.[12] Tetraethyl lead reduced "engine knock," a premature ignition of fuel in the engine

---

*Mercury also occurs in a third form: in inorganic compounds, such as mercuric sulfide (mercury ore). Most exposures to the metallic and inorganic forms of mercury are occupational exposures (Chapter 5) or stem from the use of consumer products (Chapter 7).

cylinders that makes an annoying sound and causes engine wear and a loss of power. After production began at three plants, a number of workers showed frank lead poisoning—suffering psychosis and hallucinations—and some of them died. There followed a brief hiatus in production and a hearing before the Surgeon General. Foreshadowing future events, scientists expressed concern about dispersing lead so widely in the environment when its health risks short of actual poisoning were not well understood. But political pressure won out: In 1925, a committee appointed by the Surgeon General quickly concluded that leaded gasoline did not pose a health hazard, and production resumed.[12]

This decision ultimately spread lead in the environment wherever people drove cars—for if lead is present in gasoline, it is also present in exhaust. When leaded gasoline is in use, lead is widespread in airborne particulate matter, which is gradually deposited on the ground through settling or with precipitation. Thus, inhalation exposures to airborne lead are important while leaded gasoline is in use, but decline fairly quickly after the use of leaded gasoline is discontinued. However, exposures to lead in soil or dust, mostly by incidental ingestion, continue long after leaded gasoline has been banned. The burden of lead in soil is especially heavy in urban areas. (Another important source of lead in soil is deteriorating paint, to which lead was commonly added to increase the paint's durability; see Chapter 7.) Lead has been phased out as a gasoline additive in most countries of the world—in the United States as of 1996, in the European Union nations as of 2000, and in sub-Saharan Africa and most of Latin America by 2006. As of 2006, fewer than 20 countries worldwide—in northwest Africa, the Middle East, Central Asia, and Southeast Asia—were still using leaded gasoline.[13,14]

Finally, oil contains some naturally occurring **volatile organic compounds (VOCs)**—organic compounds, such as benzene, that volatilize significantly at ordinary environmental temperatures. Other VOCs are sometimes added to gasoline to improve its performance. Some VOCs are released whenever oil or gas is burned. More are released with any gasoline that escapes unburned through the tailpipe or evaporates from the fuel tank or some other part of a vehicle, contributing to the concentration of these pollutants in ambient air—that is, air in the general outdoor environment.

Secondary Pollutants Formed in the Atmosphere: Ozone, Nitric Acid, Sulfuric Acid

Some of the pollutants listed in Table 4.1 are chemically transformed in the environment, producing **secondary pollutants** that are also important; **Table 4.2** adds these pollutants, with arrows linking precursor pollutants to secondary pollutants. Thus, for example, a chemical soup called **photochemical smog** is created through a complex series of chemical reactions among NO_x, VOCs, and other chemicals in the presence of sunlight. This brand of smog is a particular problem in warm, sunny locales such as Manila, Jakarta, Mexico City, and southern California. The **ozone** (O_3) that is a key component of photochemical smog is an important secondary pollutant. As noted in Chapter 2, the naturally occurring layer of ozone in the stratosphere is valued for the protection it provides against ultraviolet radiation. However, the ozone formed at ground level as a result of pollution is a health hazard. (The term **smog**, originally coined as a combination of *smoke* and *fog*, is sometimes used more generally to refer to any visible air pollution.)

Table 4.2   Key Sources of Major Air Pollutants, Including Secondary Pollutants, from the Burning of Fossil Fuels

Pollutant	Sources of Pollutants			
	Vehicles (gasoline, diesel)	Electric Power Plants (coal, oil)	Heating Buildings (oil, natural gas)	Manufacturing (coal, oil, natural gas)
Basic products of the combustion process				
Carbon dioxide (CO_2)	✓	✓	✓	✓
Carbon monoxide (CO)	✓			
Nitrous oxide (N_2O)	✓	✓		
Nitrogen dioxide (NO_2), Nitric oxide (NO)	✓	✓		
Sulfur dioxide (SO_2)		✓		(some)
Particulate matter (PM)	✓	✓	✓	✓
Other pollutants liberated by combustion				
Mercury (from coal)		✓		(some)
Lead (from leaded gasoline)	✓			
Volatile organic compounds (from gasoline)	✓			
Secondary pollutants formed in the atmosphere				
Ground-level ozone (O_3) in photochemical smog	✓			
Nitric acid (HNO_3)	✓	✓		
Sulfuric acid (H_2SO_4)		✓		

Note: Arrows link precursor pollutants to secondary pollutants.

Another indirect environmental effect of burning fossil fuels emerged as a divisive political issue in the 1970s. Through complex chemical reactions in the atmosphere, nitric oxide and nitrogen dioxide are gradually converted to nitrates and nitric acid, and sulfur dioxide is gradually converted to sulfates and sulfuric acid (see Table 4.2). These secondary pollutants are then deposited in precipitation—an outcome originally dubbed **acid rain** and now known more formally as **acid deposition**. In forests, acid deposition acidifies soil and can severely damage the leaves of trees. In some lakes and streams, fish species that cannot tolerate acidic waters have been completely eliminated. Acid deposition also damages buildings and statuary. However, acid deposition does not directly affect human health—in particular, "acid rain" is not so acidic that it causes harm on contact.

Power plants are often built with very tall smokestacks to disperse pollution and avoid local effects, and this can result in acid deposition in distant locations. For instance, coal-burning plants in the midwestern United States cause acid precipitation in New England and eastern Canada. Similar problems have arisen between European countries and between China and Japan, which bore the brunt of acid deposition from Chinese coal-fired power plants.

Local and Regional Health Impacts of Burning Fossil Fuels

This description of health impacts revisits the set of pollutants listed in Table 4.2, but grouped somewhat differently. It first considers the health effects of particulates and key pollutant gases—carbon monoxide, nitrogen dioxide, sulfur dioxide, and ozone—of which the last is a secondary pollutant formed in the atmosphere. It then takes up the health effects of the heavy metals mercury and lead that are liberated by the burning of fossil fuels.

Particulates and Pollutant Gases

This section describes the fate of inhaled particulates and pollutant gases in the body, their physiologic effects (mostly in the respiratory system), and their ultimate health impacts.

Fate of Particulates and Pollutant Gases in the Respiratory System

In the upper respiratory system, air inhaled through the nose passes from the nostrils through the nasal passages to the throat (**Figure 4.2**), and of course air can also be inhaled through the mouth. At the larynx, the throat gives way to the cartilaginous **trachea** (windpipe), which is considered a part of the lower respiratory system. Below the trachea, the air passages become more and more finely subdivided. The trachea divides into two **bronchi** (singular *bronchus*), which are also cartilaginous airways, surrounded by muscles, each serving one lung. The bronchi in turn divide into **bronchioles**—smaller, more flexible airways. All these elements— nose and throat, trachea, bronchi, bronchioles—form a transport system for moving air in and out of the lungs.

At rest, an adult inhales about 360 to 600 liters of air per hour (about 8.6 to 14.4 cubic meters per day).[15] Although children's lung capacity is smaller, they spend more time outdoors than adults do, exercise more, breathe more through the mouth, and tend to entrain a more intense personal dust cloud[16]—a phenomenon sometimes referred to as the "Pigpen effect," after the character in the comic strip *Peanuts*.

Gas exchange, the real business of breathing, takes place deeper in the lung. Bronchioles divide into **respiratory bronchioles**—very small conducting airways that are a sort of transitional zone—which in turn divide into **alveolar ducts**. The walls of the alveolar ducts have many outpocketings: clusters of tiny sacs called **alveoli**. A network of capillaries twines around the alveoli, enabling the exchange of gases: diffusion of oxygen from alveoli to bloodstream, and diffusion of carbon dioxide in the reverse direction. The total alveolar surface area in contact with capillaries is approximately 75 square meters—roughly the area of a tennis court.[17]

Particulates and pollutant gases enter the respiratory system with each inhaled breath. In the upper respiratory system, air flow is rapid, and the reversals between inhaling and exhaling are more turbulent than in the lower region. Like a speeding car in a tunnel, an airborne particle in

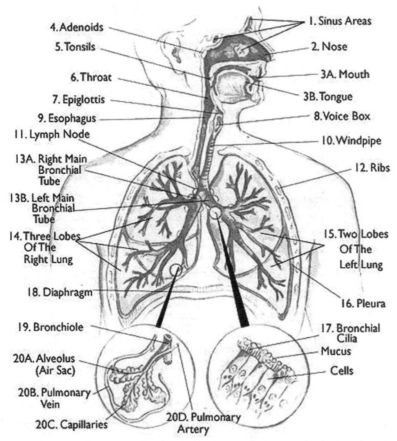

4. Adenoids
5. Tonsils
6. Throat
7. Epiglottis
9. Esophagus
11. Lymph Node
13A. Right Main Bronchial Tube
13B. Left Main Bronchial Tube
14. Three Lobes Of The Right Lung
18. Diaphragm
19. Bronchiole
20A. Alveolus (Air Sac)
20B. Pulmonary Vein
20C. Capillaries
20D. Pulmonary Artery

1. Sinus Areas
2. Nose
3A. Mouth
3B. Tongue
8. Voice Box
10. Windpipe
12. Ribs
15. Two Lobes Of The Left Lung
16. Pleura
17. Bronchial Cilia
Mucus
Cells

FIGURE 4.2 The human respiratory system. Reprinted with permission. © 2007 American Lung Association. For more information about the American Lung Association or to support the work it does call 1-800 LUNG-USA (1-800-586-4872) or log on to www.lungusa.org.

the trachea, bronchi, or bronchioles may careen into a curving wall or strike a wall head-on at a fork in the passageway. With each branching, the total surface area of the respiratory channels increases, trapping more particles. Deep in the lung, where there is less turbulence, particles may simply settle out. Once a particle lodges on an internal surface, it is not readily exhaled, but must be removed by some physiological mechanism.

Particles, which come in various shapes and densities, are classified by size using an idealized spherical diameter. The terms PM_{10} and $PM_{2.5}$ refer to particulate matter 10 microns or less in diameter (about the size of a protozoan cell) and 2.5 microns or less in diameter, respectively. As a general rule, particulates 10 microns or less in diameter are considered **respirable** (inhalable) **particulates**. Particulates between 10 and 2.5 microns come mainly from natural or mechanical sources (such as plowing, grinding, or abrasion), whereas **fine particulates** ($PM_{2.5}$) come mostly from combustion. **Ultrafine particulates** are those 0.1 microns or less in diameter. The most common source of ultrafine particulates is diesel engines—which often idle for extended periods, while truckers sleep or while school buses wait for children. Diesel exhaust particulates (DEP) also have a distinctive chemical makeup.

The fate of particulates in the body is mostly determined by their size: Smaller particles stay airborne longer and penetrate deeper before settling out (see **Table 4.3**). In essence, the smaller the particle, the more it behaves like a gas, whether in the airways or in the ambient environment.

Some coarse particles are filtered out by fine hairs lining the nasal passages. These particles may be expelled by sneezing or blowing the nose, or they may be swallowed.

Particulates 2.5 to 10 microns in diameter settle out in the trachea and bronchi, which are lined with **cilia**—tiny finger-like protrusions of the cells that line the airway. The cilia, which beat in unison, slowly propel a carpet of mucus upward toward the throat—a mechanism known as the **mucociliary escalator**. Particles deposited in this region ride this moving carpet up to the throat, from which the mucus is swallowed or spit out.

Fine particulates can reach the small airways and the alveoli. In the alveoli, macrophages (scavenger cells of the immune system) engulf some particles and remove them via the lymph system. In recent years it has become clear that ultrafine particulates can pass through the alveolar wall into the bloodstream and thus circulate throughout the body.[18]

Among the gaseous pollutants, both ozone and its precursor nitrogen dioxide penetrate the lower respiratory tract, as does sulfur dioxide if it is adsorbed to particles or aerosols. Carbon monoxide crosses the alveolar boundary into the blood, entering the general circulation.

Physiologic Effects of Particulates and Pollutant Gases

The physiologic mechanisms by which air pollutants cause toxicity are complex and interrelated, and are described here only in general terms. Overall, the organ systems most affected are the respiratory system and the cardiovascular system.

Particulate matter and the major pollutant gases from the burning of fossil fuels have direct irritating effects in the respiratory passages (**Table 4.4**).

- Particulate matter and ozone damage the cells that line the respiratory tract.[19,20] Ozone most strongly affects the cells that have cilia; as a result, ozone exposure makes the mucociliary escalator less effective. Particulates and ozone also cause local inflammation.[21,22] As described in Chapter 3, chronic inflammation of the bronchi is a feature of asthma, and asthmatics are more susceptible to this effect of air pollutants.

Table 4.3 Likely Sources and Fates of Respirable Particulates, by Size Category

Diameter (microns)	Key Sources	Penetration and Fate in Body
2.5–10	Natural and mechanical sources	Settle out in trachea and bronchi; removed via mucociliary escalator
0.1–< 2.5	Combustion	Reach small airways and alveoli; in alveoli, may be removed by macrophages
< 0.1 (ultrafine)	Combustion (especially of diesel fuel)	Can pass through alveolar wall into bloodstream

Table 4.4 Key Respiratory Effects of Common Air Pollutants

| | Effects in Respiratory System | | | |
| | Irritating Effects | | | |
Pollutant	Damage to Cells Lining the Respiratory Tract	Local Inflammation	Bronchoconstriction	Impairment of Immune Scavenger Cells in Alveoli
PM	✓	✓		✓
NO₂			(in asthmatics)	✓
SO₂			✓	
O₃	✓	✓	(in asthmatics)	

Data from: Bernstein JA. Health effects of air pollution. *J Allergy Clin Immunol*. 2004;114(5):1116–1123. Chen-Yeung MNW. Air pollution and health. *Hong Kong Med J*. 2000;6(4):390–398. Costa DL, Amdur MO. Air Pollution. In: Klaassen CD, ed. *Casarett and Doull's Toxicology: The Basic Science of Poisons*. New York, NY: McGraw-Hill; 1996:857–882. Olivieri D, Scoditti E. Impact of environmental factors on lung defences. *Eur Respir Rev*. 2005;14:51–56.

- Sulfur dioxide causes bronchoconstriction (a reduction in the diameter of the bronchi, resulting from muscle contraction),[21,22] which hampers air flow and leads to respiratory distress, especially if it occurs along with local inflammation. In people with asthma, the other common pollutant gases, ozone and nitrogen dioxide, can also increase bronchoconstriction,[22] which is a characteristic condition of this chronic disease.
- Finally, fine particulates and nitrogen dioxide can impair the functioning of the immune system's scavenger cells in the alveoli.[19] Evidence of other effects of nitrogen dioxide in healthy individuals is inconsistent,[22] and nitrogen dioxide's greatest impact on respiratory health is as a precursor to ozone.

Airborne particulates and pollutant gases also have important indirect effects on the heart; these effects occur via complex physiological pathways. For example, local lung inflammation, by increasing systemic inflammation, can increase the risk of blood clots. Air pollutants can also affect the autonomic nervous system, which controls the heart's rhythm.[23,24] Because ultrafine particulates pass through the alveolar wall into the systemic circulation, they are capable of causing inflammatory responses and health effects elsewhere in the body.[25]

Carbon monoxide, after crossing into the bloodstream in the lung, binds to hemoglobin in blood. Because carbon monoxide's affinity for hemoglobin is much greater than that of oxygen, it displaces the oxygen that hemoglobin ordinarily carries to the tissues of the body. By denying oxygen to the brain, carbon monoxide causes a loss of alertness and, at high doses, unconsciousness and death.

Health Impacts of Particulates and Pollutant Gases

At mid-20th century, three episodes of heavy, visible air pollution—in Belgium's Meuse Valley in 1930, in Donora, Pennsylvania, in 1948, and in London in 1952—focused the attention of both scientists and the general public on the hazards of air pollution. In December of 1952, London was blanketed for 5 days in a smoky, sulfurous fog.* A temperature inversion had laid a cap of warmer, less dense air over a packet of cooler, heavier air in the London basin, creating stagnant conditions. It had been a cold winter, and perhaps a million coal-burning furnaces were releasing smoke in the area. Londoners were burning high-sulfur coal in these postwar years so that the more desirable low-sulfur coal could be exported to bring cash into the economy. The resulting high concentrations of particulate matter and sulfur dioxide cast a pall over the city—in some locations, the daytime visibility was near zero for 48 hours—and a number of people later reported experiencing the taste of sulfur. Still, in the context of a long history of smoky fog, as well as the recent wartime bombings that had claimed 30,000 lives in London, people for the most part took the smog in stride.

Thus, it came as a surprise that about 12,000 deaths over the following 3 months were ultimately attributed to the London Smog. Many sudden deaths occurred at home during the smog, and hospitalizations and emergency room admissions increased sharply. Autopsies of several adults who died during the smog showed shedding of the bronchial lining, attributed to the extreme acidity of the smog. The majority of deaths were caused by pneumonia, exacerbation of emphysema or chronic bronchitis, or cardiovascular causes.

The London Smog was a turning point in public health, spurring not only research on the health effects of air pollution but also the effort to set air pollution standards in the industrialized nations. It is estimated that the concentration of total suspended particulates during the London Smog was as high as 7000 $\mu g/m^3$. Probably nearly all these particulates were respirable: in samples taken during a 1955 air pollution episode in London, 99% of the total suspended particulates were less than 2.5 μg in diameter.[26] For comparison, the current US standards for $PM_{2.5}$ are a 24-hour mean of 35 $\mu g/m^3$ and an annual mean of 15 $\mu g/m^3$. Thus, $PM_{2.5}$ concentrations during the worst of the London Smog probably approached 200 times the current US daily standard.

Even so, the concentration of total suspended particulates during the worst of the London Smog was probably only 10 to 15 times higher than current annual mean concentrations in some cities in lower-income countries (for example, 400 $\mu g/m^3$ in Delhi, India, and 800 $\mu g/m^3$ in Lanzhou, China, in 1995).[27] Indeed, a young Beijing physician visiting a US laboratory in 2006 commented that she had never before seen lung tissue that was pink, having observed only tissue blackened by particulate pollution.[28]

---

*Specifics in this description of the London Smog and its aftermath come from several sources: Bates D. A half century later: recollections of the London Fog. *Environ Health Perspect.* 2002;110(12):A735. Bell M, Davis D, Fletcher T. A retrospective assessment of mortality from the London smog episode of 1952: the role of influenza and pollution. *Environ Health Perspect.* 2004;112(1):6–8. Black J. Intussusception and the great smog of London, December 1952. *Arch Dis Children.* 2006;88:1040–1042. Davis D, Bell M, Fletcher T. A look back at the London Smog of 1952 and the half century since. *Environ Health Perspect.* 2002;110(12):A734. Dooley E. Fifty years later: clearing the air over the London Smog. *Environ Health Perspect.* 2002;110(12):A748. Whittaker A. Killer smog of London, 50 years on: particle properties and oxidative capacity. *Sci Total Environ.* 2004;334–335:435–445.

An extensive epidemiologic literature on the health impacts of air pollution has been generated in locations around the world—from the United States to Europe to Hong Kong. Ambient concentrations of particulates (variously defined), as well as NO_2, SO_2, and O_3, have all been linked to daily (acute) overall mortality and to acute cardiovascular mortality, sometimes lagged by 1 to 5 days after the air pollution measurement.[22,23,29] That is, the mortality rate for a given day may be associated with pollutant concentrations on the same day or on an earlier day.

Airborne particulates and the same three pollutant gases have also been linked to acute morbidity in the form of hospital admissions—for any respiratory disease and for **chronic obstructive pulmonary disease** (mostly emphysema and chronic bronchitis); and for any cardiovascular disease and specifically for heart failure.[22,23] Further, in urban areas around the world, the same four pollutants have been clearly shown to exacerbate asthma in those who have the disease. Asthma exacerbation has been variously assessed as an increase in symptoms (wheezing and chest tightness), increased hospital admissions or emergency room visits for asthma, increased use of emergency medications by children with asthma, and increased school absences because of asthma.[16,22,30–33]

In addition, in a large study in 6 US cities the ambient concentration of airborne particulate matter has been associated with long-term overall mortality, with lung cancer mortality, and with both acute and chronic cardiopulmonary mortality (that is, cardiovascular and nonmalignant respiratory causes grouped together).[34,35] Findings such as these show indirectly that air pollution reduces life expectancy. Later follow-up of the same study population has confirmed these associations and has documented a reduction in mortality associated with a decline over time in fine particulate concentrations.[36]

The original study of 6 cities reported more than 6 times as many deaths from cardiovascular disease as from nonmalignant respiratory disease attributed to air pollution.[34] These data are a reminder that cardiovascular disease is the leading cause of death in the US population (nearly 700,000 deaths each year), and that any factor that affects the risk of cardiovascular disease has enormous public health implications. Intuitively, it may seem that air pollution simply affects respiratory health, but in fact its effects are much broader, and in terms of numbers of deaths, air pollution's greatest impact is through cardiovascular mortality.

Because of air pollution's effects on respiratory and cardiovascular health, susceptible populations are particularly at risk. In infants, for example, both particulate matter and sulfur dioxide have been linked to low birthweight, and a number of studies have also linked particulate pollution to infant mortality[16] and to respiratory mortality in the postneonatal period.[37] Some research has been suggestive of an association between air pollution and Sudden Infant Death Syndrome (SIDS), though the evidence is not conclusive.[38]

Over the past 20 years, events have created two natural experiments that demonstrated the positive health effects of reducing air pollution. In 1990, the Irish government banned the marketing, sale, and distribution of bituminous coal in the city of Dublin. A comparison of mortality before and after the ban revealed a 15.5% drop in respiratory mortality and a 10.3% drop in cardiovascular mortality.[39] A few years later, during the 1996 summer Olympic games, traffic was tightly restricted in the greater Atlanta area. During this period, 30% lower peak daily ozone concentrations were documented, along with a dramatic decline in instances of acute care for asthma.[40]

Heavy Metals: Mercury and Lead

Two major by-products liberated by the burning of fossil fuels—the heavy metals mercury and lead—reach humans via different exposure pathways, as described earlier, but both have neurotoxic effects.

Health Effects of Methylmercury

As described earlier, elemental mercury released into the environment from the burning of coal is converted by microorganisms to methylmercury, which becomes concentrated in the tissues of large predator fish, which in turn are eaten by people. Today, this pathway accounts for most of the general population's exposure to mercury from ambient environmental sources.*

The neurological impacts of high prenatal exposure to methylmercury include mental retardation, cerebral palsy, deafness, and blindness.[41] These effects were made tragically clear in the 1960s in the area around Minamata Bay, Japan, where a local chemical company was using inorganic mercury as a catalyst in the manufacture of acetaldehyde. Unknown to the plant's operators, the process converted some of the inorganic mercury into methylmercury, which was then released with a waste stream into Minamata Bay.[42] The result was high levels of methylmercury in the sediments of the bay—and high exposures to residents of the area, for whom fish was a dietary staple. Over a period of years, an entire cohort of children exposed in utero or after birth suffered the effects of this exposure. Exposure to methylmercury as an adult can also cause sensory and motor impairments,[41] but fetal and childhood exposures are much more damaging.**

Recent epidemiologic research has documented subtle effects on neurological development of much lower exposures to methylmercury than those that occurred at Minamata. For example, one major study has been conducted in the Faroe Islands (located in the North Atlantic between Iceland and Norway), where the traditional diet includes whale meat and blubber. The range of exposures to methylmercury in the Faroe Islands overlaps with that in the United States, but includes higher exposures. Using neuropsychological testing, researchers have measured subtle impacts of prenatal methylmercury exposure in Faroese children up to age 14, including effects on language, attention, and memory, and to a lesser extent on fine motor function.[43–45]

Findings like these raise concern for low-level exposure to all pregnant women and young children. But women and children in some demographic groups are at even greater risk because of their dietary habits. Canned tuna, an inexpensive source of protein, is a staple in many households. Certain Native American groups depend heavily on fish that they catch themselves, sometimes from badly polluted waters—an unfortunate intersection of environmental pollution and traditional culture, often reinforced by poverty.[46] The US EPA and FDA have jointly

---

*In the past, a methylmercury fungicide was used to treat food grains, with tragic consequences in some populations, but this practice ceased in the 1970s.

**Exposure to elemental or inorganic mercury also causes neurological impacts, somewhat different from those described here for methylmercury.

issued recommendations on fish consumption for women who are pregnant or might become pregnant.

Health Effects of Lead

Lead is a neurotoxicant with both acute and chronic effects. Lead from leaded gasoline, and also from lead paint, is widespread in the environment, especially in soil and dust. Young children, of course, have greater incidental ingestion exposures to soil and dust than do adults, primarily through hand-to-mouth behavior. Infants in utero and young children are especially vulnerable to lead's neurotoxic effects. This is partly because their nervous systems are still developing. Children also absorb a much higher percentage of ingested lead than do adults—and absorption is further increased if a child's diet is deficient in iron and calcium. Lead is distributed throughout the body, causing a range of effects including kidney toxicity, anemia, hypertension, and reproductive effects. Because lead binds chemically at sites ordinarily occupied by calcium, it accumulates in bone and teeth, especially in children whose diets are low in calcium. Landmark health studies[47] assessed exposure by measuring lead in baby teeth that children had shed.

Today the most common biomarker used to assess children's exposure to lead is the concentration in blood, usually referred to as **blood lead level (BLL)**, measured in micrograms of lead per deciliter of blood (µg/dL). It is generally recommended that children with BLLs greater than 45 µg/dL undergo **chelation**, a painful treatment that increases the excretion of circulating lead. Because such a reduction in blood lead can mobilize lead stored in bone, multiple rounds of chelation are often required to bring down a child's blood lead level. Blood lead levels well below 45 µg/dL can also cause neurotoxic effects in children. In the United States, the Centers for Disease Control and Prevention designates a **blood lead action level**, the blood lead level at which action should be taken to reduce a child's exposure. The action level has dropped steadily through recent decades as lead's effects have been discerned at ever-lower levels. In the 1960s, the action level was 60 µg/dL, and it has been lowered several times since then:

1971: 40 µg/dL
1975: 35 µg/dL
1985: 25 µg/dL
1991: 10 µg/dL

Today there is good evidence of harm below the current action level of 10 µg/dL. Indeed, the neurotoxicity of lead is the only noncancer effect of a toxicant that is generally considered to have no threshold. The US EPA has declined to set a Reference Dose for lead because any Reference Dose would depend on the assumption that a threshold exists.

The health impact of lead exposure is often evidenced by a lower score on an intelligence test—a lower intelligence quotient, or IQ—an effect that has been documented in many studies. According to a recent review,[48] for example, each 1-µg/dL increment in blood lead level is associated with an average decrement in IQ of 0.87 points. Some recent evidence suggests that the IQ decrement per µg/dL blood lead may actually be greater at lower blood lead levels.[48] Of course, cognitive ability is more than just IQ. Lead's detrimental effects in several domains, such as memory, learning, and problem solving, are well documented.

And lead's neurological impacts are more than just cognitive. Lead exposure affects physical performance—for example, the fine motor coordination needed to develop writing skills.[49] Further, lead exposure has been tied to behavioral outcomes, including attention deficit hyperactivity disorder, oppositional behavior, and aggressive behavior.[49] In adolescent males, a higher body burden of lead has been associated with increased risk of having been adjudicated as delinquent in juvenile court.[50]

But even the simple deficit of a few IQ points becomes a sobering loss if we think at the population level rather than the individual level.[48] An individual with an IQ of 130 or higher is usually considered gifted; and an individual with an IQ of 70 or lower is usually considered to be intellectually impaired to a degree that limits his or her independence and places demands on the resources of society. Of course, these are not bright lines, and similarly, people cannot discern 5-point differences in IQ in their acquaintances. But in principle, if the BLL of everyone in a population were increased by just a few micrograms per deciliter so that everyone's IQ decreased by 5 points, then the entire bell curve for IQ would shift 5 points downward. In a population of 100 million, such a shift would substantially reduce the gifted subgroup in the population (from 6 million to 2.4 million) while increasing the cognitively impaired subgroup (from 6 million to 9.4 million).[48] This effect is shown schematically in **Figure 4.3**.

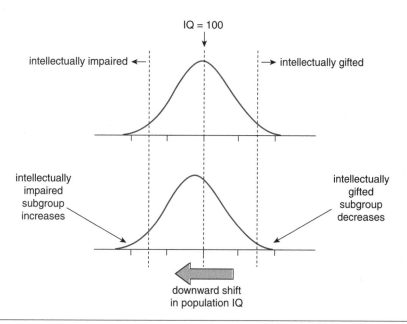

FIGURE 4.3   Decrease in intellectually gifted subgroup, and increase in intellectually impaired subgroup, with a small downward shift in population IQ. *Source*: Reprinted from *NeuroToxicology*, vol. 27; Gilbert, SG, Weiss B. A rationale for lowering the blood lead action level from 10 to 2 µg/dL. 693–701; 2006; Figure 3, with permission from Elsevier.

In fact, the burden of lead exposure is not evenly distributed across US society, but rather falls more heavily on disenfranchised groups such as lower-income groups and people of color. Disenfranchised populations are more likely to live near high-traffic roadways, to live in older, dilapidated housing, and to lack the resources to abate a lead hazard. Finally, they are less likely to have access to information about lead's hazards and how to reduce their exposures.

Such social inequities in exposure and effect can be magnified over time, in a cycle of inter-generational effects.[51] Children in lower socioeconomic groups are likely to be more exposed to lead and are also less likely to have a diet high in iron and calcium. Thus, as a group, they bear a heavier burden of lead's cognitive, physical, and behavioral impacts. These burdens make it harder for them, as adolescents and young adults, to get a good education, acquire job skills, and stay out of jail. And without these advantages, they are more likely to have pregnancies and rear children in settings where the risk of lead exposure is high. Children in higher socioeconomic groups, in contrast, generally continue to encounter conditions that further insulate them, and ultimately their children, from lead's impacts.

Global Climate Change

The most profound impact of our dependence on fossil fuels is global climate change, and the biggest driver of global climate change is carbon dioxide—a gas that is a natural constituent of the atmosphere and has no direct human health effects. Carbon dioxide has not traditionally been thought of as a pollutant. After all, we exhale it with every breath, and plants depend on it for photosynthesis. Yet carbon dioxide, in excess, has become a pollutant—much as "the dose makes the poison" in toxicology.

Anthropogenic Gases and the Enhanced Greenhouse Effect

As described in Section 2.1, carbon dioxide and nitrous oxide, both naturally occurring trace gases in the atmosphere, are known as greenhouse gases because they retain solar energy in the atmosphere, keeping the earth's climate warm enough for plants and animals to live. But with more of these gases entering the atmosphere from the burning of fossil fuels (see Table 4.2), the resulting *enhanced* greenhouse effect is proving to be too much of a good thing. Ozone from the burning of fossil fuels also makes a significant contribution to global climate change, as do methane and halocarbons, which are not associated with the burning of fossil fuels.

Carbon dioxide has the greatest impact because such large quantities are produced through the large-scale burning of fossil fuels by the industrialized nations. This impact is truly world-wide because it occurs through effects on the natural **global carbon cycle (Figure 4.4)**.

The carbon cycle is the set of processes by which carbon, the fundamental building block of life, moves from the environment through living things and back into the environment. As shown in simplified form in Figure 4.4, green plants take carbon from the atmosphere, incorporating it into glucose through photosynthesis; animals, which feed on plants, convert glucose back to carbon dioxide through cellular respiration. Carbon stored in plant and animal tissue is also returned to the environment through death and decay. (See the following sidebar titled "About Photosynthesis, Respiration, and Decay.")

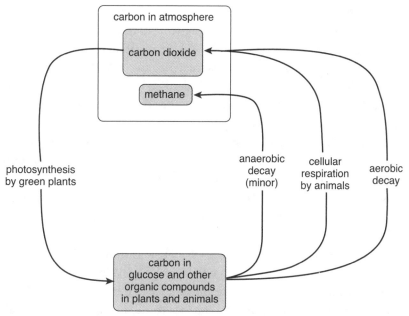

FIGURE 4.4 The global carbon cycle (excluding fossil fuels).

About Photosynthesis, Respiration, and Decay

Photosynthesis, a chemical process that occurs in the cells of green plants, uses energy (from the sun) to convert carbon dioxide (from the atmosphere) and water into glucose and oxygen.

carbon dioxide + water + energy → glucose + oxygen

Plants then convert glucose into the more complex compounds that make up their tissues.

Respiration, a chemical process that occurs in the cells of animals, accomplishes the reverse transformation. Food (actually, glucose from the digestion of food) is the body's fuel. Like combustion, *cellular respiration* converts glucose (which contains hydrogen and carbon) and oxygen into carbon dioxide, water, and energy for the body's use.

glucose + oxygen → carbon dioxide + water + energy

Unlike combustion, cellular respiration is a slow and steady process that occurs at body temperature.

Other organisms in an ecosystem, the decomposers of dead plant and animal matter, accomplish the same chemical transformation through *aerobic decay*. (To a lesser degree, decay also occurs in the absence of oxygen; in this case, methane is produced in lieu of carbon dioxide.)

Together these processes allow carbon, a fundamental nutrient, to be cycled within ecosystems.

Where do fossil fuels fit into this continuous cycling of carbon? Fossil fuels are decaying organic matter that, in effect, took a detour into long-term storage (see **Figure 4.5**). For millions of years, this stored carbon was not a part of the global circulation of carbon. But now, as fossil fuels are burned, the long-sequestered carbon is reentering the cycle in the form of carbon dioxide. Thus, the burning of fossil fuels has converted dead-end storage into a new pathway on one side of the cycle. With no compensating pathway on the other side, excess carbon is accumulating in the atmosphere in the form of carbon dioxide.

The warming effect of anthropogenic greenhouse gases is often quantified as the net gain in radiation energy that results from reducing outgoing terrestrial radiation (heat) relative to incoming solar radiation (see **Table 4.5**). The anthropogenic production of carbon dioxide is so great that this gas alone accounted for just over half of the net gain in radiation energy as of the late 1990s, despite the fact that the other gases listed are more potent in their warming effects, molecule for molecule.

In 2001, about 25% of global carbon dioxide emissions from the burning of fossil fuels were produced by the United States.[52] Some 95% of US emissions of carbon dioxide, and most anthropogenic ground-level ozone, are attributable to the burning of fossil fuels.[52] The other greenhouse gases listed in Table 4.5—nitrous oxide, methane, and halocarbons (organic compounds containing halogens, such as chlorine or fluorine)—come mainly from sources other than the burning of fossil fuels, including industry, agriculture, and community wastes.

Environmental Impacts of Global Climate Change

The notion of global warming was once controversial. Today, however, there is broad scientific consensus that the earth's climate is warming and also changing in other ways, and the term

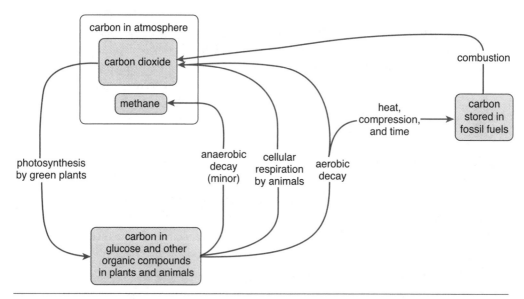

FIGURE 4.5   The global carbon cycle (including fossil fuels).

Table 4.5 Percentage of Net Gain in Energy in the Earth–Atmosphere System from Five Major Greenhouse Gases That Is Attributable to Each Gas

Greenhouse Gas	Percentage of Net Gain
Carbon dioxide	56.5
Methane	16.3
Ozone	10.2*
Halocarbons	11.6
Nitrous oxide	5.4

*The warming effect of ozone as listed here represents the net effect of an increase in tropospheric ozone (caused mostly by the burning of fossil fuels) and the depletion of stratospheric ozone (caused by certain organic chemicals; see Section 5.1).

Data from: Intergovernmental Panel on Climate Change. IPPC, 2007: Technical Summary. In: *Climate Change 2007: The Physical Science Basis*. Contribution of Working Group I to the Fourth Assessment Report of the Intergovernmental Panel on Climate Change. Cambridge, England, and New York, NY: Cambridge University Press; 2007.

global warming has been supplanted by **global climate change**. Because of the sweeping nature of this environmental question, in 1988 the World Meteorological Organization and the United Nations Environment Programme jointly established the Intergovernmental Panel on Climate Change (IPCC), an international team of scientists who regularly assess the research data on this issue.

Three basic climate-related environmental changes during the past century have been well documented[53]:

- The global surface temperature rose by approximately 0.74°C—about 1.3°F—from 1906 to 2005, and most of the warmest years have been among the most recent. These figures reflect rising temperatures of both air near the earth's surface and near-surface ocean waters.
- There has been a worldwide decline since the mid-1960s in the area covered by snow and glaciers.
- An average rise in sea level of 1.8 millimeters per year from 1961 through 2003 has been documented—almost 3 inches over the 42-year period.

These changes are related, as shown in **Figure 4.6**: Warmer surface air contributes to the melting of snow and glaciers, and this meltwater contributes in turn to the rise in sea level. Thermal expansion of surface seawater that is warming overall—despite the addition of glacial meltwater—also contributes to the rise in sea level. Finally, the warming of surface air has a circular aspect: Warmer air temperatures result in more evaporation of surface water, increasing the water vapor (a greenhouse gas) in the atmosphere.

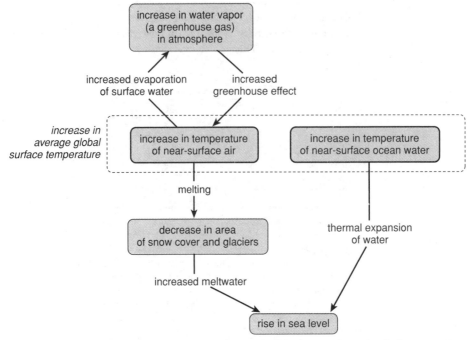

FIGURE 4.6 Connections among major climate-related environmental changes. *Data from*: Intergovernmental Panel on Climate Change. IPPC, 2007: Technical Summary. In: *Climate Change 2007: The Physical Science Basis. Contribution of Working Group I to the Fourth Assessment Report of the Intergovernmental Panel on Climate Change.* Cambridge, England, and New York, NY: Cambridge University Press; 2007.

Climate data show an increased frequency of heat waves since the mid-20th century, longer and more intense droughts since the 1970s, especially in the tropics and subtropics, and more frequent heavy precipitation events in many areas.[53] Climate scientists are currently considering whether episodes of El Niño/Southern Oscillation (ENSO) might be related to global climate change.[54]*

Scientific evidence indicates that most of the warming that has taken place since the mid-20th century is very likely attributable to increased concentrations of greenhouse gases in the atmosphere—that is, it is caused by human activity—and that changes will continue through the 21st century.[53] Using a set of climate models, each based on a set of assumptions about

---

*El Niño is a change in the surface currents in the eastern South Pacific: The usual cold, nutrient-rich current is replaced by a warm current that does not support the typically dense populations of fish. Because surface currents are driven largely by friction between air and water, this change occurs when the normal prevailing winds become much weaker or even reverse—which is caused in turn by shifts in atmospheric pressure (the Southern Oscillation). An El Niño event typically occurs every 5 to 10 years and lasts a few months, often around the New Year.

global development, IPCC has estimated the environmental impacts of a range of emissions scenarios. The most optimistic scenario assumes a world "with reductions in material intensity and the introduction of clean and resource-efficient technologies" and an emphasis on sustainability. The most pessimistic is a sort of business-as-usual scenario that assumes "very rapid economic growth" and a technological emphasis on fossil fuels.

The global average estimates for the end of the 21st century under the optimistic scenario are a temperature increase of 1.8°C and a rise in sea level of 0.18 to 0.38 meters; under the pessimistic scenario, a temperature increase of about 4.0°C and a rise in sea level of 0.26 to 0.59 meters.[55] The environmental impacts of rising sea level include increased coastal erosion, the conversion of coastal marshes to open water, and the intrusion of salt water into coastal aquifers. Although it is deemed very likely that the deep ocean thermohaline circulation will slow down, it is deemed very unlikely that there will be a dramatic shift in the global circulation of deep ocean waters before 2100[55]—an effect whose impact on climate would be truly catastrophic. Finally, scientists are increasingly concerned that the ocean's absorption of excess atmospheric carbon dioxide (not shown in Figure 4.6) will affect marine ecosystems.

Human Health Impacts of Global Climate Change

The processes that make up global climate change are complex and interrelated, and there is considerable uncertainty about exactly when, where, and to what degree specific human health impacts will occur. But many of the scenarios that have been modeled converge in predicting certain public health impacts associated with overall rising temperatures, a rising sea level, and more frequent extreme weather events.[56] If these basic changes occur, what will be the health impacts?

Higher overall temperatures will increase the range of major disease vectors[56]—most important, mosquitoes—with a corresponding increase in vectorborne diseases, including malaria. Many areas where malaria and other mosquito-borne illnesses are prevalent are in lower-income regions. There may also be an increase in waterborne and foodborne illnesses with increasing temperatures[56]—as is seen now in seasonal fluctuations—because warmer temperatures are more conducive to microbial reproduction. If geographic shifts in temperature occur, then corresponding shifts will occur in the regions where specific crops thrive;[56] this will be disruptive and is likely to affect diet and nutrition.

A rising sea level will slowly inundate low-lying coastal regions;[56] many of the most heavily populated low-lying areas are in lower-income countries. The change in sea level will affect food supplies, claiming agricultural land and disrupting breeding grounds for fish and shellfish. Saltwater intrusion into freshwater aquifers will affect drinking water supplies. The loss of habitable land will create refugees, potentially in large numbers.

Finally, more frequent extreme weather events will produce familiar impacts on a grander scale.[56] Heat waves will produce crop failures, as well as human deaths from heart attacks and heat strokes. Storms and floods will cause physical injuries and hunger (perhaps evolving into malnutrition or famine, depending on circumstances). And they will produce conditions conducive to infectious disease, including emerging infectious diseases: flooding that enhances the breeding of mosquitoes, physical disruption that increases contact with rodent vectors, overcrowding that aids the transmission of respiratory illnesses, damage to the sewage and drinking water systems that ordinarily protect against diarrheal disease. We have only to look at the devastating effects of Hurricane Katrina in 2005 in the United States—one of the world's wealthiest countries—to appreciate the health impacts and social disruption that can come in the wake of an extreme weather event.

The Kyoto Protocol on Global Climate Change

In February 2005, the Kyoto Protocol, an international agreement to reduce the world's emissions of greenhouse gases, went into effect, having been agreed to in 1997. The industrialized nations that signed the protocol agreed to reduce their collective emissions of greenhouse gases, for the period 2008 to 2012, to a level 5.2% below 1990 levels. The United States, the world's single largest emitter of greenhouse gases, had proposed that emissions be merely stabilized, rather than reduced, and did not sign the agreement.

Regulation of Air Pollution from Burning of Fossil Fuels

The first federal air pollution law in the United States was the Air Pollution Control Act of 1955. Coming just a few years after the London Smog, this early legislation mostly supported research. Two laws passed during the 1960s took tentative steps toward controlling air pollution, but it was the Clean Air Act of 1970 that set up a broad framework to do so. The US EPA was created in 1971 to implement the Clean Air Act of 1970. There have been two major sets of amendments to the Clean Air Act, in 1977 and 1990, and some other laws have addressed specific air pollution issues.

By its nature, air pollution is challenging to control. The atmosphere is not confined, like a body of water, nor does it respect boundaries drawn on maps. And although some important sources of air pollution, such as power plants, are stationary, automotive vehicles are highly mobile pollution sources.

In principle, two aspects of air pollution can be assessed: *concentrations* of pollutants in ambient air; and *emissions* of pollutants from sources. Ambient concentrations cannot be controlled directly—it is possible only to set a maximum allowed concentration in ambient air and then assess compliance with this standard. The only levers for the control of air pollution are at the source. Here there are two major options: to set a limit on emissions and then measure performance (that is, adherence to the limit); or to require specific technologies that will result in lower emissions. The US regulatory framework for air pollution uses a combination of approaches: ambient standards, performance standards for emission sources, and technology requirements for emission sources.

The US EPA sets health-based limits for the concentration in ambient air for a short list of widespread pollutants, known as **Criteria Air Pollutants**. The six Criteria Air Pollutants are carbon monoxide, NO_2, SO_2, particulate matter, lead, and ground-level ozone. All are pollutants from the burning of fossil fuels, listed in Table 4.2.* For the five Criteria Air Pollutants that are

---

*Nitric oxide is not listed separately as a criteria pollutant because it is converted to NO_2 in the atmosphere.

gases, EPA has created a measure of daily air quality called the **Air Quality Index**. Each day, for each of the five pollutants, and for local areas across the country, EPA publishes a numerical score from 0 to 500 (a lower score indicates cleaner air) and a category rating, ranging from good to hazardous. These ratings indicate the degree of health concern not only for the general population but for susceptible subgroups of the general population, and many newspapers publish the local Air Quality Index each day.

For the Criteria Air Pollutants, the EPA sets maximum allowable concentrations. These are the **National Ambient Air Quality Standards**, or NAAQS ("nax"), set at levels intended to protect human health (see **Table 4.6**). Each state, through a State Implementation Plan, is required to translate these ambient standards into emissions limits that will enable the state to meet the national standards. For purposes of monitoring and enforcement, each state is divided into geographic areas made up of adjacent counties or townships. Any area that fails to meet any of the NAAQS is designated as a "nonattainment area" for a given pollutant, and a program of control measures to bring the area into compliance must be agreed upon. Such noncompliance is not uncommon.

In addition to setting ambient standards for a small number of common pollutants, the US EPA is charged with setting emissions standards for a long list of less common but more toxic pollutants. This list of 188 Hazardous Air Pollutants (HAPs), also known as "air toxics," includes mercury and its compounds, though most HAPs are volatile organic compounds. For these chemicals, the EPA is charged with setting National Emission Standards for HAPS (NESHAPS) for stationary sources. Some are performance standards and others are technology standards; neither type is a health-based standard. For example, the standard for mercury emissions is a performance standard—emissions from all power plants are capped at a given level—though units of allowed emissions can be traded among regulated facilities as a cost-effective

Table 4.6 Current National Ambient Air Quality Standards

Pollutant	Primary Standard	Averaging Time
Carbon monoxide	9 ppm (10 mg/m^3)	8-hour
	35 ppm (40 mg/m^3)	1-hour
Lead	1.5 μg/m^3	Quarterly
Nitrogen dioxide	0.053 ppm (100 μg/m^3)	Annual
Particulate matter (PM$_{10}$)	150 μg/m^3	24-hour
Particulate matter (PM$_{2.5}$)	15.0 μg/m^3	Annual
	35 μg/m^3	24-hour
Ozone	0.08 ppm	8-hour
	0.12 ppm	1-hour
Sulfur oxides	0.03 ppm	Annual
	0.14 ppm	24-hour

Adapted from: US Environmental Protection Agency. *National Ambient Air Quality Standards (NAAQS)*. Available at: http://www.epa.gov/air/criteria.html. Accessed December 19, 2006.

way to reduce mercury emissions from the energy sector as a whole. Citing the shortage of health effects data on many chemicals, the EPA has regulated only seven air toxics to date under NESHAPS (asbestos; the metals mercury, arsenic, and beryllium; the VOCs benzene and vinyl chloride; and radionuclides). Technology standards under NESHAPs now take the form of a requirement to use either "generally available control technology" or "maximum achievable control technology."

In regulating mobile sources of air pollution—mostly cars and trucks—EPA has used a range of approaches over the years to address both criteria pollutants and others, by regulating tailpipe emissions, engine performance, and fuel. For example, EPA has set limits on tailpipe emissions of hydrocarbons, carbon monoxide, and nitrogen oxides (specified in grams of pollutant per mile driven). Further, states are required to implement programs to inspect cars to ensure that they meet these emissions limits. The agency also established overall mileage requirements for each auto manufacturer's fleet—the corporate average fuel economy standards, or CAFE ("café") standards. In recent years, as the health hazards of diesel exhaust have been documented, EPA has begun a program to reduce emissions from diesel engines.

The use of lead as a gasoline additive was gradually reduced between 1973 and 1986 as EPA phased in new limits. During this period, car manufacturers introduced catalytic converters (devices that reduce the pollutants in exhaust), which were needed to meet emissions limits—and this also speeded up the phase-out of lead because lead damaged the converters. Leaded gasoline was eliminated in the United States in 1996. The benefit of removing lead from gasoline shows clearly in **Figure 4.7**, which tracks the decline of blood lead levels in US children as leaded gasoline was phased out—a public health success story, though a belated one.

A more recent innovation is the development of "reformulated gasoline," which produces less VOC pollution when it is burned, thus reducing the formation of ozone. Use of reformulated gasoline is now required in urban areas that have serious smog problems. On the whole, the regulation of pollution from cars is a difficult challenge in the United States, where many citizens live in suburban settings, consider a large car to be a basic necessity, and show little support for higher gas prices, public transit, carpooling, or bicycle lanes.

In the US regulatory framework, acid deposition is controlled through the Clean Air Act's emissions limits on NO_2 and SO_2. The 1990 amendments set a plan for reducing total SO_2 emissions over time specifically to address the problem of acid deposition, adding a market-based system of trading emission allowances. And, reflecting the transboundary nature of this problem, the United States and Canada have agreed to a joint program to reduce emissions of NO_x and SO_x.

To date, carbon dioxide, despite its looming public health impact as a greenhouse gas, has not been regulated by the US Environmental Protection Agency on grounds that it was not an air pollutant under the Clean Air Act. In 2007, however, the Supreme Court struck down that interpretation, ruling that carbon dioxide and other heat-trapping gasses are indeed air pollutants under the law and can be regulated as such.[57] Some states have already taken action on global climate change—a California law, for example, requires the state to reduce its emissions of greenhouse gases to 1990 levels by 2020.[58] California is also a member, with four other western states, of the Western Climate Initiative, created in 2007 to develop regional strategies to reduce greenhouse gas emissions.[58]

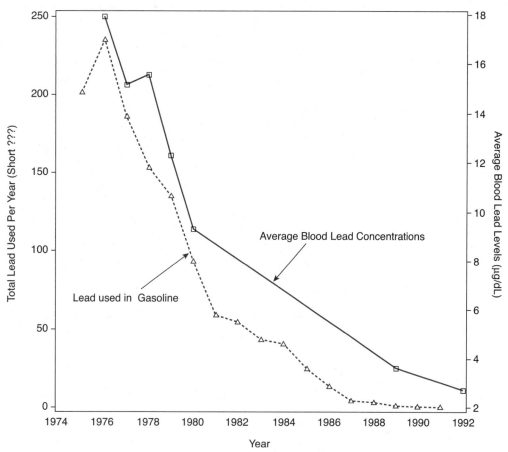

FIGURE 4.7 Decline in lead used in gasoline, and of average blood levels in US children, 1974–1992. *From*: US Environmental Protection Agency, Great Lakes National Program Office. *Great Lakes Binational Toxics Strategy Report on Alkyl-lead: Sources, Regulations and Options, 2000*. Available at: http://www.epa.gov/glnpo/bns/lead/Step%20Report/steps.pdf. Accessed April 12, 2008.

Key elements of the US regulatory framework for air pollution appear in **Table 4.7**. This table is the second in a series of similar tables that place regulatory provisions within the traditional regulatory domains of environmental health.

The Clean Air Act also gives the EPA a key role in the implementation of another piece of legislation, the National Environmental Policy Act (NEPA), signed into law in 1970. (The scope of this law extends well beyond environmental health *per se*, and for this reason it is not listed in Table 4.7). NEPA requires all federal agencies in the executive branch of government to evaluate and disclose the environmental impacts of their proposed actions—for example, building an interstate highway or cutting timber—*before* decisions are made or actions are taken. Depending on the complexity of the proposed action, this disclosure may take the form of a full **environmental impact statement** (EIS) or a more streamlined environmental assessment. Thus

Table 4.7 Overview of US Regulatory Framework for Environmental Health Hazards (2)

Environmental Health Domain	Major Laws and Key Provisions for the Control of Environmental Health Hazards
Biological hazards	Public Health Service Act (PHSA)—development of guidelines for vaccination; use of quarantine or isolation to prevent entry of infectious diseases into the United States; conduct of surveillance and investigation of outbreaks
Air pollution	*Clean Air Act (CAA)—ambient standards (NAAQS) for Criteria Air Pollutants; emissions standards for Hazardous Air Pollutants, including mercury; emission allowances for SO_2 (to control acid deposition); removal of lead from gasoline; requirement to sell reformulated gasoline in high-smog areas*
Ionizing radiation	
Alternative energy sources	
Hazardous wastes	
Occupational health	
Industrial water pollution	
Toxic chemicals	
Pesticides	
Food supply	
Sewage wastes and community water supply	
Municipal solid waste	
Consumer products	
Environmental noise	

Note: New information appears in italics.

NEPA added the explicit consideration of a new factor—environmental impacts—to the traditional criteria of technical and economic feasibility in agencies' decision-making, although the law stops short of actually requiring protection of the environment.[59]

In principle, the Environmental Protection Agency must comply with NEPA's requirements as other agencies do. However, many EPA actions—for example, under the Clean Air Act and the Clean Water Act—are exempt from NEPA's requirements in light of the fact that EPA's own procedures already achieve the same objectives. Further, as alluded to just above, EPA has an important role in the implementation of NEPA: The Clean Air Act requires EPA to review and comment publicly on environmental impact statements by all other federal agencies and evaluate the acceptability of the environmental impacts of the agencies' planned actions.

4.2 Electricity from Nuclear Fuel

In contrast to coal, which people have used as fuel for a thousand years or more, uranium has been tapped as a source of energy only in the last 60 years. Following World War II, during which nuclear weapons were developed and used, serious efforts were begun to develop peaceful applications of nuclear technology—in particular, to generate electricity. Nuclear power is derived from the controlled splitting of uranium atoms, in contrast to the uncontrolled chain reaction of a nuclear weapon.

Nuclear power was attractive on several grounds. It was "clean," producing none of the combustion products associated with coal- and oil-fired power plants. It would produce inexpensive electricity, perhaps even "too cheap to meter," in the optimistic view of the US Atomic Energy Commission in the early 1950s. And, although uranium is a nonrenewable resource, US reserves would serve for many decades. US plans for civilian nuclear power and military nuclear weapons dovetailed nicely because both were managed by the Atomic Energy Commission; for example, radioactive wastes from civilian power plants were to be reprocessed for use in both power plants and weapons.

The early optimism over nuclear power faded as the safety challenges of operating power plants and reprocessing or entombing their radioactive wastes became clear. By the early 1980s, the US nuclear power industry had reached a plateau. However, in the era of global climate change and dwindling oil reserves, nuclear power remains in the mix of energy technologies for the United States and the world.

The environmental and health impacts of using uranium as a fuel are very different from those associated with fossil fuels. This section treats the following topics:

- The nature of radiation and radioactive decay, as background needed to understand the nuclear fuel cycle
- The major stages in the nuclear fuel cycle (which, like the fossil fuel cycle, is not really a cycle)
- The health effects of ionizing radiation and specifically of radiation exposures from the nuclear fuel cycle
- The US regulatory framework for preventing or limiting exposures to ionizing radiation from the nuclear fuel cycle

An Introduction to Radiation

In simple terms, **radiation** is energy in transit, in packets, behaving either as particles or as waves. One source of radiation is the radioactive decay of atoms of certain chemical elements, such as uranium.

Radioactive Decay

Chemical elements exist as different **isotopes** (see the sidebar titled "About Atomic Structure, Chemical Isotopes, and Uranium," which follows). Certain isotopes of some chemical elements, including uranium, are unstable, or **radioactive**. To achieve a more stable configuration, an atom of a radioactive isotope ejects a part of its nucleus; this process is termed **radioactive decay**. A sample of uranium, in which many atoms are undergoing radioactive decay, emits a steady stream of such particles—that is, radiation.

The particle ejected from the nucleus of an atom during radioactive decay can be either an alpha particle or a beta particle. An **alpha particle** consists of two protons plus two neutrons. A **beta particle** is simply an electron, and with the ejection of this negative particle, a neutron in the nucleus is converted to a proton.

Thus, the ejection of either an alpha or a beta particle changes the number of protons in the nucleus, and this in turn changes the chemical element. For example, when an atom of uranium ejects an alpha particle, what is left is an atom with 90 protons. This element is thorium, and we say that uranium "decays into" thorium. Alpha decay, but not beta decay, also changes the mass number (see **Table 4.8**).

Such decays occur in chains, creating new elements in characteristic series. Table 4.8 shows the decay chain for uranium-238. The ejection of an alpha particle (two protons plus two neutrons) is reflected in the mass number, which is reduced by four; the ejection of a beta particle, in contrast, does not affect the mass number.

About Atomic Structure, Chemical Isotopes, and Uranium

At their most basic, atoms are made up of three types of particles. In the nucleus are two types of particles that on the atomic scale are relatively massive: protons, which are positively charged, and neutrons, which have no charge. Orbiting around the nucleus are the much smaller electrons, which are negatively charged.

A chemical element is defined by the number of protons in its nucleus; for example, if an atom has 92 protons, it is a uranium atom. But atoms of the same element can have *different* numbers of neutrons in the nucleus; these are different *isotopes* of the element.

Uranium as it exists in nature consists almost entirely of two isotopes. Most uranium is an isotope with 92 protons and 146 neutrons, denoted as uranium-238 (the mass number, 238, is the number of protons and neutrons in the nucleus); most of the remainder, less than 1% of naturally occurring uranium, is uranium-235, which has 92 protons and 143 neutrons.

Table 4.8 The Decay Chain of Uranium-238

Particle Ejected			Half-life			
Alpha	Beta	Radioactive Isotope	Seconds	Minutes	Days	Years
x		Uranium-238				4.47 billion
	x	Thorium-234			24.10	
	x	Protactinium-234		1.17		
x		Uranium-234				245,500
x		Thorium-230				75,400
x		Radium-226				1599
x		Radon-222			3.823	
x		Polonium-218		3.04		
	x	Lead-214		26.9		
	x	Bismuth-214		19.7		
x		Polonium-214	0.000164			
	x	Lead-210				22.6
	x	Bismuth-210			5.01	
x		Polonium-210			138.4	
		Lead-206 (stable)				

Data from: Holden N. Table of the isotopes. In: Lide D, ed. *CRC Handbook of Chemistry and Physics*. 84th (2003–2004) ed. Boca Raton, Fla: CRC Press; 2003:11-50–11-197.

The rate at which atoms undergo radioactive decay varies widely. As shown in Table 4.8, each radioactive isotope, or **radionuclide**, has a characteristic **half-life**, the time it takes for half the atoms in a sample of the element to undergo radioactive decay. Half-lives range from microseconds to billions of years. From a public health point of view, the most important radioactive elements in the uranium-238 decay chain are those with short half-lives. Atom for atom, these elements emit the most radiation in a given period of time.

Of particular concern is the decay of **radon** (highlighted in Table 4.8). Because radon is a gas, it is highly mobile in the environment and is readily inhaled. Moreover, radon has a relatively short half-life of about 4 days, and the decay of radon kicks off a series of very rapid breakdowns. In fact, the four isotopes that follow radon in the decay chain are commonly referred to as radon progeny (or, in earlier literature, radon daughters).

Electromagnetic Radiation

The release of an alpha or beta particle is often accompanied by a burst of energy. This energy is **gamma radiation**, which is a type of **electromagnetic radiation**. The energy of electromagnetic radiation travels through space in the form of waves rather than subatomic particles. Electromagnetic radiation varies in wavelength, the distance from one peak to the next (**Figure 4.8**), and the **electromagnetic spectrum** is the full set of distinct types of electromagnetic radiation, arranged in order of wavelength.

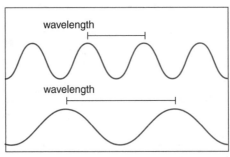

FIGURE 4.8 Electromagnetic radiation of shorter and longer wavelengths.

Because all electromagnetic radiation moves at the same speed (the speed of light), shorter-wavelength radiation has higher energy: More packets arrive in a given period of time (that is, they arrive with greater frequency). Gamma radiation is a short-wavelength, high-energy form of electromagnetic radiation (see the sidebar titled "About the Electromagnetic Spectrum," which follows).

About the Electromagnetic Spectrum

Electromagnetic radiation emitted from different sources has characteristic wavelengths. Taken together, these types of radiation make up the *electromagnetic spectrum*, which ranges from the very-long-wavelength radiation of power lines (thousands of meters) to the very-short-wavelength cosmic radiation that originates in outer space (less than one-trillionth of a meter).

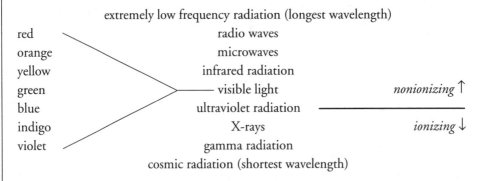

In the middle of the electromagnetic spectrum, infrared and ultraviolet radiation bracket the familiar spectrum of visible light. Sunlight is made up of infrared radiation, visible light, and ultraviolet radiation. Infrared radiation is simply heat; any object that is warmer than its surroundings gives off infrared radiation.

Ionizing and Nonionizing Radiation

In public health, it is important to distinguish between ionizing and nonionizing radiation, a functional distinction based on radiation's biological effect. **Ionizing radiation** is radiation that, when it strikes matter, has enough energy to knock an electron out of orbit, creating an ion.* Such ionization can lead to damage to the cells of the body.

All the products of radioactive decay—alpha and beta particles and gamma radiation—are ionizing forms of radiation. **Cosmic radiation** and X-rays are also ionizing. In the electromagnetic spectrum, the dividing line between ionizing and nonionizing radiation falls within the ultraviolet range (see the preceding sidebar titled "About the Electromagnetic Spectrum"). The shortest-wavelength **ultraviolet radiation**, known as UV-C, is ionizing; other ultraviolet radiation (the longer-wavelength UV-A and UV-B) is not. **Nonionizing radiation**, although it does not have enough energy to knock an electron out of orbit, can cause biological damage; both UV-B and UV-A radiation in sunlight are now recognized as risk factors for skin cancer (see Chapter 5).

The Nuclear Fuel Cycle

As it operates in the United States today, the **nuclear fuel cycle** is not actually a cycle but rather a one-way series of events, usually grouped into three stages (see **Figure 4.9**). In the first stage, often called the **front end** of the process, uranium is mined and ultimately fabricated into a form that can be used as fuel in a power plant. The middle stage is the generation of electricity at nuclear power plants. The last stage, often referred to as the **back end**, is the disposal of the radioactive wastes produced by power plants. If nuclear wastes were to be reprocessed—and some other countries do reprocess these wastes—this partial recycling would be grafted onto the current one-way flow of nuclear materials, as represented by dashed lines in Figure 4.9.

The Front End of the Nuclear Fuel Cycle

Uranium is widespread in the earth's crust. For example, it is found at low concentrations in granite and in many coal deposits. However, it is practical to mine only uranium-bearing rock in which concentrations are much higher—that is, uranium ore. Uranium ore has been removed both from underground mines and, especially in the earlier years of the industry, from surface mines. Nearly all uranium deposits in the United States are in the western states—mostly in Colorado, Utah, Arizona, and New Mexico—and historically most US uranium mining took place on Navajo tribal lands.

The mining of uranium ore releases radiation into the confined spaces of underground mines, and also into the ambient environment. Mining produces waste in the form of crushed rock, known as **mine tailings**. Of course, the line between ore that is worth mining and ore that is not worth mining is blurry (and it changes over time with shifts in the market price of uranium), and thus mine tailings contain higher concentrations of uranium than ordinary rock does.

---

*An ion is an atom that is either missing electrons or has extra electrons, and thus has a positive or negative charge.

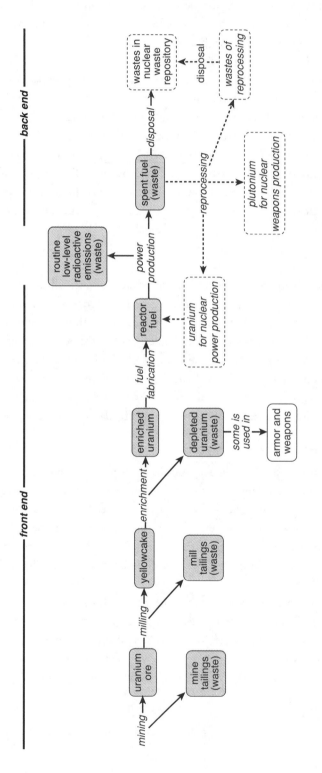

FIGURE 4.9 The nuclear fuel cycle.

Mine tailings are left in large piles on the ground surface near mines. Radon gas is released from tailings to the air, radioactive dust is carried on the wind, and rainwater leaches radioactive constituents into groundwater.

Uranium extracted by mining is next processed at a mill. Milling converts the uranium ore to a more concentrated form known as **yellowcake**, and it is yellowcake that is transported to the eastern United States for further processing. Milling also produces large volumes of depleted ore in the form of sandy sludge, known as **uranium mill tailings**.

Such waste is dumped in piles on the ground or placed in walled impoundments. Like mine tailings, mill tailings are a source of radon and radioactive dust. Nevertheless, in the past mill tailings were sometimes used for construction. For example, in the 1950s many tons of tailings piled in Grand Junction, Colorado, were given away free to builders, who used them in constructing basements and patios in the area.[60]

In the United States at present, there are 26 licensed uranium milling sites, though most are inactive because of the decline in the uranium industry. As of 1996, the 26 licensed sites represented a total of about 200 million metric tons of tailings, and 24 abandoned sites contained a total of about 26 million metric tons[61]—mostly in the western United States (**Figure 4.10**). Some of the abandoned piles have since been moved to more isolated locations, and some have been covered to reduce the release of radon and minimize leaching to groundwater.[62]

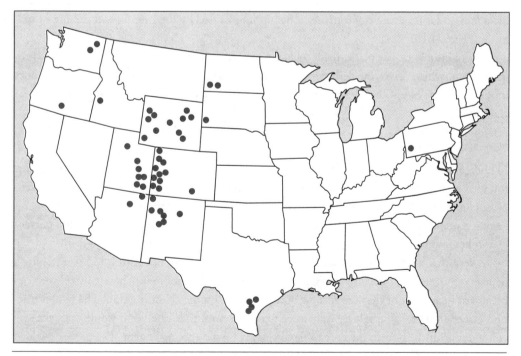

FIGURE 4.10   Locations of uranium mill tailings piles in the United States. *From*: Environmental Protection Agency. *Uranium Mill Tailings*. Available at: http://www.epa.gov/radiation/docs/radwaste/402-k-94-001-umt.htm. Accessed October 7, 2006.

In recent years, it has become common to use an acidic or alkaline solution to dissolve uranium from the ore in which it is embedded, rather than mining; this process is known as **in situ leaching**. When uranium is leached from ore in situ, yellowcake is produced in a single step, along with liquid wastes. This waste is placed in a man-made pond, and water is allowed to evaporate, leaving behind radioactive sludge. Both mining and in situ leaching take uranium out of its natural geologic setting, where human exposure to radiation is very limited, into the realm of human activity and exposure.

Most naturally occurring uranium, and therefore most of the uranium in yellowcake, is uranium-238. However, it is uranium-235 that can be used as fuel in a power reactor. For this reason, the next step in uranium processing is to increase the ratio of uranium-235 to uranium-238. This step, known as **enrichment**, is actually achieved by *removing* uranium-238 from the yellowcake. This excess uranium-238, called **depleted uranium**, has some uses—in particular, because it is extremely dense, it is used to make military armor and armor-piercing weapons—but most is treated as waste with a relatively low level of radioactivity.

The final step in preparing uranium for use in power plants is **fuel fabrication**. The enriched uranium is formed into hard pellets, which are placed inside long, thin metal tubes. These loaded tubes are the fuel rods that will be used in a nuclear power plant.

Nuclear Power Plants

At present there are 104 nuclear power plants operating in the United States (see **Figure 4.11**), most located far from the environmental disruptions caused by the mining and milling of uranium (Figure 4.10).

In a traditional power plant, fossil fuels are burned to generate heat, which is used to produce steam, which drives the turbines that generate electricity. A nuclear power plant operates in the same way, except that the heat used to produce steam is generated by a controlled nuclear chain reaction.

Normal Operations

In the core of a power reactor, tens of thousands of uranium fuel rods stand upright, surrounded by water. The core is bombarded with neutrons. Each neutron that strikes the nucleus of a uranium atom causes it to split, or fission, into two smaller atoms of different elements, releasing more neutrons along with energy (heat). Any of these neutrons that strikes the nucleus of another uranium atom causes it to split, releasing still more neutrons—and so forth.

To keep this **nuclear fission** chain reaction from cascading out of control, rods containing a neutron-absorbing material are inserted into slots among the fuel rods. These **control rods** can be moved in and out of the core to slow down or speed up the chain reaction. The fission reaction can be shut down rapidly by fully inserting the control rods, though it would still take several months for the heat in the core to be dissipated by the cooling system. The core is shielded to contain the radiation produced by the fission reactions.

In one common design, the water (as liquid or steam) circulates in a loop, passing through the reactor core and the steam turbine. The circulating water has two functions, which are really two sides of the same coin. In the core, it acts as a coolant, removing heat from the nuclear

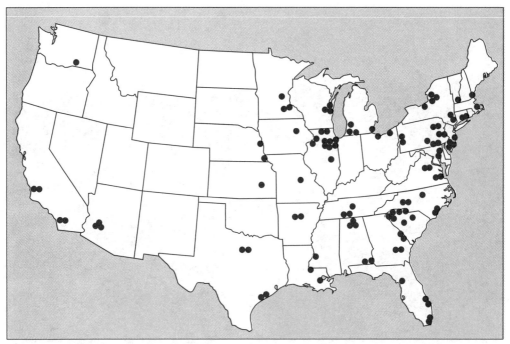

FIGURE 4.11   Approximate locations of nuclear power plants in the United States. *Data from*: US Energy Information Administration. *US Nuclear Reactors: Reactor Status List*. Available at: http://www.eia.doe.gov/cneaf/nuclear/page/nuc_reactors/reactsum.html. Accessed: October 7, 2006.

chain reaction; then, having absorbed heat in the core, it is converted to steam, which serves to drive a turbine. After passing through the turbine, the steam is cooled and condensed, returning to the core in liquid form. (This basic design is known as a boiling water rector; other designs are also used.)

It is critical to keep the core of a nuclear reactor from becoming too hot. Overheating will compromise the structural integrity of the fuel rods, which in turn will prevent the control rods from moving freely into the core, which will result in even greater overheating and damage to the fuel rods. This very dangerous cycle of effects can lead to a partial or full meltdown of the core, with the potential for large releases of radioactivity. The cylindrical or dome-shaped containment building that surrounds a nuclear reactor (two are shown in **Figure 4.12**, housing the two reactors) is designed to limit the escape of radioactivity in the event of an accident. The most visible part of a nuclear power plant, the very large cooling tower (four are shown in Figure 4.12), simply dissipates heat from the plant during normal operations and is not unique to nuclear technology.

The containment building is only the most visible safety feature of a nuclear reactor. Redundant and flexible safety features are engineered into commercial reactors. A key element is an independent emergency core cooling system that refloods the reactor core in the event that

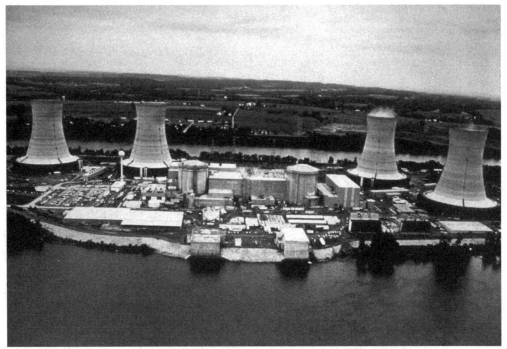

FIGURE 4.12   The Three Mile Island nuclear power plant in Pennsylvania was the site of the most serious accident at a US commercial nuclear plant. *Source*: Reprinted courtesy of CDC Public Health Image Library. ID# 1194. Content provider: CDC. Available at: http://phil.cdc.gov/phil/details.asp. Accessed August 21, 2007.

the core loses coolant—though an accident that causes physical damage to the core can render this system ineffective.

During normal operations, a nuclear power plant releases small amounts of numerous radioactive fission products into the air, including iodine-131 and strontium-90 as well as radioactive isotopes of the noble (that is, chemically inert) gases xenon and krypton.

Accidents at Nuclear Power Plants

Nuclear power is an unforgiving technology in two ways: First, if the reactor core is damaged, accidents can spiral out of control, as at the Chernobyl plant in 1986; and second, the health effects of radiation are serious and long-lasting. And, of course, nuclear power plants are subject to all the mundane factors that contribute to accidents at other industrial facilities, including bad design decisions, aging physical plants, human error, and natural disasters.

For example, at the Browns Ferry nuclear plant in Alabama in 1975, a maintenance worker using a candle to locate air leaks accidentally set fire to insulation surrounding some electrical cables. Because this accident happened in a room where cables from all over the plant converged, many components were simultaneously disabled, and a serious accident was narrowly averted.

The most serious nuclear accident in the United States, at the Three Mile Island plant in Pennsylvania in 1979, began when a valve stuck open so that coolant drained out of the core. The operators' instrument panel did not make it clear that the valve was open. It appeared to them that the core had *too much* water, so they shut off the emergency cooling pumps. Although a part of the core melted, the reactor vessel remained intact.

The design of the Soviet reactor at Chernobyl differed from that of Western reactors in important ways, including the lack of a containment building and the use of graphite to absorb neutrons in the core. At Chernobyl, a complicated series of events and human errors resulted in a power surge in the core at a time when the emergency core cooling system had been turned off as part of a test. The fuel rods melted and ruptured, rendering the control rods ineffective, and a steam explosion destroyed the reactor core. The ensuing graphite fire released large quantities of radioactive elements into the air, creating a plume that spread across Europe.

The Back End of the Nuclear Fuel Cycle

Over time, the amount of "unburned" uranium-235 in the core of an operating power reactor declines. The reactor is periodically shut down to remove spent fuel and replace it with new fuel rods. The spent fuel is extremely hot, releasing both radiation and heat. It is placed immediately in an underground storage pool at the reactor site; the pool is shielded to prevent the escape of radiation, and circulating water gradually cools the spent fuel. After about a year, spent fuel can be removed from the pool, though it is still highly radioactive.

Embedded in the spent fuel are two types of radioactive materials created by bombarding uranium with neutrons. Fission products—elements lighter than uranium—are created when neutrons *split* uranium nuclei. At the same time, if an atom *absorbs* a neutron, the atom becomes a different element, with a higher atomic number. In this way, plutonium and other elements heavier than uranium are created in the spent fuel. These heavy elements are sometimes called transuranic elements because their atomic numbers are higher than that of uranium.

As noted earlier, the original plan in the United States was to recycle the wastes of nuclear power plants, extracting "unburned" uranium-238 to be fabricated again into fuel pellets. As shown in Figure 4.9, such **reprocessing** of spent fuel would also extract plutonium to be used in making nuclear weapons—and it would create a new waste stream of highly radioactive material, now in liquid form. These liquid wastes of reprocessing would contain uranium and plutonium not captured by reprocessing, as well as the fission products and transuranic elements present in the spent fuel. This waste stream, like the original spent fuel, would require permanent storage in a repository.

In the United States, commercial reactor fuel has not been reprocessed for more than 30 years, for three reasons. First, it is not clear that reprocessing reduces the waste management challenges of nuclear power. It is also not clear that reprocessed fuel is cheaper than the newly made fuel it is intended to replace. And finally, there is some risk that reactor-grade plutonium, if obtained by terrorists or rogue nations, could be used to make a crude nuclear weapon.* A number of countries, including the United States, have charged that Iran's nuclear power program is intended for this purpose, although conclusive evidence has not emerged.

If reprocessing was the United States' Plan A for nuclear wastes, then Plan B has been to build a permanent repository (Figure 4.9, dashed lines). A federal law (the Nuclear Waste Policy Act of 1982; explained later) set this process in motion, but progress has been painfully slow. A starting list of nine sites in six states was finally whittled down to one site at Yucca Mountain in southern Nevada, approved in 2002. But construction has not yet begun, and opposition to the facility may still prevent it altogether.

Not surprisingly, not-in-my-back-yard (NIMBY) opposition to the nuclear waste site has been strong. Political opposition to the Nevada site is also rooted in a clear geographic injustice: Like the uranium tailings piles, the site is located in a part of the country not served by nuclear power. Indeed, only eight of the country's 104 operating nuclear plants are in states west of the Rocky Mountains.[63] The site's location has also raised another thorny issue: Trains would have to crisscross the country to carry spent fuel to Nevada.

On the plus side, the chosen site is on federally owned land adjacent to the Nevada Test Site. This large expanse of federally owned land is already highly contaminated with radioactive materials as a result of decades of nuclear weapons testing (see **Figure 4.13**). The population density in the immediate area is low. In this arid region, the water table is so deep that current plans call for the repository to be built 1000 feet below the surface *and* 1000 feet above the water table.[64]

If and when spent fuel finally reaches this permanent resting place, it must be sequestered for a very long time—it will take about 300,000 years for its radioactivity to become comparable to the uranium ore originally mined.[65] This very long time frame greatly amplifies the technical challenges of finding a location where the repository will not be compromised. Over so many thousands of years, hydrologic conditions may change. Earthquakes may occur. Even communicating the hazard to people in the distant future is a challenge.

In the absence of a permanent repository, spent fuel from US nuclear power plants remains in interim storage. Some is still stored in pools at reactor sites. Some spent fuel has been moved to dry storage in steel containers placed in concrete vaults at reactor sites. Spent fuel is quantified in units of metric tons of heavy metal (MTHM) present in the fuel. As of 2006, more than 50,000 MTHM of spent fuel was stored at more than 100 sites in 39 states.[66] If the present statutory cap of 70,000 MTHM on the capacity of the Yucca Mountain repository is maintained, and if the repository opens as planned in 2017, its capacity will be fully committed by the time it opens.[66]

Finally, nuclear power plants themselves, when they are decommissioned (that is, closed down), become radioactive waste. To date, 23 plants have been decommissioned or are in the process of being decommissioned.[67] After the plant's works are flushed out to remove radioactive debris, the facility can be dismantled and its components—such as the reactor vessel—

*In contrast to commercial nuclear reactors, the main purpose of military reactors is to produce plutonium to be used in weapons, and wastes from these reactors have always been reprocessed.

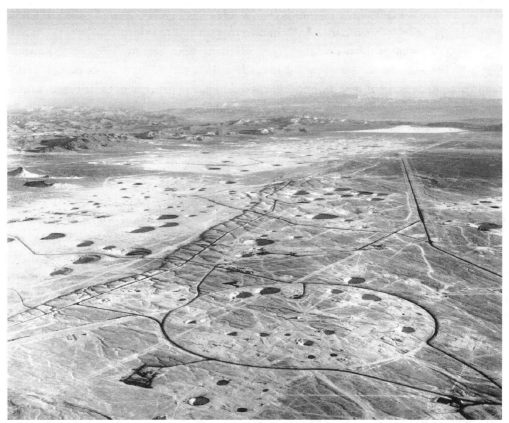

FIGURE 4.13 The Yucca Flat area of the federally owned Nevada Test Site is pockmarked with craters made by nuclear weapons tests. *Source*: Courtesy of National Nuclear Security Administration/Nevada Site Office.

shipped offsite for permanent disposal as radioactive waste. Federal regulations give plant operators the option of letting the facility stand for some years before being dismantled, to allow radioactivity to decline; decommissioning must be completed within 60 years after the plant closes. To date, most waste from decommissioned US nuclear power plants has been shipped to a commercial radioactive waste facility in Barnwell, South Carolina.

Low-Level Radioactive Wastes

In addition to leaving highly radioactive spent fuel and reactor components as wastes, nuclear power production also yields wastes with lower levels of radioactivity. These **low-level radioactive wastes** include protective gear worn by workers, used filters and tools, and residues from cleaning the cooling water used in reactors. These wastes emit much less radiation than does spent reactor fuel, the wastes of reprocessing spent fuel, or the components of decommissioned reactors. Low-level radioactive wastes are not physically hot and do not require the same shielding as high-level radioactive wastes. And the time required for most low-level wastes to decay to the point where the radiation they emit is comparable to natural background radiation can be counted in hundreds of years rather than hundreds of thousands of years.

In addition, some of the nation's low-level radioactive waste originates outside the nuclear fuel cycle. For example, some medical and research facilities use radioactive materials for sterilization of equipment, for diagnostic or treatment techniques in patients, or for testing in laboratory animals. Such activities yield radioactively contaminated waste products, such as syringes or glassware or the carcasses of test animals.

Under a federal law (the Low-Level Radioactive Waste Policy Amendments Act of 1985, discussed later), each US state became responsible for disposing of low-level radioactive wastes generated within the state. The law encourages states to form groups (called compacts), within which one state hosts a waste facility for all the compact's member states. As of January 2007, all but nine states had joined a compact;[68] however, no new facilities to store low-level radioactive wastes have been built. Only two sites—the long-established facilities in Hanford, Washington, and Barnwell, South Carolina—currently accept all classes of low-level radioactive wastes. Both these states are now in compacts; the Hanford site has already restricted its services to members of its compact, and Barnwell plans to do the same as of 2008.[69] Thus, a crisis is looming in the management of low-level radioactive wastes.

The Future of Nuclear Power

The story of nuclear power in the United States to date has been one of great expectation followed by great disappointment. As shown in **Figure 4.14**, optimism peaked in the years 1974–1976 with 217 plants in the pipeline, in operation, or retired from service. After 1976, although the number of licensed plants continued to increase for some years, cancellations steadily eroded the number of plants on order, a process hastened by the 1979 accident at Three Mile Island. As public confidence declined, construction and licensing became more drawn out and costly. From 1996 to 2007, no new nuclear plants went into service in the United States.

At present, nuclear plants provide about 20% of US electric power, and a considerably larger share in most European countries.[70] Nuclear power is currently the source of less than 3% of electricity in both China, which has substantial uranium reserves, and India, which does not.[70]

The global future of nuclear power depends partly on technological developments. A new type of reactor, known as a pebble-bed modular reactor, is now under development in South Africa. Touted as inherently safe, the reactor's core would contain many thousands of small freely moving spheres ("pebbles"), some containing grains of uranium fuel and others containing graphite, a neutron-absorbing material. Control rods would be moved among the spheres. A fusion reactor—which would derive energy from fusing the nuclei of atoms together, rather than splitting them as in a fission reactor—has been discussed for some time but remains in the distant future.

Two thirds of the world's known uranium reserves are located in ore deposits in just four countries: Australia (28%), Kazakhstan (15%), Canada (14%), and South Africa (10%); the

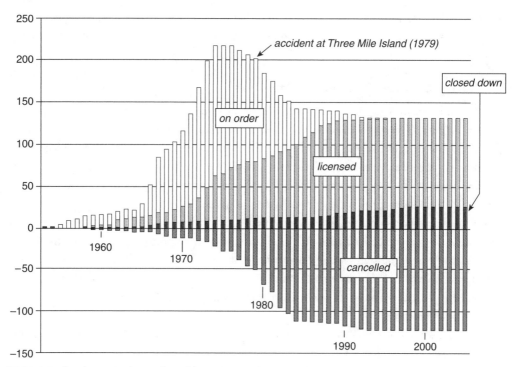

FIGURE 4.14 Number of nuclear power plants in the United States, 1953–2005. *Data from*: US Energy Information Administration. *US Nuclear Reactors: Reactor Status List*. Available at: http://eia.doe.gov/cneaf/nuclear/page/nuc_reactors/reactsum.html. Accessed October 7, 2006; and Union of Concerned Scientists, personal communication (dataset on US nuclear power plants); 2000.

United States is home to just 3% of this resource base.[71] At the current rate of electricity production, the world's known resources are estimated to be adequate for some 80 years, and similar resources, not yet discovered, could add more than 200 years to this time horizon.[71] In principle, though not yet in practice, uranium could also be extracted from tailings at gold and phosphate mines, and even from seawater—an enormous potential resource.[71] Specialized reactors have been developed to convert naturally occurring thorium into a fissile isotope of uranium (U-233, not a naturally occurring isotope),[71] and of course it would be possible to reprocess nuclear wastes already generated. It is impossible to know at present which of these potential resources will be realized as technology, costs, and health concerns are weighed in coming decades.

Health Impacts of the Nuclear Fuel Cycle

This section considers in turn the units used to measure exposure to ionizing radiation; the sources of exposure to ionizing radiation, both natural and man-made; the biological effects of ionizing radiation; and the health impacts of radiation exposures that originate in the nuclear fuel cycle. It concludes with a brief assessment of the tradeoffs in health risks of using nuclear and fossil fuels.

Measuring Exposure to Ionizing Radiation

Two sets of internationally agreed units are used to quantify exposure to ionizing radiation. The first set of units (**Grays**, abbreviated Gy) measures the intensity of a radiologic exposure: the amount of energy delivered per gram of tissue. The second set of units (**Sieverts**, abbreviated Sv) incorporates the **relative biological effectiveness (RBE)** of a radiologic exposure. That is, expressing exposure in Sieverts takes account of the fact that some types of radiation do more damage than others, per unit of energy delivered to tissue.*

Relative biological effectiveness is determined largely by the density of ionization along the path taken through tissue by a particle. An alpha particle (two protons plus two neutrons), because it is relatively massive, causes a dense track of ionizations along its path. A beta particle (an electron), which is much smaller, causes less frequent ionizations along its track. And gamma rays—mere waves of energy—pass through the body, only occasionally dislodging an electron by a direct hit.

Thus, the same dose, expressed in Grays, of alpha, beta, or gamma radiation translates into different doses expressed in Sieverts:

$$\text{dose (Gy)} \times \text{RBE} = \text{dose (Sv)}$$

As a rule of thumb (see **Table 4.9**), the RBE of alpha radiation is about 10 times that of gamma radiation, and the RBE of beta radiation is about 5 times that of gamma radiation. However, relative biological effectiveness can be affected by the type of cell or tissue and other factors.

The impact of radiation exposure also depends on whether the radiation is delivered to the interior of the body by ingestion or inhalation, or to the exterior of the body—that is, to the skin. Alpha, beta, and gamma radiation are all internal hazards—that is, they cause ionizations if they are delivered directly to vulnerable internal cells (see **Table 4.10**). As an internal exposure, alpha radiation causes the most damage because its track of ionizations is so dense; and gamma radiation causes the least damage.

If radiation exposure comes from outside the body, it's a different story. An alpha particle, with its dense track of ionizations, gives up its energy over such a short distance that it doesn't even penetrate through the layer of dead cells on the surface of the skin. Thus, alpha radiation is not hazardous as an external exposure. A sheet of paper would also shield against alpha radiation.

---

*Grays and Sieverts correspond to the **rads** and **rems** of older terminology, which is still widely used; 1 Gray = 100 rads; 1 Sievert = 100 rems. One milli-Sievert (1/1000 Sievert) is abbreviated mSv; 1 micro-Sievert (one-millionth Sievert) is abbreviated μSv. Another unit, the **Becquerel (Bq)** is not a measure of dose, but simply of radioactivity: one Becquerel = one disintegration per second. (An older unit of radioactivity is the **Curie**.)

Table 4.9   An Example Showing the Relationship between Dose in Grays and Dose in Sieverts for Alpha, Beta, and Gamma Radiation

Type of Radiation	Description	Dose in Grays	Relative Biological Effectiveness (RBE)	Equivalent Dose in Sieverts
Alpha	2 protons + 2 neutrons	2	10	20
Beta	1 electron	2	5	10
Gamma	High-energy electromagnetic radiation	2	1	2

Beta radiation passes through the skin, but does not penetrate deep into the body; a thin sheet of plastic or aluminum shields against beta radiation. Gamma radiation passes completely through the body, and a dense material like lead or concrete is needed to protect against it.

Typical Sources of Exposure to Ionizing Radiation

People are exposed on a more or less continuous basis to ionizing radiation from several natural sources, as well as from man-made sources. The major natural sources of external exposure are cosmic radiation, which originates in outer space, and terrestrial radiation—that is, radiation emitted from solid minerals, such as uranium and thorium, in rocks and soil. The major sources of internal exposure are inhalation of radon (including exposure to radon progeny) and ingestion of water and food: Plants take up radioactive elements from soil; animals eat plants; and people in turn consume both plants and animals as food.

It is not a simple matter to estimate the average share of people's exposure to ionizing radiation that comes from these natural sources. Exposure to cosmic radiation varies with altitude—exposure is greater in Denver than in Boston, for example—and local geology affects terrestrial radiation as well as radiation in water and food. Inhalation of radon (including radon progeny)

Table 4.10   Key Characteristics of Alpha, Beta, and Gamma Radiation

Type of Radiation	Description	Internal Hazard?	External Hazard?	Effective Shielding	Examples of Emitters
Alpha	2 protons + 2 neutrons	Yes	No	Dead skin cells, paper	Uranium-238, radon and progeny
Beta	1 electron	Yes	Yes	Aluminum, plastic	Strontium-90, iodine-131
Gamma	High-energy electromagnetic radiation	Yes	Yes	Lead, concrete	(Often accompanies alpha or beta)

is on average the greatest source of exposure because radon is a gas, and therefore highly mobile; and also because it begins a series of rapid breakdowns, as described previously. In the general population, exposure to radon is determined mainly by its accumulation in indoor settings[72] and thus depends not only on geology but also on building styles—for example, building materials, airtightness of construction, and the presence of basements. As a global average, radon accounts for about half of exposure from natural sources, but as shown in **Figure 4.15**, the typical range includes much higher exposures. Thus, it is not unusual for radon to be the dominant source, driving a higher-than-average total exposure.

Turning to man-made sources of ionizing radiation, the UN Scientific Committee on the Effects of Atomic Radiation (UNSCEAR) estimates the global average annual exposure to diagnostic medical X-rays at 0.4 mSv, but notes dramatic differences according to the intensity of health care. In countries with the highest intensity of health care, including the United States, average radiation exposure from diagnostic X-rays is roughly equal to the global average exposure from inhalation of radon—and the actual balance between these two sources of exposure depends on local geology, construction techniques, and health care. UNSCEAR estimated a very low global average annual exposure to ionizing radiation from nuclear weapons

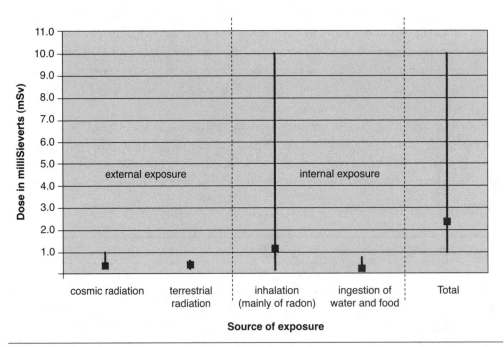

FIGURE 4.15 Estimated worldwide annual doses of ionizing radiation from natural sources (global average and typical range). *Data from*: United Nations Scientific Committee on the Effects of Atomic Radiation (UNSCEAR). *UNSCEAR 2000 Report to the General Assembly, with Scientific Annexes: United Nations*; 2000: table 1. Available at: http://www.unscear.org/unscear/en/publications/2000_1.html. Accessed October 19, 2006.

fallout (5 μS) in the late 1990s, after decades without aboveground nuclear weapons testing by the major powers.*

For certain anthropogenic exposures, global or even national averages are not useful. People who live near a nuclear power plant have somewhat elevated radiation exposures, as do those who work in nuclear power plants. Those who work in uranium mines or mills can have significant occupational exposures. And of course, for those who are in the wrong place at the wrong time, exposures from a nuclear plant accident (or a nuclear weapon) would overwhelm all other exposures and would fall outside the typical range of natural exposures shown in Figure 4.15.

Biological Effects of Ionizing Radiation

As noted earlier, all the products of radioactive decay—alpha, beta, and gamma radiation—are forms of ionizing radiation. That is, they have the capacity to create charged ions, which are biologically active, by knocking electrons out of orbit. Because much of the human body is water, ionizing radiation often strikes water in tissues, creating ions that react with cellular compounds, including DNA.

Scientists distinguish between high-level and low-level exposures to ionizing radiation. A high-level exposure is defined as a whole-body dose of 1 Sv or greater, occurring within minutes or hours. High-level exposures occur mainly in industrial accidents, including nuclear power plant accidents, or with exposure to nuclear weapons blasts.

High-level exposure to ionizing radiation causes three well-known syndromes, all caused by the death of cells, which together are known as **radiation sickness**. Cell death in the central nervous system (the brain and spinal cord) leads to stupor and loss of coordination. Cells that are forming and dividing rapidly are particularly susceptible to the effects of ionizing radiation. In the gastrointestinal tract, cells die and are sloughed off, resulting in massive destruction of the gut. And the bone marrow stops producing blood cells, leading to hemorrhage, anemia, and decreased resistance to infection. High-level exposure to ionizing radiation is frequently fatal. A dose of about 3–5 Gy is fatal to 50% of exposed adults within 60 days; a dose of about 10 Gy is 100% fatal.[73]

Chronic low-level exposure to ionizing radiation, rather than causing cells to die, causes damage to their DNA. In adults and children—including unborn children—this damage results in an increased risk of later developing cancer via mechanisms described in Chapter 2. The fetus and young child are most susceptible to ionizing radiation because more cell division and tissue differentiation are occurring in their bodies. Like other cancer risks, the risk of cancer from ionizing radiation is understood to have no threshold—that is, any dose greater than zero carries some risk. People who survive a high-level exposure to ionizing radiation are also subject to increased cancer risk afterward.

---

*The 1963 Limited Test Ban Treaty permitted underground testing but disallowed testing in the atmosphere or outer space or underwater. The 1996 Comprehensive Test Ban Treaty banned all nuclear weapons testing. These agreements were signed by the United States and other major nuclear powers; a small number of tests have been conducted since 1996 by other countries.

Intensive study of survivors of the 1945 atomic bomb blasts at Hiroshima and Nagasaki has yielded much of what we know about the risks of ionizing radiation. This large group (originally about 120,000) included both males and females of all ages, with acute whole-body exposure at various distances from the blasts. Analyses of this group have documented statistically significant associations between exposure to ionizing radiation and risk of leukemia; cancers of the breast, thyroid, ovary, bladder, lung, colon, liver, and stomach; and nonmelanoma skin cancer.[74] Because ionizing radiation's effect has no threshold, lower-level exposures also carry some risk of these cancers, although it becomes more difficult to discern a statistical association at lower doses.

Low-level exposure to ionizing radiation in utero has effects in addition to the later risk of cancer.[73] Very early in pregnancy, even low exposure can cause a failure of the embryo to implant in the uterine wall. Exposure after week 2 can cause miscarriage or, if it occurs in the third trimester, neonatal death. In addition, exposure to ionizing radiation in weeks 2 through 25 can result in major malformations or growth retardation, and exposures in weeks 8 through 25 can result in reduction of IQ, with the potential for severe mental retardation. In general, the fetus is more sensitive to exposures that occur earlier in these vulnerable periods.

Radiation Exposures and Health Effects of the Nuclear Fuel Cycle

People have exposures to ionizing radiation throughout the nuclear fuel cycle. At the front end, miners and mill workers are exposed to the natural decay products of uranium. Nuclear power plants release products of nuclear fission—at low levels as routine emissions, and at much higher levels in the event of an accident. At the back end of the nuclear fuel cycle, failures and accidents—during transportation or storage of wastes—could result in exposures to radiation from the decay of wastes containing unfissioned uranium, fission products, and transuranic elements.

The Front End

Uranium miners' and mill workers' exposures to radon and radon progeny carry a risk of cancer—in particular, excess lung cancer has been well documented among uranium miners. Studies in uranium miners and other populations also indicate a synergistic effect between radon exposure and cigarette smoking in increasing lung cancer risk.[75]

In the early decades of the industry, radon exposure was unregulated, and exposures were much higher than is allowed today. In a bleak chapter in the history of public health in the United States, early uranium miners in the Southwest during the 1940s and 1950s, many of whom were either Navajo or Hispanic, worked without ventilation or protective gear. At the time, uranium mining was known to carry a high risk of lung cancer, though the specifics of radon and radon progeny had not yet been elucidated. Later research, focusing on miners active between 1956 and the early 1990s, found that the lung cancer risk of miners with the highest radon exposure was 29 times that of miners in the least exposed group.[76] Further, in a somewhat later cohort of Navajo miners, who smoked little, nearly three quarters of lung cancer cases were attributable to their occupational exposure to radon.[77] These extraordinary risks reflect the miners' very high radon exposures compared to those of the general population. Uranium miners, like coal miners, are also exposed to silica dust and risk of physical injury.

Accidents at Nuclear Power Plants

In nuclear power plant accidents, the profile of radionuclides released varies somewhat, but typically features the fission products iodine-131 (half-life about 8 days) and strontium-90 and cesium-137 (both with half-lives of about 30 years). All three elements emit beta radiation and thus pose both an internal and external radiation hazard. Emissions from a nuclear power plant accident can also include plutonium-238 (an alpha emitter) and other transuranic elements that are by-products of nuclear fission.

When iodine-131, strontium-90, and cesium-137 are released into the environment, people are exposed mostly through ingestion of water and food. Radioactive iodine and strontium, for example, can accumulate on leafy vegetables that people eat; and when cows eat contaminated grass, iodine-131 appears in their milk. In addition, iodine-131 in gaseous form is inhaled. Precipitation brings contaminated airborne dust to earth, increasing exposures through water and food.

In the body, iodine-131 is taken up by the thyroid gland, causing thyroid cancer. In fact, iodine-131 is concentrated by the thyroid gland, such that the radiation dose to the thyroid may be more than 1000 times the average dose to the whole body.[78] (Preexisting iodine deficiency increases the uptake of radioactive iodine, and therefore iodine pills taken when an accident occurs can reduce this uptake.) Strontium-90 displaces calcium and is deposited in bone, irradiating the marrow and causing leukemia. Exposure to other radioactive isotopes produced by a nuclear accident carries an increased risk of solid tumors other than thyroid cancer.

By far the most serious accident at a civilian nuclear power plant to date occurred at the Chernobyl plant in Ukraine in 1986. The challenges of doing epidemiologic research on cancer related to the Chernobyl accident are substantial. They include patchy data on exposure in the first months and years after the accident and, more broadly, social disorganization in the wake of this devastating event. Populations were dislocated and medical care was disrupted, as were food supplies and many basic social services. These factors make it harder to conduct all types of epidemiologic study. There is also, of course, increased concern about radiation-related health effects since the accident, reflected in many changes in medical care. These changes are likely to result in more complete reporting of cases than before the accident, a source of bias in surveillance studies. In addition, most solid tumors have long latencies, so it is not surprising that it has been difficult to document associations in individual-level studies during the first 20 years after the accident, when many incipient cases are yet to be diagnosed.

Since the 1986 Chernobyl accident, a dose-related increase in thyroid cancer has been clearly documented, with young children most affected.[74,79] This is not a surprising outcome. Children are more sensitive to the effects of ionizing radiation on the thyroid than are adults,[78] and they also tend to be more highly exposed to iodine-131 because they drink more milk. There is also some evidence of an increased incidence of childhood leukemia post-Chernobyl,[80] though research results have been mixed. Exposure data for the 1979 accident at the Three Mile Island plant in Pennsylvania are patchy, as is epidemiologic evidence of increased cancer risk in the exposed population.

Overall, mechanistic data leave little doubt that ionizing radiation, however low the dose, poses a risk of cancer. The real questions are what can be discerned through epidemiology, and how to weigh the benefits of nuclear power against its hard-to-measure health impacts.

The Back End

In the absence of a permanent storage site for spent reactor fuel, it is stored at reactor sites around the country. Both cooling pools and dry casks are constructed to prevent the escape of ionizing radiation, but they are not designed to last for the radioactive lifetime of the wastes. Further, the power plant sites are not isolated from the public, and in fact many are located in heavily populated areas.

If a permanent repository is built to hold spent fuel from nuclear reactors, the most likely environmental impact over the long term is groundwater contamination, especially in the event of a geologic disturbance such as an earthquake. At the chosen location, this is unlikely in the short term but possible over the very long life of such a facility. In the nearer future, the clearest risk to the public is the potential for accidents in transporting spent fuel to the storage facility.

Trade-offs in Health Risks: Nuclear Power versus Fossil Fuels

Unlike coal- and oil-fired power plants, nuclear power plants do not contribute to conventional air pollution—that is, particulates and pollutant gases. They also do not contribute to acid rain or to the slow-moving catastrophe that is global warming. On the other hand, accidents at coal- and oil-fired plants do not carry the disastrous off-site consequences of an accident at a nuclear power plant, and fossil fuels do not leave long-lasting radioactive wastes. Both coal miners and uranium miners bear a grim burden of mortality and morbidity, not only from exposure to coal dust or radiation, but from inhalation of silica dust and from physical injuries in their dangerous work environments.

Regulation of Activities in the Nuclear Fuel Cycle

As described earlier, the Atomic Energy Commission (AEC) had mixed military and civilian roles in the years following World War II: It was responsible for developing both nuclear weapons and nuclear power. Even within the realm of civilian nuclear power, the AEC had two faces, in that it was responsible for both promoting and regulating the nascent nuclear power industry. This conflict of interest was resolved by the Energy Reorganization Act of 1974, which dissolved the AEC and created a new agency, the Nuclear Regulatory Commission (NRC), responsible only for the safety of nuclear power plants.

Under this broad mandate, the agency licenses nuclear power reactors, controlling both site permits and operating licenses, and sets emissions limits for radionuclides under normal plant operations. It oversees routine operations; plant operators are required to monitor and report on radioactive emissions. The NRC also responds to incidents or accidents at nuclear power plants and regulates the storage of spent fuel at reactor sites around the country. Finally, the NRC is responsible for preventing the theft or diversion of nuclear materials.

As described previously, a national nuclear waste repository is planned for a site at Yucca Mountain in Nevada. The Nuclear Waste Policy Act of 1982 mandated that a national repository be established and was amended 5 years later to designate Yucca Mountain as the only candidate site. If work on Yucca Mountain moves forward, four federal agencies will be involved: The Department of Energy is to design, construct, and operate the facility; the Environmental Protection Agency is to develop environmental standards; the Nuclear Regulatory Commission is to license the repository and develop regulations to implement the EPA's standards; and the Department of Transportation will be responsible for the cross-country transportation of radioactive wastes to the repository.[81] The Nuclear Regulatory Commission is also responsible for implementing the Low-Level Radioactive Waste Policy Amendments Act of 1985, described earlier, which calls for states to form compacts for the management of these wastes.

Under a 1978 set of amendments to the Atomic Energy Act, named the Uranium Mill Tailings Radiation Control Act, the EPA sets standards for the management of abandoned mill tailings sites by the Department of Energy. Active tailings sites are licensed by the Nuclear Regulatory Commission.

Key elements of the regulatory framework for the nuclear fuel cycle appear in **Table 4.11**. This table is the third in a series of similar tables that place regulatory provisions within the traditional regulatory domains of environmental health.

4.3 Alternatives to Fossil and Nuclear Fuels

In considering alternatives to fossil and nuclear fuels, it is useful to begin by asking where our energy currently comes from and how we use it. In 2005, about 85% of the energy used in the United States (measured in BTUs)* was derived from fossil sources (oil, natural gas, or coal); the remainder was roughly split between nuclear power and renewable sources.[82] US energy consumption in 2005 by the four major end use sectors is shown in **Figure 4.16**, with the uses of electric power broken out at the right. Like energy production, consumption is typically measured in BTUs—but because most energy originates from carbon-dioxide-emitting fossil fuels, the breakdown would be similar if it were assessed in terms of CO_2 emissions. Thus, Figure 4.16 gives a good picture of the climate impacts of our various activities.

Our current degree of dependence on fossil fuels is not sustainable—that is, it cannot be maintained over the long future that we would like to imagine for the human race. Instead, we will use up reserves of coal, oil, and natural gas within a few generations, and the ecological

---

*British thermal units (BTUs) are used to describe the energy content of fuels.

Table 4.11   Overview of US Regulatory Framework for Environmental Health Hazards (3)

Environmental Health Domain	Major Laws and Key Provisions for the Control of Environmental Health Hazards
Biological hazards	Public Health Service Act (PHSA)—development of guidelines for vaccination; use of quarantine or isolation to prevent entry of infectious diseases into the United States; conduct of surveillance and investigation of outbreaks
Air pollution	Clean Air Act (CAA)—ambient standards (NAAQS) for Criteria Air Pollutants; emissions standards for Hazardous Air Pollutants, including mercury; emission allowances for SO_2 (to control acid deposition); removal of lead from gasoline; requirement to sell reformulated gasoline in high-smog areas
Ionizing radiation	*Energy Reorganization Act (ERA)—safety requirements for operating nuclear power plants, including licensing, emissions limits, storage of wastes* *Nuclear Waste Policy Act (NWPA)—requirements to build and regulate a repository for radioactive wastes, including spent reactor fuel* *Uranium Mill Tailings Radiation Control Act —standards for management of abandoned mill tailings*
Alternative energy sources	
Hazardous wastes	
Occupational health	
Industrial water pollution	
Toxic chemicals	
Pesticides	
Food supply	
Sewage wastes and community water supply	
Municipal solid waste	
Consumer products	
Environmental noise	

Note: New information appears in italics.

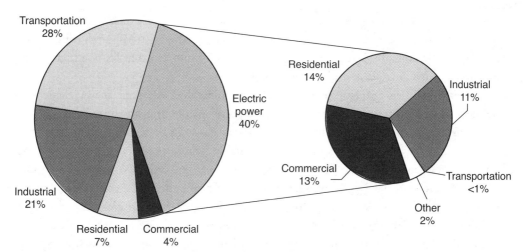

FIGURE 4.16   Energy consumption, by end use, in the United States, 2005. *Data from*: US Energy Information Administration. *Annual Energy Review 2005*, 2006: tables 2.1a and 8.9. Available at: http://www.eia.doe.gov/emeu/aer/. Accessed November 25, 2006.

impacts, including the effects of global climate change, will far outlive these resources. A reliance on nuclear fuels, on the other hand, might be considered sustainable *if* we assume that new technologies will be developed to safely make use of a variety of nuclear resources. Whether nuclear technologies, given their complexity and cost, will be accessible to lower-income countries is another question—and uranium deposits, like fossil fuel resources, are unevenly distributed around the world. Clearly, the energy path taken by the industrialized countries in the 19th and 20th centuries—a path that depends principally on fossil fuels—will not be open to many lower-income countries striving to gain the benefits of modern development in the 21st century.

Some energy sources are not just sustainable, but **renewable**; that is, the energy source is either continually renewed in nature (for example, wind or water) or can readily be renewed through human effort (for example, by planting trees to replace those burned as fuel). The major renewable energy sources are wind power, water power (*hydropower*), underground heat sources (*geothermal energy*), solar energy, and trees and other plant fuels (collectively called *biomass fuels*).

Many renewable energy technologies, unlike today's major energy sources, lend themselves to a decentralized energy sector, although they can also be incorporated into centralized systems. In the industrialized nations, the infrastructure for producing and distributing energy forms a complex interconnected system. Reserves of the major fossil fuels—coal, oil, and gas—are concentrated geographically, and large quantities must be moved to locations where power is to be generated. The transport of coal takes advantage of ordinary railroad lines, but oil and gas must be moved via dedicated pipelines, terminals, and tankers. Nuclear materials must also be transported and processed, and though the quantities involved are much smaller, the safety and security issues are pressing. As noted earlier, electricity is a highly transportable form of energy. Precisely because of this feature, electric plants are tied into an extensive power grid of interconnected generating plants and transmission lines.

Such large-scale energy systems are inherently vulnerable. All their major elements—pipelines, oil and gas terminals, tankers, electric power plants, transmission lines—are susceptible to disruption. The centralized power system has long been criticized as inherently "brittle."[83] That is, the system is designed to reliably handle predictable problems rather than to be resilient in the face of the unexpected. Even an ordinary event—a lightning strike, an everyday mistake, or a software failure—can ripple through a complex and brittle system in unexpected ways. In 2003, for example, some trees that had grown up in a right-of-way came into contact with electrical power lines in Ohio. The result was a cascading blackout that left 50 million people in the eastern United States and Canada without power for up to 3 days.[84]

In contrast to fossil fuels and nuclear power, renewable energy technologies use resources that are local and widely available—though not available evenly across all locations. Both power production and environmental impacts are more dispersed, and this makes it somewhat easier to achieve an equitable sharing of benefits and burdens. With coordination and some redundancy at the local and regional scale, such technologies can form flexible and resilient power networks.

This discussion of alternatives to fossil and nuclear fuels begins by considering ways to use less energy—in a sense, the most fundamental alternative to energy from any source. It then considers the major alternatives to nuclear fuels and familiar fossil fuels (listed in **Table 4.12**):

- Renewable energy options that harness the energy of the sun or earth without the use of fuels
- Alternative fuels derived from plant matter (biomass)
- New fuels derived from fossil sources
- The hydrogen fuel cell, an emerging energy technology that today relies on fossil sources but that in the future might draw on renewable sources

This discussion is much briefer than the descriptions of fossil fuels and nuclear power, reflecting the general lack of human health hazards from these more benign technologies. The section concludes with a description of US regulatory supports for alternatives to fossil and nuclear fuels.

Energy Conservation and Efficiency

Many aspects of the middle-class American lifestyle are extravagant in terms of energy consumption, even if they fit within individual budgets. **Energy conservation**—simply reducing the amount of energy we consume—and **energy efficiency**—getting more out of the energy we do consume—are twin strategies for reducing vulnerability to potential shortages and to the cost increases that will certainly occur in the future. In homes and offices, for example, we can

Table 4.12 Major Alternatives to Nuclear Fuels and Traditional Fossil Fuels

| Technology | Energy Source | |
	Renewable	Nonrenewable
Nonfuel technologies	Wind power Hydropower Solar energy Geothermal energy	

Alternative fuels	Biomass:
	  wood and brush
	  crop residues
	  dung
	Biomass fuels:
	  biogas
	  ethanol
	  biodiesel	

Nontraditional fossil fuels		Compressed natural gas (methane) Liquefied natural gas (methane) Liquefied petroleum gas (propane) Methanol (derived from fossil fuel)
New energy conversion technologies	Potential hydrogen fuel cell of the future (hydrogen obtained from water and using energy from renewable source)	Hydrogen fuel cell of today (hydrogen from hydrocarbon fuels)

conserve energy by setting our thermostats lower in the winter and higher in the summer, and turning off lights and computers when they aren't being used.

To increase energy efficiency, buildings should be well insulated, and windows in older buildings should be replaced with modern windows that dramatically reduce energy losses. Mechanical systems—heat, air conditioning, hot water—should be efficient and well maintained. Energy-efficient devices—from appliances to electronics to light bulbs—are now available and can replace inefficient devices as they wear out. All these things require an initial outlay of money, of course, and older buildings will be upgraded only over a period of years. On its website, the US EPA provides extensive information about energy conservation, and the agency gives an "Energy Star" rating of the energy efficiency of many appliances and windows.

According to the EPA, the typical US household can save up to 30% of its annual energy bill by investing in Energy Star appliances and products such as compact fluorescent light bulbs, which use about 70% less energy than traditional bulbs and last up to 10 times longer. Unfortunately, each bulb contains about 5 mg of elemental mercury;[85] if the bulb breaks, mercury is released in a powdery residue. Thus these energy-efficient bulbs pose a hazard (and a cleanup challenge) if broken accidentaly; moreover, they should not be discarded as ordinary trash.[85]

The potential gains from both energy conservation and increased energy efficiency are particularly apparent in the transportation sector. For example, the sprawling pattern of urban and suburban development that is common in US cities, along with limited mass transit (or a complete lack of mass transit) in many urban areas, contributes to our dependence on cars. Research has shown that about 25% of all trips in the United States are under 1 mile, yet 75% of those short trips are made by car.[86]

In 2003, Americans logged 2.5 trillion vehicle-miles, and 4 trillion passenger-miles, in light vehicles—that is, cars, station wagons, sport utility vehicles (SUVs), vans, and pickup trucks.[87] This averages out to more than 10,000 miles for every man, woman, and child and is about 130 times the total passenger-miles by rail, including intercity rail (Amtrak), commuter rail, and rail transit systems in urban areas. These figures also indicate that the average number of people traveling in a car is less than two—in other words, many trips are made solo.

The fundamental inefficiency of our reliance on cars is exacerbated by the low fuel economy of the US fleet of light vehicles. The lure of the large vehicle remains strong. As shown in **Figure 4.17**, over the last 30 years—a period during which the United States' decreasing energy security has been widely publicized—the share of the US light vehicle market held by SUVs has increased steadily, and even within this class there has been a shift to larger vehicles.[87] Meanwhile, the market share held by cars has steadily declined, and within this class too, there has been a shift to larger models.

After a modest improvement in the average fuel economy of new light vehicles in the late 1970s and early 1980s, fuel economy has barely held steady: Overall average fuel economy for

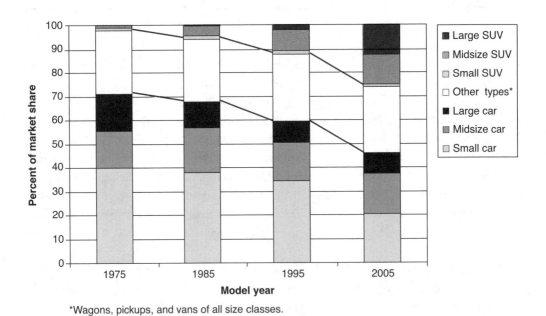

FIGURE 4.17 Market shares of light vehicles in the United States, by size class and model year, 1975–2005. *Data from*: US Department of Energy, Oak Ridge National Library. *Transportation Energy Data Book: Edition 25*, 2006: table 4.9. Available at: http://cta.ornl.gov/data/download25.shtml. Accessed August 22, 2007.

US light vehicles was 22.1 miles per gallon for the 1987 model year, and 21.0 miles per gallon for the 2006 model year. Over the same period, average horsepower in the US light vehicle fleet nearly doubled, from 118 to 219.[88] In contrast, in European countries much smaller and more fuel-efficient cars have been widely accepted.

Although the US buying public has generally resisted such fuel-efficient compact and sub-compact cars, it is beginning to embrace hybrid technologies. The **hybrid car** makes use of both a gasoline-powered combustion engine and electric power. The hybrid is an attempt to find a marketable balance between the electric car's high energy efficiency and zero emissions (but short range because of the limitations of relying on a battery) and the combustion engine's greater power and range.

In some hybrids, the two systems operate in parallel; in other configurations, the technologies are integrated. For example, in a flexible hybrid configuration like that shown in **Figure 4.18**), the source of energy to the transmission varies as needed to optimize performance; it may come from any of the following sources:

- The combustion engine directly, as in a traditional car
- An electric motor (*a*) being powered by the combustion engine via a generator (*b*)
- An electric motor (*a*) powered by an electric battery (*c*) that was previously charged by the generator (*b*) powered by the combustion engine

Plug-in hybrid cars are also coming into use: The car can be plugged into an electric outlet to recharge the battery—for example, overnight.

Freedom from Fuels

Wind power, hydropower, solar energy, and geothermal energy are renewable sources of energy that are freely available in nature (Table 4.12). For the most part, these technologies capture some available energy as it passes by, in contrast to technologies that extract energy from fuel. Of course, building and maintaining renewable energy facilities require inputs of materials and energy. But otherwise, these technologies do not rely on a supply of fuel.

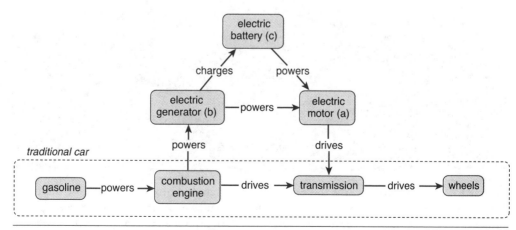

FIGURE 4.18 Schematic configuration of a hybrid car.

Wind power captures the energy of moving air. When wind strikes the blades of a wind turbine (the modern version of a windmill), it causes the shaft of the turbine to turn, converting the wind's kinetic energy into mechanical energy. The shaft is connected to a generator, which converts the mechanical energy into electrical energy.

Traditionally, the mechanical energy was not converted to electricity but was put to use directly. For example, before rural areas in the great plains of the United States had electric power, many farms and ranches had windmills that pumped groundwater up to the ground surface (**Figure 4.19**). Wind power can still be used on a micro scale to provide either mechanical energy or electricity.

However, wind turbines are now often installed in rows (as shown on the cover of this textbook) or rectangular grids; such groupings are called **wind farms**, and contribute electricity to a power grid. Modern wind turbines can be hundreds of feet tall, and are streamlined in shape and usually white in color (see **Figure 4.20**). Wind turbines cause zero environmental pollution, in the usual sense of the term. But they do make noise. At a distance of 1000 feet the sound of a wind farm is sometimes compared to that of a home refrigerator, or of a car on a highway some distance away. Given that wind farms are sited in windy locations, the "whooshing" sound of the whirling blades is sometimes masked by the sound of wind in trees and around buildings. Though some people find the sound of a wind farm irritating, others find it soothing.

A wind farm occupies a sizeable area, either on land or offshore. Wind turbines are thus prominent features of a local landscape; in fact, if they are located on land, they are often sited

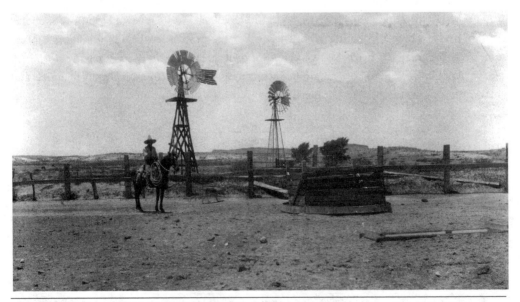

FIGURE 4.19 Windmills like the ones in this undated photo from Presidio County, Texas, are typical of traditional 19th- and 20th-century construction. *Source*: Reprinted courtesy of US Geological Survey; ID# 2247. Undated photo by G.K. Gilbert. Available at: http://libraryphoto.cr.usgs.gov/. Accessed September 13, 2007.

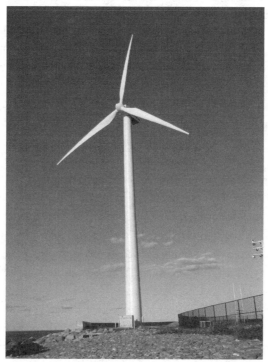

FIGURE 4.20 This modern wind turbine is one of two now generating electricity for the coastal town of Hull, Massachusetts.

on ridges to capture wind energy most efficiently. Again, reactions are mixed: Some people feel that wind turbines cause "visual pollution"; others find their simple functionality elegant and visually pleasing.

Unlike people, birds in flight appear to have difficulty seeing wind turbines. This is because, although modern turbines rotate slowly, the blades are long and therefore the tips move at up to 150 miles per hour, making them difficult to see.[89] As a result, birds sometimes fly directly into the blades and are killed. Designers are working to minimize this hazard—for example, testing the visibility of patterned blades[89]—but it seems likely that wind turbines will always pose some risk to birds.

On the other hand, the general perception of this risk is exaggerated—early reports of the problem came from a site with unusual turbines and large populations of birds of prey, such as hawks and eagles. The National Wind Coordinating Committee (a collaborative that includes representatives from electric utilities, wind developers, environmental organizations, and others) has estimated that 10,000 to 40,000 birds are killed in the United States each year by wind turbines, compared to 50 million to 80 million killed by vehicles, and some 100 million (if not many more) that fly into buildings or windows.[90] Most of the birds killed by wind turbines are the most common species, including house sparrows, European starlings, and pigeons.[90] Further, wind power is not unique in posing a risk to birds—oil pollution kills some birds every year, but public attention focuses on the problem only when there is a major spill such as the 1989 grounding of the oil tanker *Exxon Valdez* in Alaska. In 2006, the Massachusetts Audubon Society supported a wind farm proposed for Nantucket Sound off the state's shoreline, noting that the potential harm to birds was outweighed by the ecological benefits of using a renewable energy source.[91]

Like wind power, **hydropower** can be used on a micro scale—for example, a water wheel can power a small mill that grinds grain into flour or a turbine that generates electricity. Small hydro plants are usually "run-of-river" operations—that is, they operate either with no dam at all or with a small diversion that holds perhaps a day's backup supply of water.

Unlike a small hydro plant, a large hydroelectric plant relies on a strong, predictable, and even adjustable flow of water. This is achieved by storing a large volume of water behind a dam (see **Figure 4.21**), and then releasing it at a rate that supports the generation of power as it is needed.* Thus, large-scale hydropower, though it meets the definition of a renewable, alternative energy option, does more than simply capture some of the freely available energy of a watercourse as it passes by. A large hydro plant, like a coal-fired power plant, is tied into a centralized power grid.

Like a small hydropower facility, a large hydropower plant produces no emissions; but even so, it can take a heavy environmental and social toll. For example, China has recently completed construction of the massive Three Gorges Dam on the Yangtze River; by 2009, the reservoir will be full and the dam's turbines will be operational. The dam will provide electrical power for millions, mostly in China's cities, and it will help to control flooding and manage irrigation; locks will allow ships to reach locations that were previously inaccessible. But the reservoir will flood more than 1000 towns and villages (along with several archaeological sites) and displace more than a million people, many of them farmers being moved to urban areas. Downstream farmers are concerned that lands below the dam will no longer receive the rich silt left by flooding, while engineers are concerned about the accumulation of silt behind the dam. Finally, there have been charges of corruption and shoddy construction of the dam, which is located in a seismically active region, raising the specter of a catastrophic failure—which, given the size of this dam, would bring a public health disaster.

Ultimately, both water power and wind power derive from the sun—solar energy causes snowmelt and also evaporation of water, feeding the rainfall that fills rivers and streams; and differences in the solar heating of air masses cause the movements that we call wind. But the sun's energy can also be harnessed directly. Oddly enough, using **solar power** directly is more challenging. For one thing, sunlight is intermittent and variable—it is available only during the day, the number of daylight hours varies with location and season, and the sun is sometimes obscured by clouds. In addition, unlike a rushing river or a stiff wind, sunlight is a diffuse, low-intensity energy source.

---

*It is also possible, in certain locations, to capture energy from tidal movements near coastlines or in estuaries.

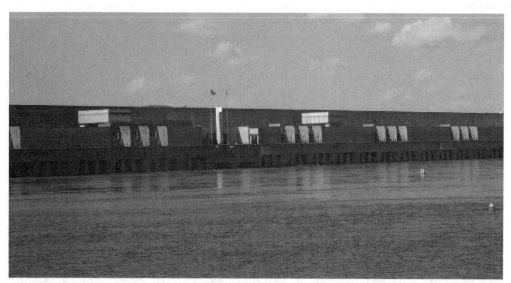

FIGURE 4.21 The water stored behind this dam will be used to generate electric power.

For this reason, a relatively large area is needed to collect enough solar energy to be useful. For small-scale heating of domestic water or indoor space, flat solar collection panels (usually installed on the roof) can be used to absorb the sun's radiation and heat a fluid, which then circulates through a heating system. Such systems are widespread on rooftops in Israel, for example.[92] On a large scale, an array of solar collectors can be used to gather and concentrate the sun's energy, and then generate electricity by heating water (or another fluid), creating steam that drives a turbine. However, such a large-scale approach is feasible only in high-sunlight locations.

Finally, the **photovoltaic cell** (also called a **solar cell**) is a device that converts sunlight directly into electrical energy. Photovoltaic cells capture only a small percentage of the solar energy that falls on them, but they can be combined in modular fashion to form arrays of any size. To date, the practical challenges of solar energy, along with the economics of the energy market, have not favored large-scale adoption of solar technologies in the industrialized countries.

Geothermal energy is the earth's internal heat energy—emerging in the form of hot water and steam at geysers or steam vents. Hot water and steam can be carried in pipes and circulated through buildings to heat interior spaces. This heat source can be used only where local geology makes it possible—in Iceland, Japan, and New Zealand, for example—and the steam or water is usually transported over short distances. Less commonly, steam from a geothermal source is used to drive a turbine that generates electricity.

Alternative Fuels

Biomass energy is simply energy stored in plant material or animal dung (**biomass**). It originates as the energy in sunlight; through photosynthesis, this energy is stored in plants. If plant material such as wood or crop residues is burned, this energy is released. Biomass fuels produce a small quantity of energy for the quantity of fuel burned, compared to, for example, natural gas. On a larger scale, plant materials can be burned to produce steam, which in turn is used to generate electricity via a turbine. In the United States, this occurs mostly at pulp and paper mills because they both produce large quantities of wood waste and need power for industrial processes.[93]

Using various complex technologies, vehicle fuels can be derived from biomass (or mixes including organic wastes from municipal waste streams). Such **biomass fuels** can be gaseous (for example, *biogas*, which is about 60% methane) or liquid. Biogas can be burned directly in some industrial processes, but if it is to be used as natural gas it must be purified, and if the natural gas is to be used as a fuel for vehicles, it must be compressed to make a liquid fuel. *Ethanol* (an alcohol fuel) is a liquid, as is *biodiesel* fuel. Biodiesel fuel, made from animal fats and vegetable oils (including used cooking oil from restaurants), burns more cleanly than diesel fuel does. Mixed with standard diesel fuel, it can be used in most diesel engines. The key advantage of such biomass-derived fuels over fossil fuels is that they are "carbon-neutral." That is, the carbon released as carbon dioxide from the combustion of biomass fuels was captured from the atmosphere by plants through photosynthesis only a short time before, much as in the carbon cycle shown in Figure 4.4.

All biomass fuels face a fundamental limitation as an energy option. If these fuels are to be produced on a large scale, then fuel crops—such as sugar cane or corn—will need to be grown on a large scale as raw material. Any plan for such "energy plantations" would require vast tracts of land, as well as enormous quantities of water. Indeed, at a global scale, such a strategy would require that very large areas of land now used for food crops be converted to energy crops.[93] The US Department of Agriculture reports that the production of ethanol is already claiming an increasing share of the US corn crop, and that this shift will probably reduce the share that is exported to other countries as food.[94]

Finally, though biomass fuels are considered alternative fuels from the perspective of the world's dependence on fossil fuels, this does not mean that they are benign as fuels. Perhaps half the world's population, mostly in rural areas of lower-income countries, uses biomass fuels for heating and cooking. The fuels used in this way include wood, charcoal, peat, straw, brush, and the dung of cattle or other herbivores—all fuels that are much less expensive than oil or gas (or electricity), commonly used in industrialized countries.[95] These biomass fuels are typically burned in simple stoves or open fires indoors, resulting in high concentrations of particulates and irritant gases in indoor air. For example, researchers have reported 24-hour average particulate concentrations (PM_{10}) of 200 to 5000 μg/m^3 indoors, and as high as 50,000 μg/m^3 near stoves.[96] Research has also documented higher exposures for girls and women because they spend more time near the fire as they engage in cooking.[97] Such exposures contribute to the global mortality burden from acute respiratory infections in young children, and maternal exposure has also been linked to low birthweight.[98,99]

Nontraditional Fossil Fuels

Some nontraditional fossil fuels are blends of fossil fuel and a biomass fuel—for example, mixed diesel and ethanol or mixed gasoline and ethanol. Other nontraditional fuels for vehicles are de-

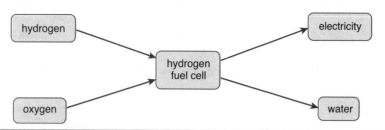

FIGURE 4.22 A conceptual model of a hydrogen fuel cell.

rived from fossil fuels: compressed natural gas and liquefied natural gas (both methane), liquefied petroleum gas (propane), and the alcohol fuel methanol, derived from coal or natural gas.
These alternatives to gasoline and diesel produce less pollution—but also less energy—per gallon consumed. Although some alternative fuels, from fossil or biomass sources, have found a
niche in the energy market, it has proved challenging to integrate them into a marketplace
dominated by familiar fuels and products designed to use them.

The Hydrogen Fuel Cell

Finally, the **hydrogen fuel cell** (see Table 4.12 and **Figure 4.22**) relies on a simple chemical reaction in which hydrogen (provided as fuel) and oxygen (from the atmosphere) are combined to
produce electricity (a flow of electrons) and, as a by-product, water. Thus, the fuel cell technology
itself is environmentally benign. The key questions are: Where does the hydrogen fuel come
from? And how much energy does it take to produce the hydrogen fuel?

Although the concept of the hydrogen fuel cell is simple, obtaining hydrogen fuel is not. In
particular, although we are surrounded by hydrogen, it is not present as hydrogen gas but
rather in chemical compounds, many of which are fossil fuels (hydrocarbon fuels). Today, hydrogen for fuel cells is derived mostly by stripping hydrogen atoms from natural gas, whose
production, like that of all fossil fuels, creates pollution. In the future, it may become practical
to obtain hydrogen from water, which would produce no pollution. But the timeline for developing such technology is unclear. At a more mundane level, the use of hydrogen fuel cells
raises difficult engineering challenges: The hydrogen gas must either be greatly compressed or
else deep-chilled to a liquid form; and an entire infrastructure of storage facilities, distribution
tankers, and fueling stations will be required.

Finally, whatever the source of the hydrogen, the energy required to produce the hydrogen
fuel is greater than the energy that is obtained when the fuel cell is put to use. Thus, the hydrogen fuel cell makes sense only if the energy used to produce the hydrogen comes from a source
that we can use freely—that is, a source, such as water power, that is continually renewed in nature. Iceland has begun to use geothermal energy to produce hydrogen for fuel cells that power
buses, as the first step toward large-scale use of this technology.[100]

Regulatory Support for Alternatives to Fossil and Nuclear Fuels

The Energy Policy Act of 2005 (EPAct), enacted as a comprehensive update of US energy
strategy, includes some supports for alternative energy sources. For example, it provides for tax

credits against the corporate income tax of energy producers that generate electricity from wind, biomass, solar power, geothermal energy, and tidal energy. It also requires the federal government to obtain 7.5% of its power from renewable sources by 2011, but this is not an ambitious goal and there is no parallel requirement for electric utilities to increase their use of alternative energy sources.

The law provides grants to state and local governments to buy hybrid vehicles and to help school districts reduce the diesel emissions of their school buses. It supports research on the use of hydrogen as a fuel. At the individual level, the act offers tax credits against the personal income tax of those who buy hybrid vehicles or cars that use alternative fuels. Tax credits are also available for certain home improvements that reduce energy consumption, such as insulation, replacement windows, and some solar heating systems.

The law also provides substantial support for traditional energy sectors, with the twin goals of expanding nuclear power and increasing domestic production of fossil fuels. These goals are in keeping with the current administration's generally supportive stance toward these energy sectors (see, for example, the report of Vice President Cheney's task force on national energy policy[101]).

Key elements of the regulatory framework for the US energy strategy appear in **Table 4.13**. This table is the fourth in a series of similar tables that place regulatory provisions within the traditional regulatory domains of environmental health.

Table 4.13 Overview of US Regulatory Framework for Environmental Health Hazards (4)

Environmental Health Domain	Major Laws and Key Provisions for the Control of Environmental Health Hazards
Biological hazards	Public Health Service Act (PHSA)—development of guidelines for vaccination; use of quarantine or isolation to prevent entry of infectious diseases into the United States; conduct of surveillance and investigation of outbreaks
Air pollution	Clean Air Act (CAA)—ambient standards (NAAQS) for Criteria Air Pollutants; emissions standards for Hazardous Air Pollutants, including mercury; emission allowances for SO_2 (to control acid deposition); removal of lead from gasoline; requirement to sell reformulated gasoline in high-smog areas
Ionizing radiation	Energy Reorganization Act (ERA)—safety requirements for operating nuclear power plants, including licensing, emissions limits, storage of wastes
	Nuclear Waste Policy Act (NWPA)—requirements to build and regulate a repository for radioactive wastes, including spent reactor fuel
	Uranium Mill Tailings Radiation Control Act—standards for management of abandoned mill tailings
Alternative energy sources	*Energy Policy Act (EPAct)—modest supports for alternative energy sources*
Hazardous wastes	
Occupational health	

Table 4.13   *(Continued)*

Environmental Health Domain	Major Laws and Key Provisions for the Control of Environmental Health Hazards
Industrial water pollution	
Toxic chemicals	
Pesticides	
Food supply	
Sewage wastes and community water supply	
Municipal solid waste	
Consumer products	
Environmental noise	

Note: New information appears in italics.

Study Questions

1. Explain how the use of fossil fuels results in human exposures to heavy metals, comparing the sources and impacts of methylmercury and lead.

2. One important lever in the effort to control global climate change is an overall reduction in emissions from the burning of fossil fuels. What do you think are fair and realistic expectations of the world's industrialized and lower-income countries in this effort?

3. Summarize the factors, related to both exposure and hazard, which combine to make naturally occurring radon a concern as a risk factor for lung cancer in uranium miners (or in the general population in some geologic regions).

4. Describe social disparities, past and present, in the burden of health risks from the nuclear fuel cycle in the United States.

5. Make an argument in favor of either a centralized disposal facility for high-level radioactive wastes or a decentralized approach to managing these wastes in the United States.

6. Gather some information on two or three hybrid sedans available in the United States. Calculate the approximate number of gallons of fuel you would save per year if you drove one of these hybrid cars rather than your own car—and then calculate the impact of driving 30% fewer miles per year under both scenarios. If you already own a hybrid, or if you don't own a car, do this exercise for a nonhybrid car owned by someone you know.

References

1. US Energy Information Administration. *Annual Energy Review 2005.* Available at: http://www.eia.doe.gov/emeu/aer/pecss_diagram.html. Accessed November 25, 2006.

2. Buckley GL. The environmental transformation of an Appalachian valley, 1850–1906. *Geograph Rev.* 1998;88(2):175–198.

3. US Energy Information Administration. *Coal Production in the United States: An Historical Overview, 2006.* Available at: http://www.eia.doe.gov/cneaf/coal/page/coal_production_review.pdf. Accessed June 3, 2008.

4. US Energy Information Administration. *Coal Transportation: Rates and Trends, 2004.* Available at: http://www.eia.doe.gov/cneaf/coal/page/trans/ratesntrends.html. Accessed January 25, 2007.

5. AFL-CIO. *Death on the Job: The Toll of Neglect.* Washington, DC; 2006. Available at: http://www.aflcio.org/issues/safety/memorial/doj_2007.cfm. Accessed April 14, 2008.

6. Stephan C. *Coal Dust Explosion Hazards, 1998.* Available at: http://www.msha.gov/S&HINFO/TECHRPT/P&T/COALDUST.pdf. Accessed April 10, 2008.

7. Haight J. Occupational health risks in crude oil and natural gas extraction. In: Cleveland C, ed. *Encyclopedia of Energy.* Elsevier; 2004:477–487.

8. Federal Energy Regulatory Commission, Office of Energy Projects. *Existing and Proposed North American LNG Terminals (map and list), 2006.* Available at: http://www.ferc.gov/industries/lng/indus-act/terminals/exist-prop-lng.pdf. Accessed February 18, 2007.

9. US Energy Information Administration. *Coal Reserves Information Sheet.* Available at: http://www.eia.doc.gov/neic/infosheets/coalreserves.htm. Accessed November 25, 2006.

10. US Energy Information Administration. *Basic Petroleum Statistics.* Available at: http://www.eia.doc.gov/neic/quickfacts/quickoil.htm. Accessed November 25, 2006.

11. US Energy Information Administration. *World Proved Reserves of Oil and Natural Gas, Most Recent Estimates.* Available at: http://www.eia.doc.gov/emeu/international/rserves.html. Accessed November 25, 2006.

12. Needleman H. Clamped in a straitjacket: the insertion of lead into gasoline. *Environ Research.* 1997;74:95–103.

13. United Nations Partnership Program. *Partnership Newsletter.* Available at: http://www.unep.org/pcfv. Accessed February 7, 2007.

14. Global Lead Advice and Support Service. *Countries Where Leaded Petrol Is Possibly Still Sold for Road Use.* Available at: http://www.lead.org.au/fs/fst27.html. Accessed February 7, 2008.

15. Witschi HR, Last JA. Toxic responses of the respiratory system. In: Klaassen CD, ed. *Casarett and Doull's Toxicology: The Basic Science of Poisons.* 5th ed. New York, NY: McGraw-Hill; 1996:443–460.

16. Trasande L, Thurston G. The role of air pollution in asthma and other pediatric morbidities. *J Allergy Clin Immunol.* 2005;115:689–699.

17. Vander A, Sherman J, Luciano D. *Human Physiology.* 6th ed. New York, NY: McGraw-Hill; 1994.

18. Nemmar A, Hoet PH, Vanquickenbourne B, Dinsdale D, Thomeer M, Hoylaerts MF, et al. Passage of inhaled particles into the blood circulation in humans. *Circulation.* 2002;105:411–414.

19. Olivieri D, Scoditti E. Impact of environmental factors on lung defences. *Eur Respir Rev.* 2005;14:51–56.

20. Costa DL, Amdur MO. Air pollution. In: Klaassen CD, ed. *Casarett and Doull's Toxicology: The Basic Science of Poisons.* 5th ed. New York, NY: McGraw-Hill; 1996:857–880.

21. Bernstein JA. Health effects of air pollution. *J Allergy Clin Immunol.* 2004;114(5): 1116–1123.

22. Chen-Yeung MNW. Air pollution and health. *Hong Kong Med J.* 2000;6(4):390–398.

23. Routledge H, Ayres J, Townend N. Why cardiologists should be interested in air pollution. *Heart.* 2003;89:1383–1388.

24. Vermylen J, Nemmar A, Nemery B, Hoylaerts MF. Ambient air pollution and acute myocardial infarction. *J Thrombosis Haemostasis.* 2005;3:1955–1961.

25. Delfino R, Sioutas C, Malik S. Potential role of ultrafine particles in associations between airborne particle mass and cardiovascular health. *Environ Health Perspect.* 2005;113(8):934–946.

26. Whittaker A. Killer smog of London, 50 years on: particle properties and oxidative capacity. *Science Tot Environ.* 2004;334–335:435–445.

27. Davis D, Bell M, Fletcher T. A look back at the London Smog of 1952 and the half century since. *Environ Health Perspect.* 2002;110(12):A734.

28. Heiger-Bernays W. Personal communication; 2006.

29. Brook R, Franklin B, Cascio W, Hong Y, Howard G, Lipsett M, et al. Air pollution and cardiovascular disease: a statement for healthcare professionals from the Expert Panel on Population and Prevention Science of the American Heart Association. *Circulation.* 2004;109:2655–2671.

30. Peden D. Influences on the development of allergy and asthma. *Toxicology.* 2002;181–182:323–328.

31. Sunyer J, Spix C, Quenel P, Ponce-de-Leon A, Ponka A, Barumandzadeh T, et al. Urban air pollution and emergency admissions for asthma in four European cities: the APHEA Project. *Thorax.* 1997;52:760–765.

32. Chew F, Goh D, Ooi B, Saharom R, Hui J, Lee B. Association of ambient air-pollution levels with acute asthma exacerbation among children in Singapore. *Allergy.* 1999;54: 320–329.

33. Thompson A, Shields M, Patterson C. Acute asthma exacerbations and air pollutants in children living in Belfast, Northern Ireland. *Arch Environ Health.* 2001;56(3): 234–241.

34. Dockery D, Pope C, Xu X, Spengler J, Ware J, Fay M, BG, et al. An association between air pollution and mortality in six US cities. *N Engl J Med.* 1993;329(24):1753–1759.

35. Pope CA, Thun MJ, Namboodiri MM, Dockery DW, Evans JS, Speizer FE, et al. Particulate air pollution as a predictor of mortality in a prospective study of US adults. *Am J Respir Crit Care Med.* 1995;151:669–674.

36. Laden F, Schwartz J, Speizer F, Dockery D. Reduction in fine particulate air pollution and mortality. *Am J Respir Crit Care Med.* 2006;173:667–672.

37. Sram R, Binkova B, Dejmek J, Bobak M. Ambient air pollution and pregnancy outcomes: a review of the literature. *Environ Health Perspect.* 2005;113(4).

38. Tong S, Colditz P. Air pollution and sudden infant death syndrome: a literature review. *Paediatr Perinat Epidemiol.* 2004;18:327–335.

39. Clancy L, Goodman P, Sinclair H, Dockery D. Effect of air-pollution control on death rates in Dublin, Ireland: an intervention study. *Lancet.* 2002;360:1210–1214.

40. Friedman M, Powell K, Hutwaner L, Graham L, Teague W. Impact of changes in transportation and commuting behaviors during the 1996 Summer Olympic Games in Atlanta on air quality and childhood asthma. *JAMA.* 2001;285(7):897–905.

41. National Research Council. *Toxicological Effects of Methylmercury.* Washington, DC: National Academy Press; 2000.

42. Clarkson T. The three modern faces of mercury. *Environ Health Perspect.* 2002;110 (suppl 1):11–23.

43. Grandjean P, Weihe P, White R, Debes F, Araki S, Yokoyama K, et al. Cognitive deficit in 7-year-old children with prenatal exposure to methylmercury. *Neurotoxicol Teratol.* 1997;19(6):417–428.

44. Grandjean P, Budtz-Jorgensen E, White R, Jorgensen P, Weihe P, Debes F, et al. Methylmercury exposure biomarkers as indicators of neurotoxicity in children aged 7 years. *Am J Epidemiol.* 1999;150(3):301–305.

45. Debes F, Budtz-Jorgensen E, Weihe P, White R, Grandjean P. Impact of prenatal methylmercury exposure on neurobehavioral function at age 14 years. *Neurotoxicol Teratol.* 2006;28:536–547.

46. US Environmental Protection Agency, Great Lakes National Program Office. *Great Lakes Binational Toxics Strategy Report on Alkyl-lead: Sources, Regulations and Options, 2000.* Available at: http://www.epa.gov/glnpo/bns/lead/Step%20Report/steps.pdf. Accessed April 12, 2008.

47. Needleman H, Gunnoe C, Leviton A, Reed R, Peresie H, Maher C, et al. Deficits in psychologic and classroom performance of children with elevated dentine lead levels. *N Engl J Med.* 1979;300(13):689–695.

48. Gilbert SG, Weiss B. A rationale for lowering the blood lead action level from 10 to 2 μg/dL. *NeuroToxicology.* 2006;27:693–701.

49. Wigg NR. Low-level lead exposure and children. *J Pediatr Child Health.* 2001;37: 423–425.

50. Needleman H, McFarland C, Ness RB, Fienberg SE, Tobin MJ. Bone lead levels in adjudicated delinquents: a case-control study. *Neurotoxicol Teratol.* 2002;24:711–717.

51. Schell LM, Ravenscroft J, Cole M, Jacobs A, Newman J, Akwesasne Task Force on the Environment. Health disparities and toxicant exposure of Akwesasne Mohawk young adults: a partnership approach to research. *Environ Health Perspect.* 2005;113(12): 1826–1832.

52. US Environmental Protection Agency. *Inventory of US Greenhouse Gas Emissions and Sinks: 1990–2004, 2006.* Available at: http://yosemite.epa.gov/oar/globalwarming.nsf/content/ResourceCenterPublicationsGHGEmissionsUSEmissionsInventory2006.html. Accessed April 14, 2008.

53. Intergovernmental Panel on Climate Change. IPPC, 2007: Summary for policymakers. In: *Climate Change 2007: The Physical Science Basis.* Contribution of Working Group I to the Fourth Assessment Report of the Intergovernmental Panel on Climate Change. Cambridge, England, and New York, NY: Cambridge University Press; 2007.

54. Intergovernmental Panel on Climate Change. IPPC, 2007: Historical overview of climate change science. In: *Climate Change 2007: The Physical Science Basis.* Contribution of Working Group I to the Fourth Assessment Report of the Intergovernmental Panel on Climate Change. Cambridge, England, and New York, NY: Cambridge University Press; 2007.

55. Intergovernmental Panel on Climate Change. IPPC, 2007: Technical summary. In: *Climate Change 2007: The Physical Science Basis.* Contribution of Working Group I to the Fourth Assessment Report of the Intergovernmental Panel on Climate Change. Cambridge, England, and New York, NY: Cambridge University Press; 2007.

56. Intergovernmental Panel on Climate Change. IPPC, 2007: Summary for policymakers. In: *Climate Change 2007: Impacts, Adaptation and Vulnerability.* Contribution of Working Group II to the Fourth Assessment Report of the Intergovernmental Panel on Climate Change. Cambridge, England, and New York, NY: Cambridge University Press; 2007.

57. Greenhouse L. Justices say EPA has power to act on harmful gases. *New York Times,* April 3, 2007.

58. California Air Resources Board. *Greenhouse Gas Emissions Inventory and Mandatory Reporting.* Available at: http://www.arb.ca.gov/cc/ccei.htm. Accessed February 22, 2007.

59. Black H. Imperfect Protection: NEPA at 35 Years. *Environ Health Perspect* 2004:112(5) A292-A295.

60. Ripley A. Radioactive building sand stirs dispute. *New York Times,* September 27, 1971.

61. US Environmental Protection Agency. *Uranium Mill Tailings.* Available at: http://www.epa.gov/radiation/docs/radwaste/402-k-94-001-umt.htm. Accessed October 7, 2006.

62. US Department of Energy, Office of Environmental Management. *Uranium Mill Tailings Remedial Action.* Available at: http://web.em.doe.gov/bemr96/umtra.html. Accessed October 7, 2006.

63. US Energy Information Administration. *US Nuclear Reactors: Reactor Status List.* Available at: http://www.eia.doe.gov/cneaf/nuclear/page/nuc_reactors/reactsum.html. Accessed October 7, 2006.

64. US Department of Energy, Office of Civilian Radioactive Waste Management. *Overview: Yucca Mountain Project, 2006.* Available at: http://www.ocrwm.doe.gov/fact sheets/doeymp0026.shtml. Accessed December 20, 2006.

65. Ryskamp JM. *Nuclear Fuel Cycle Closure, 2003*. Available at: http://nuclear.inl.gov/docs/papers-presentations/nuclear_fuel_cycle_3-5-03.pdf. Accessed October 23, 2006.

66. Statement of Edward F. Sproat III, Director for the Office of Civilian Radioactive Waste Management, US Department of Energy, before the Subcommittee on Energy and Air Quality, Committee on Energy and Commerce, US House of Representatives, September 13, 2006.

67. US Nuclear Regulatory Commission. *Fact Sheet: Decommissioning Nuclear Power Plants*. Available at: http://www.nrc.gov/reading-rm/doc-collections/fact-sheets/decommissioning.pdf. Accessed October 7, 2006.

68. US Nuclear Regulatory Commission. *Low-Level Waste Compacts*. Available at: http://www.nrc.gov/waste/llw-disposal/compacts.html. Accessed December 26, 2007.

69. American Geological Institute. *Low-Level Nuclear Waste Disposal Update (10-4-02)*. Available at: http://www.agiweb.org/gap/legis107/lowlevel_waste.html. Accessed December 26, 2007.

70. US Energy Information Administration. *International Energy Outlook 2006*. 2006. Available at: http://www.eia.doe.gov/oiaf/ieo/ieographic_data.html. Accessed October 7, 2006.

71. Herring J. Uranium and thorium resource assessment. In: Cleveland C, ed. *Encyclopedia of Energy*. Elsevier; 2004.

72. United Nations Scientific Committee on the Effects of Atomic Radiation (UNSCEAR). *UNSCEAR 2000 Report to the General Assembly, with Scientific Annexes: United Nations; 2000*. Available at: http://www.unscear.org/unscear/en/publications/2000_1.html. Accessed October 19, 2006.

73. US Centers for Disease Control and Prevention. *Prenatal Radiation Exposure: A Fact Sheet for Physicians, 2005*. Available at: http://www.bt.cdc.gov/radiation/pdf/prenatalphysician.pdf. Accessed April 14, 2008.

74. National Academy of Sciences. *Biological Effects of Ionizing Radiation (BEIR) VII: Health Risks from Exposure to Low Levels of Ionizing Radiation*. Washington, DC: National Academies Press; 2005.

75. Frumkin H, Samet J. Radon. *CA: Cancer J Clinicians*. 2001;6(51):337–344.

76. Gilliland FD. Radon progeny exposure and lung cancer risk among non-smoking uranium miners. *Health Physics*. 2000;79(4):365–372.

77. Gilliland FD. Uranium mining and lung cancer among Navajo men in New Mexico and Arizona, 1969–1993. *J Occup Environ Med*. 2000;42(3):278–283.

78. Williams D. Cancer after nuclear fallout: lessons from the Chernobyl accident. *Nature Reviews: Cancer*. 2002;2:543–549.

79. Moysich K, Menezes RJ, Michalek AM. Chernobyl-related ionising radiation exposure and cancer risk: an epidemiological review. *Lancet: Oncol*. 2002;3(5):269–279.

80. Noshchenko AG, Zamostyan PV, Bondar OY, Drozdova VD. Radiation-induced leukemia risk among those aged 0–20 at the time of the Chernobyl accident: a case-control study in the Ukraine. *Int J Cancer*. 2002;99:609–618.

81. US Nuclear Regulatory Commission. *High-Level Waste Disposal: What We Regulate*. Available at: www.nrc.gov/waste/hlw-disposal.html. Accessed December 20, 2006.

82. US Energy Information Administration. *Annual Energy Review 2005*. 2006. Available at: http://www.eia.doe.gov/emeu/aer/. Accessed April 10, 2008.

83. Lovins AB, Lovins LH. *Brittle Power: Energy Strategy for National Security*. Andover, Mass: Brick House Publishing; 1982.

84. US–Canada Power System Outage Task Force. *Interim Report: Causes of the August 14th Blackout in the United States and Canada*. 2003. Available at: http://www.nrcan-rncan .gc.ca/media/docs/814BlackoutReport.pdf. Accessed January 21, 2004.

85. US Environmental Protection Agency. *Mercury-Containing Light Bulb (Lamp) Frequent Questions*. Available at: http://www.epa.gov/bulbrecycling/faqs.htm. Accessed May 28, 2008.

86. Frumkin H. Urban sprawl and public health. *Public Health Rep*. May–June 2002;117: 201–212.

87. US Department of Energy, Oak Ridge National Laboratory. *Transportation Energy Data Book*. 25th ed. 2006. Available at: http://cta.ornl.gov/data/download25.shtml. Accessed August 22, 2007.

88. US Environmental Protection Agency. *Light-Duty Automotive Technology and Fuel Economy Trends: 1975 through 2006*. 2006. Available at: http://www.epa.gov/oms/cert/ mpg/fetrends/420r06011.pdf. Accessed April 14, 2008.

89. Morrison ML, Sinclair K. Environmental impacts of wind energy technology. In: Cleveland C, ed. *Encyclopedia of Energy*. Elsevier; 2004.

90. National Wind Coordinating Committee. *Avian Collisions with Wind Turbines: A Summary of Existing Studies and Comparisons to Other Sources of Avian Collision Mortality in the United States*. National Wind Coordinating Committee; 2001. Available at: http://www.nationalwind.org/publications/wildlife/avian_collisions.pdf. Accessed April 14, 2008.

91. Daley B. Audubon review supports wind farm. *Boston Globe*, March 29, 2006.

92. Israel Ministry of Foreign Affairs. *Solar Energy in Israel*. 2002. Available at: http://www .mfa.gov.il/MFA/Facts%20About%20Israel/Science%20-%20Technology/Solar% 20Energy%20in%20Israel. Accessed February 1, 2007.

93. Kammen DM. Renewable energy: taxonomic overview. In: Cleveland C, ed. *Encyclopedia of Energy*. Elsevier; 2004:385–412.

94. US Department of Agriculture, Economic Research Service. *Ethanol Reshapes the Corn Market*. 2006. Available at: http://www.ers.usda.gov/AmberWaves/April06/pdf/ EthanolFeatureApril06.pdf. Accessed April 14, 2008.

95. Maxwell N. Environmental injustices of energy facilities. In: Cleveland C, ed. *Encyclopedia of Energy*. Elsevier; 2004.

96. Ezzati M, Kammen DM. The health impacts of exposure to indoor air pollution from solid fuels in developing countries: knowledge, gaps, and data needs. *Environ Health Perspect*. 2002;110(11):1057–1068.

97. Ezzati J, Saleh H, Kammen D. The contributions of emissions and spatial microenvironments to exposure to indoor air pollution from biomass combustion in Kenya. *Environ Health Perspect.* 2000;108(9):833–839.

98. Smith K, Samet J, Romieu I, Bruce N. Indoor air pollution in developing countries and acute lower respiratory infections in children. *Thorax.* 2000;55:518–532.

99. Mishra V, Dai X, Smith K, Mika L. Maternal exposure to biomass smoke and reduced birth weight in Zimbabwe. *Ann Epidemiol.* 2004;14:740–747.

100. Natural Resource Defense Council. *Building the Hydrogen Boom.* Spring 2005. Available at: http://www.nrdc.org/onearth/05spr/frontlines.asp. Accessed January 29, 2007.

101. National Energy Policy Development Group. *National Energy Policy: Reliable, Affordable, and Environmentally Sound Energy for America's Future.* 2001. Available at: http://www.whitehouse.gov/energy/National-Energy-Policy.pdf. Accessed April 14, 2008.

Producing Manufactured Goods

Learning Objectives

After studying this chapter, the reader will be able to:

- Define or explain the key terms throughout the chapter

- Characterize the uses, common sources of environmental exposure, and toxicity of these groups of synthetic organic chemicals: organic solvents, phthalate plasticizers and bisphenol A, PCBs, dioxins and furans, PBDEs, and PFCs

- Describe in simple terms the effect of chlorofluorocarbons in the stratosphere and the implications for human health

- Appreciate the toxicity of certain metals to workers and others

- Summarize briefly the current status of nanotechnology and what is known about its potential risks to human health

- Discuss the occupational exposures to and health effects of major physical hazards: asbestos, cotton dust, mechanical hazards, noise, and light during the biological night

- Appreciate that certain occupational exposures cause asthma

- Give examples of social disparities in exposure to industrial hazards, both within the United States and internationally

- Describe key approaches to managing the public health risks associated with industry

- Describe the US regulatory framework for managing the public health risks associated with industry

In the prosperous decades that followed World War II, many people in North America and Europe were able to acquire more material goods. Especially in the United States, this period saw a rapid change from an ethic based on thrift and self-denial to expectations of convenience and instant gratification. Whereas an earlier generation's motto had been "use it up, wear it out, make it do," a new generation yearned for "the good life." In the 1950s, the symbols of the good life were a house, a car, a washing machine, and a television. By the start of the 21st century, consumerism had reached new heights, and "the good life" had become "lifestyles" that encompassed large suburban homes, sport utility vehicles, luxury housewares, and an astounding array of electronic devices for computing, communications, and entertainment.

Of course, these products do not spring magically into existence. Each one has a history: Raw materials are obtained and then transformed through manufacturing. As already described, nothing ever really goes away—and so all these processes create wastes, as well as hazards to workers, and sometimes even to consumers. In the mid-20th century, smokestack industries and air pollution dominated the landscape of many US cities and towns (see **Figure 5.1**). Today, the icon of industrial pollution is the 55-gallon drum of chemical waste (see **Figure 5.2**).

Modern consumers are increasingly insulated from the realities of industrial pollution. For example, eight times as many Americans now work in service industries as work in manufacturing,[1] and more and more manufacturing is moving to lower-income countries. To many residents of an industrialized country who buy and use a product, that product's footprint—in environmental destruction or pollution, in consumption of nonrenewable energy resources, in workers' illnesses and injuries—may be largely invisible.

This chapter provides the story behind the manufactured products of modern society, describing the major chemical and physical hazards associated with manufacturing and its pollution. It describes the uses and health effects of several groups of synthetic organic chemicals (Section 5.1) and a number of metals (Section 5.2) and explores the potential risks of emerging nanotechnologies (Section 5.3). The chapter then describes a set of physical hazards that especially affects workers (Section 5.4) and identifies asthma-causing agents in the workplace (Section 5.5). Section 5.6 notes social disparities in the burden of industrial pollution in the ambient environment, and the chapter concludes with a description of the US regulatory framework for chemicals and chemical pollution (Section 5.7).

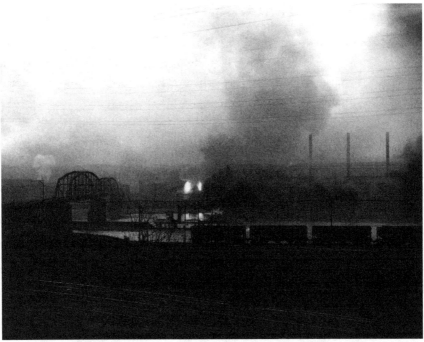

FIGURE 5.1　Polluted air blankets a US city in 1946. *Source*: Reprinted courtesy of CDC Public Health Image Library. ID# 8998. Content provider: CDC/Roy Perry. Available at: http://phil.cdc.gov/phil/details.asp. Accessed August 21, 2007.

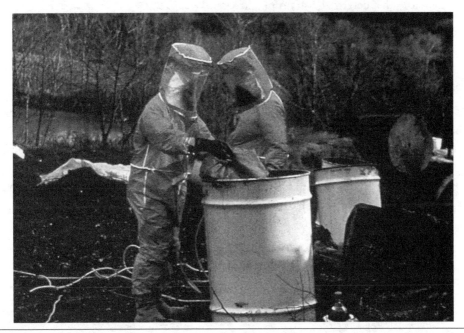

FIGURE 5.2　Workers wear protective gear as they handle hazardous wastes. *Source*: Reprinted courtesy of CDC Public Health Library. ID# 1530. Content provider: CDC. Available at: http://phil.cdc.gov/details.asp. Accessed October 3, 2007.

5.1 Synthetic Organic Chemicals

In the United States today, thousands of **organic chemicals** are in use. The great majority of these chemicals are man-made and are produced from petroleum. The capacity to make such **synthetic organic chemicals** from oil, a hydrocarbon resource, rests on carbon's unique flexibility in forming stable bonds.

In an oil refinery, the constituents of crude oil are separated into lighter and heavier fractions, which are then used to make many products, including various fuels (for example, gasoline, diesel fuel, jet fuel, kerosene); nonfuel products (for example, lubricating oils, greases, petroleum jelly, asphalt); and chemicals that become raw materials for the production of other chemicals in the chemical industry.[2] Thus, some of what we think of as chemical manufacturing takes place at oil refineries, and some at separate chemical plants.

Synthetic organic compounds have been designed and produced for many uses. Among these are many products so familiar that we might not even think of them as chemicals: soaps and detergents; cosmetics and toiletries; plastics and synthetic rubbers; inks and dyes; paints, coatings, polishes, and adhesives; pharmaceuticals; and even explosives. Because there are far too many synthetic organic chemicals to consider individually, this discussion focuses on some groups that are both common and pose a risk to human health:

- Organic solvents
- Chemicals used in the production of plastics
- A set of environmentally persistent toxic substances
- Chemicals that deplete the stratospheric ozone layer

Another important group of toxic chemicals, pesticides, is discussed in the context of agriculture and food (see Chapter 6).

Organic Solvents

Organic solvents are chemicals that dissolve other substances. They are useful in many cleaning applications in industry and are also used in synthesizing other chemicals. Solvents have a wide variety of chemical structures. However, many widely used solvents fall into one of two groups, both of which are low-molecular-weight, volatile chemicals (see **Table 5.1**). One group is simple hydrocarbons in which the carbon atoms are arranged in a ring. Four common solvents in this group—benzene, toluene, ethylbenzene, and xylene, commonly referred to together as

Table 5.1   Some Widely Used Organic Solvents

Nonchlorinated Solvents	Chlorinated Solvents
Benzene	Trichloroethylene (TCE)
Toluene	Tetrachloroethylene (PCE)
Ethylbenzene	1,1,1-trichloroethane (TCA)
Xylene	

BTEX ("bee-tex")—are often derived from petroleum at the refinery and are used as feedstocks in the production of other chemicals.

In the other group of widely used solvents, the carbon atoms are arranged in a chain rather than in a ring, and one or more of the hydrogen atoms has been replaced with a chlorine atom. This group of chlorinated (chlorine-containing) solvents includes trichloroethylene (TCE) and other compounds that have environmental breakdown products similar to TCE's—including tetrachloroethylene (commonly known as perchloroethylene, or PCE) and 1,1,1-trichloroethane (TCA; also known as methyl chloroform), among others.

Industrial solvents of all types are released into the environment, mainly by the industries that make them and the industries that use them. Petroleum refineries, for example, release large quantities of BTEX,[2] and the chemical industry is also an important source of solvent contamination because solvents are used as intermediaries in producing other chemicals. In other industries, chlorinated solvents are widely used to clean or "degrease" metals in the manufacture of electronic components—which today are found in products ranging from automatic coffeemakers to airplane navigation systems. And, with the explosion of the computer industry and other electronics-related industries during the last decades of the 20th century, chlorinated solvents are among the most common contaminants of groundwater in the United States.[3] Many solvents are moderately soluble in water and can be transported over long distances, making cleanup a difficult challenge.

In the textile industry, solvents are widely used in dying and dry cleaning,[4] resulting in occupational exposures at a large number of small businesses. At one time, highly toxic benzene was used as a dry cleaning agent (see **Figure 5.3**). Over time, benzene was largely replaced by trichloroethylene in dry cleaning, and TCE in turn has been largely replaced by tetrachloroethylene (PCE), now used at dry cleaning businesses in almost every city and town. However, some cleaners also offer water-based cleaning methods that do not damage fabrics which cannot be washed in a home washing machine.

Most solvents affect the central nervous system. Acute high-level exposures cause symptoms such as dizziness, loss of coordination, confusion, and unconsciousness; and chronic lower-level exposures can lead to memory loss or other intellectual impairment.[5] Long-term exposure to many solvents damages the liver, kidneys, or both; benzene also causes anemia.[5] Among the solvents mentioned earlier, WHO's International Agency for Research on Cancer lists benzene in Group 1 (carcinogenic to humans); benzene is well known to cause leukemia in people.[6] IARC places TCE and PCE in Group 2A (probably carcinogenic to humans), and ethylbenzene in Group 2B (possibly carcinogenic to humans).

Phthalate Plasticizers and Bisphenol A

Plastics are a set of synthetic organic chemicals familiar in items we use every day; **plasticizers** are the chemicals used in manufacturing plastics to make them flexible (the word *plastic* means malleable or pliable). As a result, the chemicals used as plasticizers, called **phthalates**, are present in plastic products. Even plastics that seem fairly hard need some flexibility so that they can sustain an impact without shattering. Another chemical, **bisphenol A**, is also widely used in the production of certain plastics. For example, polycarbonate plastic bottles, including some baby

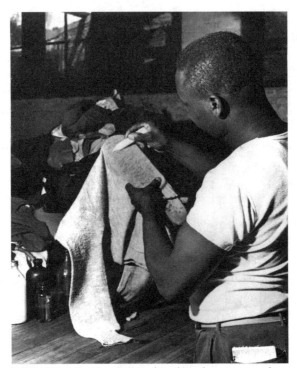

FIGURE 5.3 In 1950, this dry cleaning worker used benzene to spot-clean a garment. *Source*: Reprinted courtesy of CDC Public Health Image Library. ID# 9453. Content provider: CDC/Barbara Jenkins, NIOSH. Available at: http://phil.cdc.gov/phil/details.asp. Accessed August 21, 2007.

bottles and refillable water bottles, may contain small amounts of both phthalates and bisphenol A. Bisphenol A is also used to make the linings of food and drink cans. A number of such products are now being withdrawn from the market.

Phthalates and bisphenol A are classed as semivolatile compounds—although less volatile than VOCs, they do slowly move from a plastic product into the air. Similarly, though these chemicals are not highly water-soluble, they slowly mobilize from a plastic container into a liquid held in the container. Phthalates are somewhat lipophilic and bioaccumulate in fish; however, they do not biomagnify across higher levels in ecosystems, because higher animals metabolize and excrete them.[7]

Different chemicals in the phthalate family are used for different purposes.[7,8] A higher-molecular-weight phthalate, di(2-ethylhexyl)phthalate (DEHP), is present in polyvinyl chloride (PVC) plastic. This very common plastic material is used in many products, including water pipes, flooring, upholstery, credit cards, and plastic shower curtains. PVC plastic is also used in food packaging and intravenous bags used for blood or other medical products. Di-isononyl phthalate (DiNP) is used in many plastic toys. Other, lower-molecular-weight plasticizers—

di-butyl phthalate (DBP), diethyl phthalate (DEP), and dimethyl phthalate (DMP)—are found mostly in household or cosmetic products that are spreadable or sprayable. These phthalates are found in hair spray and nail polish, lotions and perfumes, glue and insect repellent, insecticides, and coatings on pharmaceuticals.

More than 3 million metric tons of phthalates are produced globally each year, and they are ubiquitous in the environment.[7,8] As a result of the wide use of phthalates in products, people living in industrialized nations are routinely exposed to these chemicals at low levels.[7,8] In fact, the most recent exposure study of a nationwide sample of Americans documented biomarkers of phthalate exposure (phthalate metabolites) in the urine of males and females of all ages and ethnic groups.[9]

Phthalates and bisphenol A are considered **endocrine disruptors**, or **endocrine-disrupting compounds**—that is, chemicals that interfere in some way with the body's hormone system. Endocrine disruptors can mimic the effect of a hormone, or block its effect, or even influence the body's production of the hormone. The term **environmental hormone** is also sometimes used to refer to endocrine-disrupting chemicals in the environment, and the term **xenoestrogen** refers to environmental chemicals with effects similar to those of the female hormone estrogen.*

In laboratory studies, both DEHP and DINP cause developmental toxicity in animals, and the body system most sensitive to their effects is the immature male reproductive system.[7] Data from animals also show clearly that phthalates both cross the placenta and are present in milk,[7] indicating the potential for high exposure in utero and in infancy. Based on limited evidence, links have been hypothesized between phthalate exposure and low sperm count in the adult male, as well as certain developmental disorders in humans—for example, cryptorchidism (undescended testis) or hypospadias (wrongly placed opening of the urethra) in the infant male.[10] A recent epidemiologic study documented a link between higher maternal phthalate exposure during pregnancy and a smaller distance between the anus and the genitals in the newborn male infant.[11] (Such a reduction is considered a marker of feminization because anogenital distance is typically shorter in females than in males; however, a normal distance for male infants has not been established.)

At least two subgroups of the general population are of concern because they may have high phthalate exposures: any person receiving an intravenous drip for an extended period; and infants and young children because they suck or chew on plastic pacifiers, bottle nipples, and teething toys. Thus, critically ill male infants are of particular concern because they are both susceptible and highly exposed.[12] In the United States, phthalates have been removed from plastic items that are intended to be put in an infant's mouth, and DINP, which is less toxic than DEHP, is being substituted in toys for older children.[7] Similarly, the European Union has banned certain phthalates in products for children.[8]

---

*The pharmaceutical diethylstilbestrol (DES), administered to pregnant women from the late 1940s through the 1960s (because it was believed to prevent miscarriage), was an early endocrine disruptor. Among other effects, it has been linked to reproductive abnormalities in the sons, daughters, and even granddaughters of the women who took the drug.

Finally, mechanistic evidence is emerging of a link between exposure to environmental chemicals and obesity, and there is limited evidence of such a link in studies in rodents and humans. Prenatal exposure to bisphenol A has been linked to early weight gain and adult obesity in rodents.[13] Exposure to tributyl tin, an organic tin compound used in PVC plastics and fungicides, has been linked to increased lipid accumulation in rodents.[14] In people, a national cross-sectional study showed that obese men (as measured by waist circumference) were more likely to have high concentrations of phthalate metabolites in their urine,[15] after controlling for potential confounding variables. Findings like these await confirmation in long-term epidemiologic studies—and diet, exercise, and genetics remain important predictors of obesity—but laboratory scientists have begun to use the term *obesogen* to refer to a chemical that causes weight gain.

Persistent Toxic Substances

At the opposite end of the physical-chemical spectrum from organic solvents are a set of organic compounds known for their persistence in soil and sediment. Most originate as man-made chemicals, created for specific purposes, but some are unanticipated by-products of industrial chemical processes. These persistent compounds bioaccumulate in animal tissues and biomagnify through an ecosystem's food chain. As a result of these traits, these chemicals have become ubiquitous in the global environment: They have spread throughout the world in soil carried by wind and water, and also in the bodies of birds and aquatic animals that are long-distance travelers.

Several groups of persistent chemicals are now known to be toxic to people, and these are the chemicals of concern here. The descriptive term **persistent toxic substances** is used in this text; other labels, some of which have regulatory meaning, have been used to refer to overlapping sets of chemicals.* The persistent toxic substances described here are halogenated compounds; that is, they contain an element from the group known as **halogens**, which includes chlorine, fluorine, bromine, and iodine. As a group, the halogens are highly reactive, and this accounts for both their usefulness in organic chemistry and their potential to cause harm in the body. In fact, chlorine does not occur naturally in organic compounds in mammals, and it has been argued that the chemical industry violated a "biological taboo" in introducing synthetic chlorinated compounds into ecosystems.[16]

The first generation of synthetic halogenated hydrocarbons were high-molecular-weight chlorinated compounds. Within this group, polychlorinated biphenyls (PCBs) are a set of chemicals that were used mainly to insulate electrical devices. Dioxins and furans,** a large

---

*The term *persistent organic pollutants* (POPs) originates with the Stockholm Convention (see text). Another term, *persistent, bioaccumulative, and toxic* (PBT) *chemicals*, has been used more recently by the US EPA to designate a set of chemicals of regulatory concern. This list has some overlap with the POPs list, but includes other organic chemicals as well as the heavy metals lead and mercury. Both terms are often used more loosely, as descriptive rather than regulatory names. A more recent coinage, *ubiquitous bioaccumulative toxins*, captures the implications of persistence; however, the term *toxin* typically refers to a substance produced naturally by a plant or animal.
**The term *dioxins and furans* is shorthand for polychlorinated dibenzo-*p*-dioxins (PCDDs) and polychlorinated dibenzofurans (PCDFs).

group of structurally related chlorinated compounds, were never manufactured but have been created as by-products of various chemical processes. In recent years, two other groups of persistent toxic substances have emerged as causes of concern. These halogenated chemicals are not chlorinated but rather contain bromine or fluorine. Polybrominated diphenyl ethers (PBDEs) have been used mostly as flame retardants in fabrics, electronic devices, and furniture; and perfluorochemicals (PFCs) have been widely used in nonstick coatings.

The Stockholm Convention on Persistent Organic Pollutants, which originated as an initiative of the United Nations Environment Programme, is an international agreement on controlling a set of chemicals designated as persistent organic pollutants and commonly referred to as POPs. The agreement was adopted in 2001 at a meeting in Stockholm, entered into force in 2004, and has been ratified by 153 countries. The United States, though it was a signatory to the Convention, has not yet ratified it. The list of chemicals comprises PCBs, dioxins and furans, along with DDT and eight other organochlorine pesticides (aldrin, chlordane, dieldrin, endrin, heptachlor, hexachlorobenzene, mirex, and toxaphene; see Chapter 6). Countries that have ratified the agreement agree to eliminate or reduce the release of these chemicals—sometimes referred to as the "dirty dozen"—into the environment.

Polychlorinated Biphenyls, Dioxins, and Furans

Polychlorinated biphenyls (PCBs) are a large family of related man-made compounds—there are 209 distinct PCBs, which were produced by the Monsanto Corporation and sold mainly as seven different mixtures, under the trade name Arochlor. These compounds have high molecular weights and are oily liquids or solid waxy substances. As a group, PCBs are chemically stable and nonflammable, and have low electrical conductivity. Because of these properties, they were widely used as insulating fluids in electrical equipment, such as transformers, and General Electric (GE) was Monsanto's main customer for PCBs. PCBs were manufactured in the United States from 1930 through 1977.[17] Globally, about 1.5 million metric tons of PCBs were produced, and perhaps 20% to 30% of this amount ultimately found its way into the environment.[18]

Although PCBs were used in closed systems, they entered the wider environment in large quantities as industrial wastes. For example, two General Electric manufacturing plants in New York released up to 1.3 million pounds of PCBs into the Hudson River between 1947 and 1977; the EPA's ongoing cleanup effort extends over a 200-mile stretch of the river.[19] The sediments of many rivers and lakes, including the Great Lakes on the US–Canadian border, are contaminated with PCBs from industrial releases. Accidental releases still occur from time to time when aging PCB-laden equipment fails—or burns in a fire, releasing PCBs to the atmosphere.

The manufacture of PCBs also created as by-products a family of chemicals called dioxins. Dioxins are a group of structurally related compounds, as are the furans, which are chemically similar to dioxins and often occur with them. The most toxic of the dioxins and furans is 2,3,7,8-*tetrachlorodibenzo-p-d*ioxin, or TCDD. Dioxins, furans, and PCBs behave similarly in the environment and have been found to have mostly similar health effects.

Dioxins occur as by-products not only in the production of PCBs, but also of various other chemical processes involving chlorinated organic compounds. For example, dioxins were chemical by-products in the manufacture of an herbicide—a chemical used to kill unwanted plants—known as 2,4,5-trichlorophenoxyacetic acid (2,4,5-T). As a result, dioxins were present as contaminants in 2,4,5-T. This herbicide in turn was one of two major ingredients in a defoliant (dubbed Agent Orange after its color-coded container) used by the US military during the Vietnam War. A defoliant is a substance that causes the leaves to fall off plants, and defoliants are sometimes used in war to deny cover to enemy combatants. The US military sprayed Agent Orange widely in Vietnam from 1962 to 1971.[20] As a result, both US soldiers and many Vietnamese were exposed to the dioxin that contaminated this herbicide.

Dioxins also appear in the waste streams of the pulp and paper industry, whenever chlorine is used in the production processes. And dioxins can be produced when chlorinated plastic materials are burned. In a modern waste incinerator, temperatures are usually kept high enough to minimize the production of dioxin. However, any uncontrolled burning of ordinary household waste—or, for that matter, any fire in a home or office building—produces dioxins.

Dioxins have also been released into the environment through accidents. In 1972 and 1973, for example, waste oil—later found to be contaminated with dioxin—was spread on dirt roads to control dust in the town of Times Beach, Missouri, mysteriously sickening children and animals. The town was evacuated a decade later, when soil samples taken in 1982 showed high concentrations of dioxin.[21] In 1999, elevated concentrations of PCBs in chicken feed—ultimately traced to recycled fat used by the feed manufacturer—sickened birds at several poultry farms in Belgium; for a short time, contaminated meat reached the food supply.[22]

Acute exposure to PCBs or dioxins causes **chloracne**, a painful and disfiguring skin condition that can last for months or for more than 15 years.[23] Chloracne has been documented in accident victims—for example, those who consumed rice oil contaminated by PCBs in a Japanese factory in 1968;[24] and those who lived near a chemical plant in Seveso, Italy, in 1976, when an explosion released a cloud containing dioxins and their chemical precursors.[23] Chloracne came to public attention recently with the dioxin poisoning in 2004 of the Ukrainian political leader Viktor Yushchenko.[25]

Today the general population has ongoing low-level exposure to PCBs and dioxins—mostly from eating fish, meat, and dairy products because these chemicals are persistent in sediments and soil and become magnified in animal tissues. Indeed, studies in industrialized nations have documented that everyone carries low levels of dioxins and furans in his or her tissues.[18] Although PCBs are no longer in production, workers can be exposed when handling older electrical equipment.

In humans and other mammals, PCBs, TCDD, and many other dioxins and furans have several health effects in common because these effects are mediated through a single biological mechanism with wide-ranging impacts.* Effects of TCDD documented in animals include liver

---

*Chemicals in this group exert their effects by binding to the aryl hydrocarbon (Ah) receptor protein; on the basis of this shared biological mechanism, these chemicals are sometimes referred to together as dioxin and dioxin-like compounds (Webster TF, Commoner B. Overview: the dioxin debate. In: Schechter A, Gasiewicz T, eds. *Dioxins and Health*. 2nd ed. New York, NY: John Wiley and Sons; 2003:1–53).

damage, immunotoxicity, birth defects, reduced fertility, endometriosis, and cancer.[18] In studies of nonhuman primates, chronic PCB exposure has been shown to lower birthweight, affect memory and learning, and affect the immune and endocrine systems.[26] IARC classifies PCBs in Group 2A (probably carcinogenic to humans) and TCDD in Group 1 (carcinogenic to humans).[6]

Epidemiologic study of everyday exposures to PCBs and dioxins is challenging because these exposures are relatively low and are likely to occur along with exposures to other chemicals. However, several studies in the United States and Europe provide some evidence that these compounds affect human neurological development, especially with in utero exposure.[18]

Polybrominated Diphenyl Ethers

Polybrominated diphenyl ethers (PBDEs) are a large group of related compounds with structures somewhat similar to those of PCBs and dioxins. However, in contrast to PCBs, whose use was industrial, and dioxins, which are accidental by-products, PBDEs are produced for use as flame retardants in a wide range of products. Flame retardants slow the ignition and spread of fire, with the goal of reducing deaths and injuries. The large-scale synthesis of these chemicals is a relatively recent phenomenon; the global market demand for PBDEs was more than 67,000 metric tons in 1999, up from 40,000 metric tons in 1990.[27]

In a PBDE molecule, bromine atoms are substituted for hydrogen atoms. PBDE compounds are named according to the number of bromine substitutions; most commercially produced PBDEs are penta-, octa-, or deca-BDEs (that is, with 5, 8, or 10 bromine substitutions). Overall, PBDEs are relatively high-molecular-weight compounds; they are generally not volatile, instead accumulating in dust or sediment; and they are lipophilic.[27]

PBDEs are used mostly in consumer products—penta-BDEs are used mostly in fabrics (for example, in children's pajamas) and foams (for example, in mattresses). The octa- and deca-BDEs are used in plastics, both in consumer products—for example, the plastic housings of televisions, computers, and other electronic devices—and in building materials.[28] PBDEs are not chemically bound to these plastic or textile materials, and thus they can move out of these products.[27] For example, PBDEs can enter the indoor environment from consumer products in use and can enter the ambient environment when products are discarded.

PBDEs are now widespread in the environment. They have been measured in fish, shellfish, or fish-eating birds in the Baltic Sea, North Sea, Arctic Ocean, and Pacific Ocean,[29] and in seals and Beluga whales in North American waters.[30] They have also been measured in human beings. For example, a 1999 study found that the concentration of a set of PBDEs in the breast milk of Swedish women had doubled every 5 years over the preceding 25 years.[31]

The human health risks of PBDEs at the low doses to which most people are exposed are unclear.[30] The chemical structure of PBDEs is similar to that of thyroid hormones, and thyroid disruption is considered the most likely human health effect of these compounds.[30] PBDEs may be estrogenic, and some may act by a dioxin-like mechanism.[29] Mice exposed to PBDEs show learning and motor deficits.[30] As yet, the evidence on the carcinogenicity of these chemicals is too limited to make any judgment of their possible cancer risk.[30] As the toxicity of the penta-, octa-, and deca-PBDEs has become clearer, the production of these chemicals is being phased out in the United States, and has been banned in the European Union—but other brominated flame retardant chemicals appear likely to replace them.

Perfluorochemicals

A set of fluorine-containing chemicals called **perfluorochemicals** (PFCs) has been widely used since the 1950s in the production of coatings for carpets and fabrics, packaging materials for fast foods, and many other commercial applications.[32] Most familiar to consumers are brand-name products that repel water or stains or sticky food—Scotchgard and Stainmaster (made by 3M) and Teflon and Gore-Tex (made by DuPont).

These products are not themselves made of PFCs; however, manufacturing processes have released PFCs into the environment in waste streams over a long period. In 2000, based on evidence that PFCs were present in its workers' blood and were toxic to laboratory animals, 3M began a 2-year phaseout of its PFC products and informed the US EPA of its concerns.[33,34]*

It has since become clear that at least three chemicals in this group—perfluorooctane sulfonic acid (PFOS), perfluorooctanoic acid (PFOA), and perfluorohexane sulfonic acid (PFHxS)—are widespread in the US population. In a recent analysis of blood samples taken in the 2001–2002 National Health and Nutrition Examination Survey (NHANES) of Americans age 12 or older, these three chemicals were detected in pooled blood samples from each of 24 subgroups defined on age, sex, and ethnicity.[32] In an earlier study, the same scientists reported a low prevalence of exposure to perfluorochemicals among adults in Peru,[32] where products containing these chemicals are less widely used. A recent study in Japan of perfluorochemicals in umbilical cord blood at birth found PFOS in 30 of 30 blood samples and PFOA in 3 of 30 samples,[35] suggesting that prenatal exposure is not uncommon in the urban area studied.

Certainly, PFCs are widely distributed in the natural environment. PFOS has been detected at low levels in the tissues of fish, fish-eating birds (including bald eagles), and marine mammals (including dolphins and seals) at locations in North America, Europe, and the Arctic and Pacific Oceans,[36,37] with higher concentrations reported in animals in more industrialized areas. When 3M scientists discovered PFOS in the livers of *unexposed* laboratory rats, they traced the source to fish meal that was an ingredient in the commercial rat chow.[38]

PFOS and PFOA are not lipophilic, yet they persist in the human body for long periods. In a study of nine retired 3M chemical workers, the mean half-life of PFOS in the body was estimated to be about 8.7 years.[38] PFOS and PFOA tend to bind to protein in the blood and circulate through the body. In fact, they may be repeatedly removed by the liver, excreted into the intestine in bile, and then reabsorbed from the intestine. (This is a well-known toxicokinetic process called enterohepatic cycling.)

---

*In 2005, the EPA obtained a civil administrative penalty of more than $10 million against DuPont for violations of federal laws related to its production of PFOA (US Environmental Protection Agency. *E. I. Dupont De Nemours and Company Settlement 12/14/05*. 2005. Available at: http://www.epa.gov/compliance/resources/cases/civil/tsca/dupont121405.html. Accessed February 11 2007).

Information on the human health effects of PFCs is limited. A simple study of 3M workers in Alabama, in which researchers calculated a standardized mortality ratio, reported a statistically significant 25-fold increased risk of death from bladder cancer among long-time male workers who had been highly exposed to PFCs on the job (3 deaths observed, 0.12 expected based on mortality in the general population of Alabama).[38] In laboratory studies of rodents, prenatal exposure to PFOS and PFOA has been associated with elevated mortality and reduced growth.[39] In addition, PFOS exposure has been associated with reduced levels of circulating thyroid hormone in rodents.[39]

In light of the health concerns around perfluorochemicals, some have questioned the wisdom of using consumer products that are manufactured using these chemicals.[40] DuPont's Teflon and Gore-Tex are still made using PFOA; Teflon is potentially of concern because it is used to coat cookware, which is used to prepare food at high temperatures. DuPont's position is that the quantities of PFOA that might be present in Teflon are too minute to be of concern under normal conditions of use,[41] and the US EPA agrees that current information "does not indicate that the routine use of household products poses a concern."[42]

Ozone-Depleting Chemicals

Yet another group of synthetic organic chemicals can affect human health indirectly, by depleting the stratospheric ozone layer. As noted in Chapter 2, this layer of more concentrated ozone in the stratosphere absorbs some of the ultraviolet radiation in sunlight, protecting people and other animals from extremes of ultraviolet radiation.

As described earlier (see the sidebar titled "About the Electromagnetic Spectrum" in Section 4.2), ultraviolet radiation is a type of electromagnetic radiation (energy traveling through space in the form of waves). The shorter the wavelength of electromagnetic radiation, the higher its energy. Radiation in the ultraviolet range is conventionally classified according to wavelength as UV-A (longest), UV-B, and UV-C (shortest). The shortest-wavelength, highest-energy UV-C radiation is ionizing—that is, it has enough energy to knock an electron out of orbit. Fortunately, UV-C radiation in sunlight is the most effectively screened out by the stratospheric ozone layer, even in its depleted state. UV-B and UV-A radiation are not ionizing, but they do cause biological harm—specifically, skin cancer—via a different biological mechanism. Both UV-A and UV-B are less effectively screened out by stratospheric ozone than is UV-C radiation.

Depletion of the Stratospheric Ozone Layer

Oxygen exists in three forms—as a single atom (O), as the familiar oxygen molecule (O_2) that animals use for respiration, and as ozone (O_3). In the stratosphere, all three forms are present in a state of dynamic equilibrium, such that ozone is constantly being created and destroyed. Certain chemicals, including chlorine—which is naturally present in the stratosphere at low concentrations—are involved on the destruction side of the equation.

In the era of synthetic organic chemicals, human beings have created large quantities of synthetic chemicals containing chlorine. When long-lasting chlorine-containing gases are released to the air, they accumulate in the troposphere, and over time are transported by air movements to the stratosphere, where they take on a more chemically reactive form.[43] This infusion of reactive chlorine upsets the natural balance in stratospheric chlorine chemistry, and the result is a net loss of ozone. The loss of stratospheric ozone has been more extreme over the South Pole (creating the "ozone hole") because of its unique weather conditions. Eventually, reactive chlorine gases are transported back to the troposphere, where they are removed from the atmosphere by precipitation.[43]

The predominant cause of stratospheric ozone depletion has been a family of chemicals called chlorofluorocarbons (CFCs), a subgroup of halocarbons that contain chlorine, fluorine, and carbon in different combinations. These chemicals have been used mainly as refrigerants in air conditioners, as blowing agents in the creation of foam products, and as propellants in aerosol spray products. CFCs seemed the perfect chemicals: They have many uses; they are nontoxic and odorless; they are not flammable or corrosive; and they are chemically stable, producing no toxic breakdown products. Yet precisely because CFCs are chemically stable, they last for many years in the lower atmosphere, with some eventually moving into the stratosphere. Two chlorinated solvents, carbon tetrachloride and methyl chloroform, play a lesser role in ozone depletion, as do some brominated compounds. Unfortunately, the ozone-depleting halocarbons also act as minor greenhouse gases.

Health Effects of Ultraviolet Radiation

A large volume of epidemiologic research shows that three types of skin cancer—basal cell carcinoma, squamous cell carcinoma, and malignant melanoma—are associated with exposure to the sun,[44] although some specifics about the mechanism of carcinogenesis remain unclear. Both squamous cell carcinoma and basal cell carcinoma originate in cells of the outer skin layer, the epidermis—squamous cells are the most superficial cells, and basal cells are deeper in the epidermis. Malignant melanoma is a cancer of melanocytes, cells in the skin that produce pigment (melanin).

Squamous and basal cell carcinoma are much more common than malignant melanoma, but malignant melanoma is far more fatal. For example, each year in the United States there are about 800,000 to 900,000 new cases of basal cell carcinoma, and about 200,000 to 300,000 new cases of squamous cell carcinoma, but only about 60,000 new cases of malignant melanoma. Yet malignant melanoma accounts for about 8,000 deaths per year, compared to 1,000 to 2,000 deaths from nonmelanoma skin cancers combined.[45]

Fair skin color is a risk factor for all three types of skin cancer, especially for malignant melanoma.[44] The effect of sun exposure is also reflected in incidence patterns of squamous and basal cell cancer: Incidence is higher at lower (sunnier) latitudes, and these cancers occur more frequently on exposed parts of the body.[44] High exposure to sunlight early in life appears to pave the way for later skin cancer.

Cancer is not the only health effect associated with exposure to ultraviolet radiation. Exposure of the eyes to ultraviolet radiation in sunlight is associated with an increased risk of cataracts.[46] The World Health Organization estimates that up to 20% of cataracts worldwide are attributable to exposure to ultraviolet radiation[47]—a risk that could be substantially reduced with relatively simple preventive measures. Finally, exposure to UV radiation can suppress the functioning of the immune system, making people more susceptible to infectious diseases.[48]

In view of all these hazards of exposure to natural ultraviolet radiation, it is important to remember that UV radiation also triggers the synthesis of vitamin D, an essential nutrient, in the skin. In this way, exposure to sunlight is healthful, and overprotection from the sun, especially in higher-latitude locations, can deprive the body of a natural source of vitamin D.

5.2 Toxic Metals

As a group, metals—elements that are shiny, are solid at room temperature (mercury is an exception), can be melted or formed using heat, and conduct electricity and heat—have proven extremely useful to human beings. Among the 30 or more metals that are routinely used in modern industry, 6 are described here (lead, mercury, arsenic, cadmium, chromium, beryllium), chosen for their substantial public health impacts.* Of these metals, two—lead and mercury—were discussed earlier in the context of fossil fuels. All but beryllium have high atomic weights and are commonly known as heavy metals.

Lead

As described in Chapter 4, lead has profound impacts on the neurological development of the fetus, infant, and young child, and the use of an organic lead compound, tetra-ethyl lead, in gasoline caused widespread public exposure. In the industrialized countries today, most adult exposure to lead occurs in occupational settings and is exposure to inorganic lead. Lead smelter workers, for example, are exposed to inorganic lead (see **Figure 5.4**), although the acute awareness of lead's toxicity has led to generally effective controls on exposure in the United States and other industrialized countries today. Workers in demolition activities, on the other hand, may have uncontrolled exposures to lead without knowing it.[49]

Inorganic lead has central nervous system effects—on memory and attention, for example—and chronic exposure can also damage peripheral nerves, causing symptoms known as "wrist drop" and "foot drop."[49,50] Exposure to inorganic lead also causes renal toxicity, high blood pressure, and miscarriage and stillbirth.[49,50]

Mercury

As described in Chapter 4, elemental (metallic) mercury present in coal, when released into the environment, can be converted to an organic form, methylmercury, which bioaccumulates in ecosystems and to which people are exposed mainly from eating fish. Most manufacturing workers' exposures are to either elemental mercury or inorganic mercury compounds (in which

---

*Information about arsenic, cadmium, chromium, and beryllium comes mostly from three sources, which provide many of the same specifics: Grandjean P. Health significance of metal exposures. In: Wallace RB, Doebbeling BN, eds. *Maxcy-Rosenau-Last Public Health and Preventive Medicine.* New York, NY: Appleton & Lange; 1998. Goyer RA. Toxic effects of metals. In: Klaasen CD, ed. *Casarett and Doull's Toxicology: The Basic Science of Poisons.* New York, NY: McGraw-Hill; 1996. US Agency for Toxic Substance and Disease Registry. *ToxFAQs for Arsenic, ToxFAQs for Cadmium, ToxFAQs for Chromium,* and *ToxFAQs for Beryllium.* All available at: http://www.atsdr.cdc.gov/toxfaq.html.

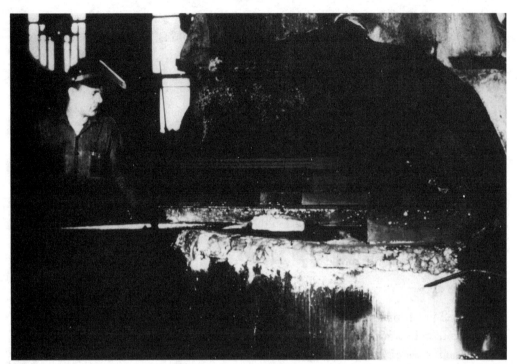

FIGURE 5.4   A laborer works with molten metal in a lead smelting plant in Cincinnati, Ohio, at mid-20th century. *Source*: Reprinted courtesy of CDC Public Health Image Library. ID# 9527. Content providers: CDC/Barbara Jenkins. Available at: http://phil.cdc.gov/phil/details.asp. Accessed August 21, 2007.

elemental mercury is combined with elements other than carbon). High-level inhalation exposure to mercury causes characteristic effects including excitability, delirium, and hallucinations.[51] In the 19th and early 20th centuries, this set of symptoms was familiar in hatters—makers of gentlemen's felt hats—who used inorganic mercury (specifically, mercuric nitrate) in processing the felt. This syndrome was brought vividly to life in the Mad Hatter of Lewis Carroll's *Alice in Wonderland*.

Arsenic

Though arsenic may be most familiar as an acute poison, in fact it is widespread in the earth's crust. Its local abundance in the earth varies widely, and in some areas is great enough to contaminate groundwater to a level that affects health. In some areas of northern New England, for example, groundwater is naturally high in arsenic. In Bangladesh, where there has been an effort in recent decades to reduce people's consumption of sewage-tainted surface waters by switching to deep groundwater, it has become clear that some groundwater contains arsenic at concentrations high enough to cause acute health effects. For a time, arsenic was used in the United States in a preservative (copper chrominated arsenic) for pressure-treated wood—in decks and play structures, for example—but this practice has been phased out for residential uses.

Arsenic is released into the ambient environment mostly by metal smelters (especially copper smelters), by the burning of coal, and in tannery wastes. Arsenic is also an ingredient in pesticides that were widely used in the past, though much less commonly today. Workers in smelters or tanneries are exposed to arsenic, and neighbors of industrial facilities or hazardous waste sites may also be exposed. Arsenic has neurotoxic effects, and chronic exposure to arsenic is associated with skin cancer (basal and squamous cell carcinoma) and cancers of the lung, liver, bladder, kidney, and prostate. IARC classifies arsenic in Group 1 (carcinogenic to humans).

Cadmium

Cadmium, which often occurs with zinc or lead in the earth's crust, is widespread in the environment, largely as a result of air pollution from the mining and smelting of these metals. Cadmium is used in metal plating and is present in the wastes of this industry. Workers in the mining, smelting, or metal-plating industries, among others, can be exposed to cadmium, as can those who live near industrial facilities or hazardous waste sites.

Exposure to cadmium is associated with chronic obstructive pulmonary disease and chronic kidney disease; the latter may cause skeletal changes causing extreme bone pain—an unusual condition known by its Japanese name, *itai-itai* ("ouch-ouch") because of an outbreak in Japan during the 1940s. Cadmium exposure has been clearly associated in epidemiologic studies with lung cancer. IARC classifies cadmium and cadmium compounds in Group 1 (carcinogenic to humans).

Chromium

Chromium occurs in several different forms. Chromium-III (trivalent chromium) is a common form and an essential trace nutrient; chromium-VI (hexavalent chromium) is rare in nature but more used in industry, and is highly toxic. Chromium-VI is produced in industrial processes including chrome plating, leather tanneries, and preserving of wood (in copper chrominated arsenic, as noted earlier). Workers in these facilities, as well as people living near hazardous waste sites, can be exposed. Hexavalent chromium damages the skin and has been linked to lung cancer. IARC classifies chromium-III in Group 3 (not classifiable as to carcinogenicity to humans) and chromium-VI in Group 1 (carcinogenic to humans).

Beryllium

Most exposure to beryllium occurs in the workplace; unlike the other metals described here, beryllium is not a common metal. It is extremely strong and lightweight and is used mainly in high-tech industries. Beryllium has been used to make fluorescent light bulbs; today it is used mainly in the space and aircraft industries. Occupational exposure to beryllium can lead to acute or chronic lung disease, as well as lung cancer. Chronic beryllium disease is a debilitating lung condition that bears some resemblance to lung diseases caused by dust and fibers, with scarring of lung tissue and severely impaired breathing. IARC classifies beryllium and beryllium compounds in Group 1 (carcinogenic to humans).

5.3 Nanotechnology

Nanoparticles, also called **nanomaterials**, are engineered particles less than 100 nanometers in diameter. That is, nanoparticles are in the same size range as the air pollutants known as ultra-fine particulates (0.1 microns = 100 nanometers). **Nanotechnology** takes advantage of the fact that the physical and chemical properties of a given material are often different on a nanoscale, opening the door to a new world of products made from many different substances, including carbon-based materials and various metals. These technologies are being developed for indus-trial processes and a range of medical applications, including imaging methods, anti-cancer therapies, and drug delivery systems.[52] The use of nanotechnology in consumer products is also increasing rapidly and being marketed enthusiastically. For example, companies now advertise nanoscale titanium dioxide as an ingredient of sunscreens and other cosmetics, and nanosilver as an antibacterial agent in socks and slippers—and even in an antibacterial coating on food and water bowls for pets.

Because nanotechnology is so new, the health effects of nanoparticles have not yet been ex-tensively studied. However, because engineered nanoparticles are similar to the more-studied ultrafine particles from environmental sources, it is reasonable to anticipate that they may have some similar health effects.[52] Like ultrafine particulates in air pollution, nanoparticles penetrate deep into the lungs and can pass through the alveolar wall into the general circulation, perhaps making normal host defenses ineffective.[53] Because of the large surface-area-to-volume ratio of these tiny particles, they are considered highly reactive and likely to induce an inflammatory re-sponse, with the potential to cause health effects throughout the body.[53,54] Finally, some com-mercial nanoparticles are nano*tubes* that could be more toxic because of their long, thin shape.[53] In sum, a great deal is yet to be learned about the health effects of nanoparticles—but what is known about inhalation exposure, dermal uptake, and systemic health effects suggests that some caution is warranted in adopting this new technology.

5.4 Physical Hazards

As described in Sections 5.1 and 5.2, industry creates and uses a range of synthetic organic chemicals and metals, which present hazards to workers, the general population (nearby or far-away), and even users of industry's products. In addition, several physical hazards are most prominent in the workplace, though some also affect people outside the occupational setting:

- Airborne fibers and dusts
- Mechanical hazards that cause physical injury
- Excessive noise, causing hearing loss and other health effects
- Shift work that exposes workers to light during the nighttime hours

Fibers and Dusts

As described in Chapter 4, the term *particulate*, as used in environmental health, embraces not only irregularly shaped particles or dusts (classified by size as idealized spheres), but also long, thin fibers; and *fibrosis* is a general term for scarring of the lungs in response to a physical irritant, with the formation of excessive fibrous tissue and a loss of flexibility that impairs breathing. Although the general population is exposed to particles from the burning of fossil fuels, it is workers who have typically sustained the highest exposures to particles and fibers. As noted previously, miners are commonly exposed to naturally occurring silica (quartz) dust in the earth's crust, and coal miners are also exposed to coal dust. Asbestos fibers and cotton dust, described here, are also important respiratory hazards to workers, and the public has some exposure to asbestos in building materials and various products.

Asbestos Fibers and Synthetic Substitutes

Asbestos is a mineral fiber that is insulating, durable, and noncombustible. As a result, it has been widely used in building insulation and in products, such as brake linings, where resistance to combustion is essential. Asbestos has been known for centuries, but it was only in the 20th century that it began to be mined on a large scale. There are three major types of asbestos—chrysotile, amosite, and crocidolite asbestos—and other minor types. Large deposits of asbestos are located in South Africa, Canada, and elsewhere around the world.

Exposure to asbestos became widespread during the 20th century, and its effects have been experienced in an ever-widening circle that begins with miners who extract asbestos from the earth. Workers have been exposed in industries that manufacture asbestos products—making brake linings or insulation products to be used in buildings, for example. Other workers have been exposed by using asbestos products on the job: auto repair workers, construction workers, and shipbuilding workers, among others. In the past, it was common for workers to carry fibers home on their clothing and bodies, exposing their families.

By the late 1800s, it was known that exposure to asbestos damaged the lungs, and by 1930 the term **asbestosis** was being used in medical journals to describe a debilitating **fibrotic lung disease**.[55] By the 1940s and 1950s, asbestosis was well known to the Johns-Manville Company and other companies that manufactured asbestos, although they concealed this information from both workers and government.[55] This deception culminated in a tangle of litigation and bankruptcies in the 1960s and 1970s.

Today asbestos is well documented as a cause not only of asbestosis, but also of lung cancer and mesothelioma. The lung cancer risks of asbestos exposure and cigarette smoking are synergistic—that is, the risk of exposure to both together is greater than the sum of their individual risks.[56] Long, thin asbestos fibers penetrate deep into the lungs, reaching the alveoli, and some even pass through lung cells to penetrate the chest cavity. Similarly, ingested fibers can ultimately reach the abdominal cavity. Asbestos fibers that escape the lungs or gastrointestinal tract can cause **mesothelioma**, a cancer of the pleura (the membranes that coat the outsides of the chest organs and the inside of the chest cavity) or the peritoneum (a similar membrane in the abdominal cavity). Mesothelioma is caused almost exclusively by exposure to asbestos,[57] and for this reason it is considered virtually a marker of exposure to asbestos—in public health terms, a **sentinel illness**. Mesothelioma is nearly always fatal.

More than 30 years after the first regulation of asbestos, deaths from its signature illnesses, asbestosis and mesothelioma, continue to rise, as shown for asbestosis in **Figure 5.5**. In 1999,

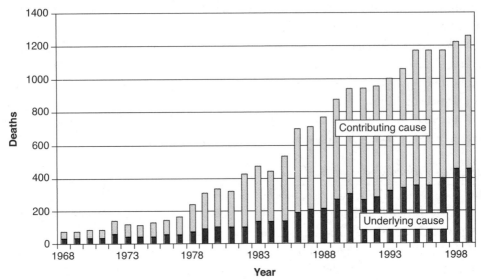

FIGURE 5.5 Annual deaths in the United States 1968–1999 with asbestosis as underlying or contributing cause. *Data from*: US Centers for Disease Control and Prevention. *Work-Related Lung Disease Surveillance Report 2002*, 2002. Available at http://www.cdc.gov/niosh/docs/2003-111/2003-111.html. Accessed April 12, 2008.

about 2500 deaths from mesothelioma were reported in the United States.[58] Asbestos-related lung cancer, though less fatal than mesothelioma, is more common.[56]

Although the regulation of asbestos lagged behind the medical understanding of its hazards, controls have been in place since the 1970s in the United States (see Section 5.7), as well as in other industrialized nations. Sadly, the manufacture of asbestos products has shifted to lower-income countries, where researchers project that more than 1 million asbestos-related deaths may occur; a movement to ban asbestos has recently gained a toehold in India.[59,60]

Various man-made mineral fibers, including fiberglass, glass wool, and ceramic fibers, have replaced asbestos in most uses since the health hazards of asbestos became clear. IARC has categorized various such fibers in Group 2B (possibly carcinogenic to humans) or Group 3 (not classifiable as to carcinogenicity to humans).[6]

Cotton Dust

Historically, cotton mill workers in the industrialized countries were exposed to high concentrations of airborne cotton dust, resulting in a fibrotic lung disease called **byssinosis**, also known as **brown lung**. Despite its name, cotton dust may contain not only cotton but also bacteria or fungi, soil, pesticides, and other contaminants. Byssinosis was well known to workers in the 1940s, but US industry downplayed the health risks and resisted regulation for many years; exposures declined dramatically after a federal standard was promulgated in 1978. In 1995, the Occupational Safety and Health Administration (OSHA) estimated that

35,000 individuals alive at that time were disabled by byssinosis;[61] CDC estimates that byssinosis was the underlying cause, or a contributing cause, of about 10 deaths per year in 2000–2002.[62]

In lower-income countries that are undergoing rapid industrialization, byssinosis is a common occupational disease. In China, for example, a cumulative incidence of byssinosis of 24% over a 15-year period (1981–1996) was documented among textile workers.[63] In India, the prevalence of byssinosis has been estimated at 30% and 38% in two different groups of textile mill workers.[64]

Mechanical Hazards

As just described, workers may be exposed to a range of synthetic organic chemicals, metals, dusts, and fibers. Yet hazards of a mechanical nature are a more visible cause of injury and death on the job. In 2004, for example, 5703 US workers suffered fatal work-related injuries—an overall annual rate of 4.1 fatalities per 100,000 workers. Most injuries are not fatal: In 2004, there were about 700 nonfatal occupational injuries for every death.[65] Some specific occupations with high risk of job-related death are shown in **Table 5.2**.

Three large industrial sectors together accounted for nearly half of all fatal occupational injuries in the United States in 2004: construction (21.5%), transportation and warehousing (14.5%), and agriculture, forestry, and fishing (11.6%). Overall, men are at higher risk of death from occupational injuries than are women: Although men make up 54% of workers, they account for 93% of all deaths from work-related injury.

A breakdown of work-related deaths by manner of death (**Figure 5.6**) shows that the largest share of fatal occupational injuries occurs in transportation incidents. Perhaps surprisingly, violence accounts for 14% of job-related deaths.

Table 5.2 Fatality Rates in Selected Dangerous Occupations, 2004

Occupation	Fatality Rate (deaths per 100,000 workers in 2004)
Logging workers	92.4
Fishermen (and women)	86.4
Structural iron and steel workers	47.0
Refuse collectors	43.2
Farmers and ranchers	37.5
Roofers	34.9
All miners	28.3

Data from: US Department of Labor, Bureau of Labor Statistics, Census of Fatal Occupational Injuries. *National Work-Related Fatality Report, 2004.* Available at: http://www.bls.gov/iif/oshcfoi1.htm. Accessed April 1, 2007.

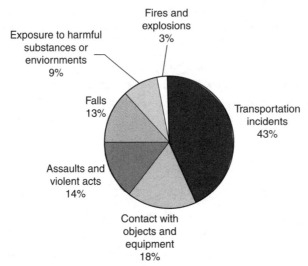

FIGURE 5.6   Breakdown of occupational fatalities in the United States, by manner of death, 2005. *Data from*: US Department of Labor, Bureau of Labor Statistics, Census of Fatal Occupational Injuries. *National Work-Related Fatality Report, 2005.* Available at: http://www.bls.gov/iif/oshcfoil.htm. Accessed April 12, 2008.

Less dramatic than acute outcomes such as deaths and mechanical injuries are the chronic impacts of exposures to vibration or repetitive work. A worker who uses a jackhammer experiences vibration throughout his or her body, but especially in the hands and arms. Over time, such vibration can damage nerves and blood vessels in the fingers, with a loss of strength in the grip.[66] Workers who do repetitive tasks—on a production line or keyboard, for example—may experience musculoskeletal disorders, including tendinitis or carpal tunnel syndrome, in which inflamed tissues press on nerves, causing pain and weakness in the hands.[67] Back pain, which can be related to many different activities, is a common concern among workers.

Noise

Noise is sometimes defined as unwanted sound (see the following sidebar titled "About Sound"), but a more useful definition from the public health perspective is sound that can damage hearing or otherwise harm health. The complexities of the human ear are beyond the scope of this text, but in simple terms, structures in the middle ear and inner ear translate sound from waves in air into vibrations of tiny bones, then into waves in fluid, and finally into nerve impulses. Most loss of hearing through aging and also through exposure to excessive noise occurs through damage to the tiny hair cells in the inner ear that translate physical energy into nerve impulses.

The **volume threshold** (measured in **decibels**) at which sound can be perceived is different at different frequencies; hearing loss appears as an upward shift in the threshold at which sound of

About Sound

Sound is a form of physical energy, like vibration or radiation. Sound energy radiates outward from a source in waves, much as waves spread out when a rock is dropped into water. Sound has two important characteristics—frequency and intensity—and what we perceive as "loudness" has to do with both of these traits. *Frequency* is the number of complete wave cycles per unit of time, and higher frequency corresponds to higher pitch. Frequency is measured in Hertz (Hz; cycles per second). *Intensity* corresponds to the amplitude of the waves (the distance between trough and peak), and greater amplitude corresponds to greater pressure. Intensity is measured in decibels (dB). The decibel scale is logarithmic: A 1-decibel increase in sound represents a 10-fold increase in the intensity of the sound. Because most environmental sounds are made up of many different sound frequencies, composite decibel scales, which weight frequencies in different ways, are used to assess them. The scale most often used in assessing human perception of environmental noise is known as the A-weighted decibel (dBA) scale. The decibel scale measures sound relative to the hearing threshold of a healthy young person.

a certain frequency can be perceived (**threshold shift**). In a hearing test, a tone at a given frequency is produced at increasing volume to establish the decibel level at which a person first perceives it.

It has been known for many years that noise can damage hearing. A person who has a short-term exposure to a very loud noise (such as an exchange of gunfire at close range) may experience a threshold shift—often temporary, but sometimes permanent. A ringing sensation in the ears, known as **tinnitus**, is also common after such an exposure. **Figure 5.7** presents the decibel levels of some common sounds.

Cumulative exposure to noise over a longer period can cause permanent hearing loss. Those who work in noisy environments—from ground crews at airports to rock musicians to those who work with heavy machinery—are at risk of noise-induced hearing loss. A study of occupational noise-induced hearing loss in Michigan found that about 51% of all cases worked in manufacturing, 15% in construction, and 10% in transportation.[68] And noise affects more than just hearing. Occupational exposure to noise has been linked to high blood pressure and to increased secretion of stress hormones known as catecholamines, which initiate the fight-or-flight response.[69,70]

Light during the "Biological Night"

Finally, the International Agency for Research on Cancer recently designated "shift-work that involves circadian disruption" as a Group 2A carcinogen (probably carcinogenic to humans).[71] The term **circadian** refers to the cycles of roughly 24 hours that occur in various physiological

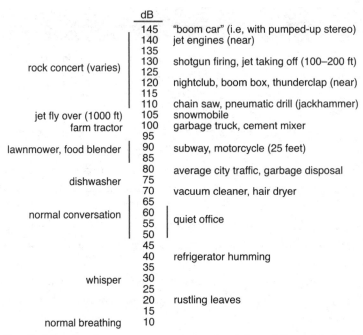

	dB	
	145	"boom car" (i.e, with pumped-up stereo)
	140	jet engines (near)
	135	
rock concert (varies)	130	shotgun firing, jet taking off (100–200 ft)
	125	
	120	nightclub, boom box, thunderclap (near)
	115	
	110	chain saw, pneumatic drill (jackhammer)
jet fly over (1000 ft)	105	snowmobile
farm tractor	100	garbage truck, cement mixer
	95	
lawnmower, food blender	90	subway, motorcycle (25 feet)
	85	
	80	average city traffic, garbage disposal
dishwasher	75	
	70	vacuum cleaner, hair dryer
	65	
normal conversation	60	quiet office
	55	
	50	
	45	
	40	refrigerator humming
	35	
whisper	30	
	25	
	20	rustling leaves
	15	
normal breathing	10	

FIGURE 5.7   Decibel levels of some common sounds. *Adapted from*: National Institute on Deafness and Other Communication Disorders. *Common Sounds*. Available at: http://www.nidcd.nih.gov/staticresources/health/education/teachers/CommonSounds.pdf. Accessed February 7, 2008.

processes, reflecting organisms' adaptations to the fundamental cycle of day and night. IARC's designation was made on the basis of evidence from both studies of the human health effects of working the night shift and studies in laboratory animals exposed to light at night. Taken as a whole, the research links exposure to light at night with suppression of the hormone melatonin (whose production normally peaks during nighttime sleep), leading to increased incidence or growth of tumors, and with the inactivation of certain genes involved in the body's daily time-keeping, resulting in tumor promotion.[71] In some employment sectors, including the health care, manufacturing, mining, transportation, communications, and hospitality sectors, more than 30% of employees work night shifts at least some of the time.[71]

5.5 Asthma-Causing Agents in the Workplace

Certain hazards from each of three groups described earlier—organic compounds, metals, and physical agents such as dusts or fibers—are known as causes of occupational asthma (that is, asthma caused by an exposure at work) among industrial workers. The most common cause of occupational asthma among industrial workers is a set of chemicals called isocyanates.[72] They are used as paint-hardening agents, to which paint sprayers are exposed in various work settings, and also as the raw materials for polyurethane foam and various adhesives and coatings.[73] Metals reported to cause occupational asthma include aluminum (used in soldering) and chromium and nickel (used in electroplating).[72] Wood dust has also been reported as a cause of occupational asthma; those exposed include sawmill workers, carpenters, and workers in the furniture industry.[72]

5.6 Social Disparities in Exposure to Industrial Pollution

A large research literature has shown social disparities in exposure to industrial pollution in the United States: both a greater burden on people of color than on whites, and a greater burden on the poor than on the well-to-do. As described previously, Navajo workers and communities have historically borne the brunt of environmental pollution and occupational hazards associated with US uranium mining. More than half of US coal is mined in two of the country's poorest states, West Virginia and Kentucky.[74-76] Several studies have documented differential exposure of African Americans to industrial hazards. An influential 1975 study of coke oven workers, for example, showed that African American men were more likely to hold undesirable jobs at the top of the oven, and this was reflected in their higher exposures to the hazardous chemicals being driven off as fumes.[77]

Outside the occupational setting, several early studies of social disparities in exposure to environmental hazards, in the 1970s, focused mainly on urban air pollution after the passage of the Clean Air Act in 1970;[78-84] most uncovered both economic and racial disparities. A later nationwide study found that for the 1970–1984 period, poor and nonwhite populations had higher exposures to total suspended particulates, and that the race gap was wider and more consistent than the income gap.[85] Still another analysis focused on interactions between race and poverty, documenting wide disparities in exposure to industrial air pollution between poor nonwhite populations and nonpoor white populations.[86]

Subsequent attention to social disparities in exposure to environmental hazards has focused more on the disposal of hazardous wastes. In the late 1970s, waste oil contaminated with PCBs was illegally dumped along more than 200 miles of roads in several counties in North Carolina. The state, faced with disposing of a large quantity of PCB-contaminated soil, selected a site—over protest—in a locale with high poverty and a mostly African American population. The planned waste site went through, but a North Carolina congressman called for the US General Accounting Office* (GAO) to examine the question of bias in the siting of hazardous waste landfills. The GAO's 1984 report, a seminal document in the nascent social movement for environmental justice, documented that three of the four large offsite hazardous waste landfills in the southeastern states were sited in poor, largely African American communities.[87] The GAO study spurred a nationwide assessment by social activists, published in 1987. This document, also a touchstone of the environmental justice movement, reported that zip codes hosting hazardous waste sites had a higher proportion nonwhite population and, less strikingly, lower income than other zip codes.[88]

---

*The GAO, renamed the General Accountability Office in 2004, is the investigative arm of Congress.

In the wake of these early reports, the last two decades have produced many studies, most documenting a differential burden of active and abandoned hazardous waste sites, industrial pollution, or industrial facilities on poor and nonwhite communities in the United States.[89,90] A recent analysis at a national scale, using spatial methods and census data from both 1990 and 2000, documented a decrease in the proportion of the population made up of people of color, as well as a decline in the proportion of the population living in poverty, with increasing distance from a hazardous waste facility (see **Figure 5.8**).[91]

Today, the continuing movement for environmental justice defines this concept broadly, seeking to redress social inequities in the burden of environmental pollution and industrial facilities, especially unjust burdens on people of color. The concept of environmental justice also includes equitable access to such positive environmental factors as clean water, the cleanup and redevelopment of contaminated industrial sites (sometimes called **brownfields**), or public transportation in urban settings, as well as participation in decision making by government.

With some environmental health risks being shifted to lower-income countries, environmental justice is also a concern on the international scale. As described earlier, the world's lower-income countries are expected to feel the impacts of global climate change more heavily than are the industrialized countries that have generated most of the greenhouse gases to date. Exposures to asbestos and cotton dust, now dramatically decreased in the industrialized coun-

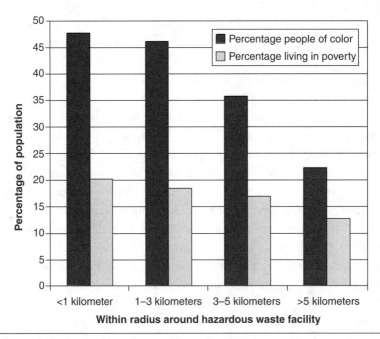

FIGURE 5.8   Demographic disparities in residential proximity to hazardous waste facilities in the United States, 1990. *Data from*: Bullard R, Mohai P, Saha R, Wright B. *Toxic Wastes and Race at Twenty: 1987–2007*: United Church of Christ, Justice and Witness Ministries; 2007: table 3.1. Available at: http://www.ejrc.cau.edu/TWART%20Final.pdf. Accessed April 17, 2008.

tries, are on the upswing in lower-income countries. And some industrialized countries, including the United States, are sending some hazardous wastes overseas for processing. This practice of exporting materials for recycling creates jobs in lower-income countries, but many are hazardous jobs with little or no protection for workers.

For example, **shipbreaking**—the dismantling of oceangoing vessels to obtain scrap metal—now occurs mostly on the shores of India and Bangladesh, where there is a market for scrap metal and its price is kept low by the lack of protections for workers. Approximately 25,000 workers at Chittagong in Bangladesh and about 40,000 at Alang in India manually dismantle ships that are run aground on the beach at high tide (see **Figure 5.9**).[92] In 2000, about 600 to 700 ships were being dismantled annually, and unless worker protections are imposed in these countries, the practice is likely to continue as a steady stream of ships reach retirement age.[92] Workers labor without protective gear and using equipment that is not maintained. They suffer falls and physical injuries and are exposed to noise, heat, explosion, fire, and smoke; asbestos; lead and mercury; organic tin compounds formerly used as antifouling agents in marine paints; PCBs; and dioxins from burning of plastics.[93] It takes about 6 months to take apart a ship by hand, as opposed to about 2 weeks in a mechanized US facility in years past.[92]

In much the same way, many used computers, after being placed in recycling programs by their owners, are sold in batches and end up being manually dismantled by unprotected workers in lower-income countries. (Many more are simply disposed of as trash or stockpiled.) Like the outsourcing of shipbreaking, this practice is driven by the cost of protections for workers in the United States and other industrialized nations. In China, on the other

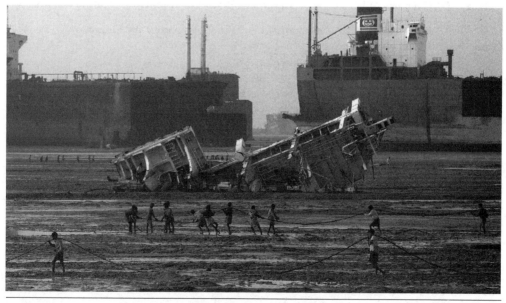

FIGURE 5.9 Manual laborers break down beached ships on the shore of Bangladesh.
© 2008 Pierre Claquin. Used with permission.

hand, entire villages serve as recycling centers—working without protection, men, women, and children sweep out toner, burn wires whose plastic coating releases dioxins, melt away lead solder over small fires, and grind and melt down plastic parts.[94]

As of 2007, the United States had not ratified the Basel Convention on Hazardous Wastes, an international agreement that provides a basis for managing the trade in hazardous wastes. One hundred sixty-nine other nations, including the United Kingdom, Germany, and other European nations, have ratified the convention.

5.7 Regulation of Industrial Pollution

The US regulatory framework for the control of industrial pollution of the environment, including hazards in the industrial workplace, is an amalgam of laws that have been passed, amended, and reamended over a period of decades. It seems most useful to describe this framework by moving "upstream" in a conceptual sense—beginning with provisions that seek to remediate the effects of past practices and ending with approaches that try to head off future hazards. Key elements of the US regulatory framework for industrial pollution appear in **Table 5.3**. This table is the fifth in a series of similar tables that place regulatory provisions within the traditional regulatory domains of environmental health.

Cleanup of Abandoned Hazardous Waste Sites

The law known colloquially as **Superfund** was originally passed in 1980 as the Comprehensive Environmental Response, Compensation, and Liability Act (CERCLA; "circla"), and then

Table 5.3 Overview of US Regulatory Framework for Environmental Health Hazards (5)

Environmental Health Domain	Major Laws and Key Provisions for the Control of Environmental Health Hazards
Biological hazards	Public Health Service Act (PHSA)—development of guidelines for vaccination; use of quarantine or isolation to prevent entry of infectious diseases into the United States; conduct of surveillance and investigation of outbreaks
Air pollution	Clean Air Act (CAA)—ambient standards (NAAQS) for Criteria Air Pollutants; emissions standards for Hazardous Air Pollutants, including mercury; emission allowances for SO_2 (to control acid deposition); removal of lead from gasoline; requirement to sell reformulated gasoline in high-smog areas
Ionizing radiation	Energy Reorganization Act (ERA)—safety requirements for operating nuclear power plants, including licensing, emissions limits, storage of wastes Nuclear Waste Policy Act (NWPA)—requirements to build and regulate a repository for radioactive wastes, including spent reactor fuel Uranium Mill Tailings Radiation Control Act—standards for management of abandoned mill tailings

Table 5.3   *(Continued)*

Environmental Health Domain	Major Laws and Key Provisions for the Control of Environmental Health Hazards
Alternative energy sources	Energy Policy Act (EPAct)—modest supports for alternative energy sources
Hazardous wastes	*Comprehensive Environmental Response Compensation and Liability Act ("Superfund") / Superfund Amendments and Reauthorization Act (CERCLA / SARA)—identify, assess health risks of, and remediate abandoned hazardous waste sites*
	Resource Conservation and Recovery Act (RCRA)—"cradle-to-grave" manifest system for hazardous wastes; standards and permits for hazardous waste storage or disposal facilities; provisions to promote hazardous waste minimization (source reduction) and recycling of hazardous wastes
Occupational health	*Occupational Safety and Health Act (OSHAct)—ambient standards (Permissible Exposure Limits) for workplace air; employers must provide Materials Safety Data Sheets (MSDSs) to workers*
Industrial water pollution	*Clean Water Act (CWA)—ambient standards (Ambient Water Quality Criteria, or AWQC) for about 150 pollutants; technology requirements and permitting system for discharges to ambient water from industry*
Toxic chemicals	*Toxic Substances Control Act (TSCA)—premanufacture notice for new chemicals; EPA can restrict manufacture, distribution, or use if new chemical poses unreasonable risk*
	Emergency Planning and Community Right-to-Know Act (EPCRA)— local and state emergency response commissions; yearly chemical reporting requirements for manufacturing facilities; data available as Toxics Release Inventory; facilities must provide Materials Safety Data Sheets (MSDSs) to local commissions
	Pollution Prevention Act (PPA)—support for source reduction/waste prevention as preferable to treatment or disposal of wastes
Pesticides	
Food supply	
Sewage wastes and community water supply	
Municipal solid waste	
Consumer products	
Environmental noise	

Note: New information appears in italics.

substantially amended in 1986 as the Superfund Amendments and Reauthorization Act (SARA). This legislation was a response to the widespread problem of hazardous wastes originating from inactive or abandoned industrial sites (see **Figure 5.10**). On the basis of the Superfund legislation, US EPA identified abandoned hazardous waste sites and created a national register of such sites, known as the **National Priorities List**.

Superfund created procedures to assess and remediate the pollution at sites, set criteria for identifying parties to be held financially responsible for the site cleanup, and established a fund (the "Superfund") to pay for cleanup if no responsible party could be identified. More fundamentally, however, the Superfund process, by first seeking to hold polluters responsible for cleanup costs, exemplified what is known as the **polluter-pays principle**. This idea, that the parties responsible for pollution should pay for the costs of remediation, has long been supported by an international body, the Organisation for Economic Co-operation and Development (OECD), whose members include the United States and most European countries.

The human health risk posed by each site is estimated based on the health effects of the chemicals that are present and the potential for human exposure, using site risk assessment procedures like those described in Chapter 2. However, the process has been slow and funding variable. As of January 2007, work had been completed at 317 sites and was in process at 1240 sites

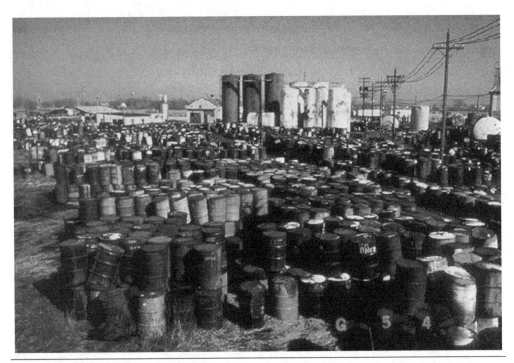

FIGURE 5.10   Drums of toxic wastes litter a Superfund site in this undated photo. *Source*: Reprinted courtesy of CDC Public Health Image Library. ID# 1193. Content provider: CDC. Available at: http://phil.cdc.gov/phil/details.asp. Accessed September 26, 2007.

(although EPA considers the physical construction work complete at 1010 of these sites). Sixty-one additional sites have been proposed for the list.[95]

Controls on Current Discharges of Manufacturing Wastes

Several major laws govern the handling of manufacturing wastes—most of which are liquids or sludges—as they are produced. Although fumes and dusts to which workers are exposed on the job are not usually referred to as "wastes," they are indeed by-products of the industrial process, and in this sense the workplace itself is an outlet for the wastes of industry. Thus, this section first describes regulation of workplace hazards, and then regulation of industrial discharges to the ambient environment.

Hazards in the Workplace

Federal requirements for the protection of workers stem from the Occupational Safety and Health Act (OSHAct) of 1970, which requires employers to provide a workplace free of "recognized hazards that are causing or are likely to cause death or serious physical harm" to employees.[96] This requirement is known as the general duty clause of the OSHAct. The law applies to most employers, but excludes the self-employed as well as family-only farm operations. The law created the Occupational Safety and Health Administration (OSHA), responsible for promulgating and enforcing occupational health standards, and the National Institute for Occupational Safety and Health (NIOSH), responsible for conducting research on occupational hazards and recommending standards to OSHA.

Federal regulations include protections for a wide range of mechanical hazards. Other than mechanical injuries, inhalation exposures are generally of greatest concern in the workplace—and steps to reduce inhalation exposures often reduce the potential for dermal and incidental ingestion exposures. Most occupational health standards take the form of a **Permissible Exposure Limit** (PEL), which is a concentration of a contaminant in air. OSHA can set up to three distinct types of PELs for a given contaminant: the PEL-TWA (time-weighted average) is a limit on the time-weighted average concentration over an 8-hour work day; the PEL-STEL (short-term exposure limit), intended to protect workers at times when the concentration exceeds the overall daily average, is a limit on the concentration to which workers can be continuously exposed during a 15-minute period (with no more than four such periods per day); and the PEL-C (ceiling) is a concentration that must not be exceeded at any time during the workday.[97]

NIOSH produces three types of Recommended Exposure Limits (RELs) that parallel the OSHA standards: the REL-TWA, REL-STEL, and REL-C. Although Recommended Exposure Limits published by NIOSH are intended as the basis for Permissible Exposure Limits promulgated by OSHA, historically there has been little connection between the two. OSHA, under pressure to set standards quickly after both agencies were established in 1970, promulgated in 1971 a set of interim PELs. Most of these standards were drawn directly from values published in 1968 by the American Council of Governmental Industrial Hygienists (ACGIH), a private organization made up mostly of industrial hygienists in state and local governments. In ACGIH terminology, these concentrations were known as **Threshold Limit Values** or TLVs and, like PELs and RELs, were designated as time-weighted averages, short-term exposure limits, or ceilings.

The process designed to replace these interim standards with permanent ones has essentially failed. In 1989, OSHA, which had promulgated only a few Permissible Exposure Limits since 1971, again adopted as PELs a large group of updated TLVs published by ACGIH—despite the fact that NIOSH had by this time published Recommended Exposure Limits for numerous chemicals. OSHA's 1989 PELs were challenged by the AFL-CIO and vacated by a federal court in 1992, leaving in force the 1971 PELs.[97]

The OSHAct requires that an employer first attempt to meet an exposure limit by modifications of the work environment, such as ventilation. Only if changes to the workspace prove inadequate to meet the PEL can workers be required to wear **personal protective equipment**, such as goggles, ear protectors, or respirators. Workers sometimes find such gear hot, clumsy, and uncomfortable, and do not always comply with a requirement to use it—and this is part of the rationale for requiring modifications to the work environment as a first step.

Although mechanical hazards often are obvious to workers, chemical hazards may not be. For this reason, workers are specifically guaranteed access to information about chemical hazards in their workplace. Manufacturers and importers of chemicals must produce a summary of their health effects in the form of a **Materials Safety Data Sheet (MSDS)**, and employers are required to provide MSDSs to workers, along with training about the chemicals to which they are exposed.

Discharges to Air

Industrial discharges of chemicals to outdoor air are regulated under the Clean Air Act. As described in Chapter 4, ambient standards have been established for a small set of Criteria Air Pollutants related mostly to the burning of fossil fuels, and emissions standards have been set for a few Hazardous Air Pollutants, which are less common but more toxic. Emissions from manufacturing facilities are subject to both sets of standards.

Discharges to Water

Today's Clean Water Act began life in 1948 under another name and has been shaped by major amendments in 1977 and 1987. The Clean Water Act originally had a lofty goal: to reduce discharges to all US lakes and rivers to zero by 1985. Although this goal was not achieved, any discharge into a body of water does require a permit. The provisions of the Clean Water Act deal not only with industrial pollution but also with municipal sewage wastes (see Chapter 7). Drinking water quality is regulated under a separate law.

Under the Clean Water Act, the federal government sets standards for ambient water quality and also sets general requirements for the technology that must be used to achieve the standards. To date, Ambient Water Quality Criteria have been set for about 150 pollutants, including both metals and synthetic organic compounds. The law requires that industrial facilities use "best available technology" to control discharges. The regulatory framework of the Clean Water Act distinguishes between two types of water pollution sources. The first type, called a **point source**, releases waste at a specific location—for example, a pipe releasing industrial wastes, or a sewage outfall. Pollution sources that cover a large area, such as abandoned coal mines, agricultural fields, or paved urban areas, are called **nonpoint sources**.

State governments set permit requirements for individual discharge sources such that the federal ambient standards and technology requirements will be met, and the states also enforce compliance with the permits. This permitting system is known as the National Pollutant Discharge Elimination System.

Land Disposal of Hazardous Wastes

Hazardous wastes from industry are regulated under the Resource Conservation and Recovery Act (RCRA; "rickra"), originally passed in 1976 and substantially amended in 1984. RCRA's provisions apply to any waste that meets one of two criteria. It may be a type of waste listed by EPA: wastes from a set of common industrial or manufacturing processes; wastes from specific industries, including petroleum refining and the manufacture of pesticides; and certain unused chemical products when they are discarded (again, pesticides are an example). Or, it may meet the definition of a **hazardous waste** under RCRA: any waste that is ignitable, corrosive, reactive (chemically unstable), or toxic, as defined by specific criteria.

RCRA incorporates two major types of requirements. First, it requires the use of a "cradle-to-grave" manifest system to track hazardous wastes from the point of generation through transportation and ultimately storage, treatment, or disposal. Second, RCRA sets performance standards and permitting procedures for **hazardous waste landfills** and underground storage tanks. RCRA also includes provisions to promote the recycling of hazardous wastes and to minimize their production. RCRA's provisions deal not only with industrial wastes, but also with municipal trash (see Chapter 7). In addition, RCRA regulates the underground disposal of liquid wastes, mostly from the oil and gas industries, by injection into deep wells.

Regulation of the Manufacture and Use of Chemicals in Industry

In principle, the 1976 Toxic Substances Control Act (TSCA; "tosca") empowers EPA to control toxic chemicals in production and commerce, before they become wastes—a precautionary approach. A company that wishes to manufacture a new chemical must submit a notice to EPA 90 days before manufacturing begins, providing information about the chemical and its effects. EPA can gather additional information about the chemical, and can then restrict the manufacture, distribution, or use of a chemical if it poses an "unreasonable" risk to human health or the environment relative to the benefits it offers.

However, as of 2006, EPA had required testing of fewer than 200 of the 20,000 chemicals added to the TSCA inventory since the law went into effect and had issued regulations to limit or ban the production of only five chemicals (or sets of chemicals).[98] There were about 62,000 chemicals in the original TSCA inventory. The painfully slow pace of this work reflects the challenge of showing unreasonable risk while respecting the confidentiality of companies' trade secrets, as well the inadequacy of EPA's resources for this task. TSCA predates the boom in nanotechnology, and EPA is currently working to develop rules that will clarify whether a given nanomaterial is to be considered a new or existing chemical substance under the law.

The Montreal Protocol on Substances that Deplete the Ozone Layer was opened for signatures in 1987 and went into force in 1989. Subsequent modifications, most recently in 1999, have made controls more stringent. A total of 191 nations, including the United States and other industrialized countries as well as lower-income countries, have now signed the agreement. The Montreal Protocol sets country-specific limits on the production and consumption of specific chemicals in terms of their ozone-depleting potential. The total atmospheric burden of ozone-depleting gases has begun to decline, and substantial recovery of stratospheric ozone is expected by about the middle of the 21st century.[43] Despite the long timeline for success, the Montreal Protocol is a working example of international cooperation on an environmental health problem of global scale.

Securing the Public's Right to Information About Chemical Wastes

When Superfund—a law to clean up after corporations that disposed of toxic wastes irresponsibly—was reauthorized in 1986, it incorporated the Emergency Planning and Community Right-to-Know Act (EPCRA; this act is Title III of the Superfund Amendments and Reauthorization Act). The provisions of this act are not about the control of industrial releases to the environment; rather, the act simply calls for information about industrial releases to be made public. The idea was that such openness would lead to more responsible behavior by manufacturers simply by breaking the cycle of corporate secrecy and disregard for consequences.

Passage of the law was motivated partly by a 1984 industrial accident at a Union Carbide plant in Bhopal, India, in which thousands of people living near the plant were killed or horribly injured by the release of a cloud of highly toxic gas, methyl isocyanate. This event sparked public outrage against Union Carbide both in the United States and internationally, increasing awareness of both industrial pollution and social disparities in its impacts.

EPCRA called for the establishment of state and local emergency response commissions to plan for, and respond to, industrial accidents. The law also set up ongoing reporting requirements for manufacturing facilities. Each year, facilities must report (in pounds) the quantities of a long list of chemicals that they have released to air or water, or placed on land, or transferred offsite. This database, called the **Toxics Release Inventory** (**TRI**), is publicly available online in a format that allows the user to generate custom reports—for example, reports of quantities of specific chemicals released by specific facilities. EPCRA also requires manufacturers to submit Materials Safety Data Sheets (which, as already described, must be made available to workers) to the local emergency response commission. The requirement on manufacturers to go public with information about the makeup and toxicity of their wastes has led to reductions in waste streams.

Pollution Prevention and the Precautionary Principle

As the preceding discussion makes clear, US environmental laws and regulations have had many positive effects on public health. Though most US environmental regulation does not reflect a truly precautionary stance, the Pollution Prevention Act of 1990 explicitly provided support for **source reduction** (also called **waste prevention**), naming it as the preferred option over treating or disposing of wastes. The act also created the Office of Pollution Prevention in the US Environmental Protection Agency, which manages pollution prevention initiatives and encourages the same in private corporations.

It is sometimes less difficult politically to move forward with precautionary approaches at a more local level. For example, some local and state governments have set regulations to encourage the substitution of water-based cleaning methods for dry-cleaning methods that use solvents. A 2006 California law sets regulations and mechanisms to reduce the state's production of greenhouse gases.[99] Another California measure, passed in 1986, requires the governor to publish annually a list of chemicals known to cause cancer or reproductive toxicity—and also requires California businesses to give warnings if their activities cause exposures to these chemicals.[100] Massachusetts passed a law in 1989, the Toxics Use Reduction Act, that sets goals for reducing the production of toxic wastes in the state, and, as a means to achieve this goal, requires firms to document plans to use less toxic chemicals in industrial processes.[101] The state's Toxic Use Reduction Institute has been effective in promoting the use of alternatives to toxic chemicals through research and training services and technical support.

Study Questions

1. What are the distinctive features of the workplace as a setting where exposure to chemical and physical hazards occurs?
2. In your view, do people have a right to both a healthy working environment and a healthy ambient environment? Why?
3. Look up some recent articles on nanotechnology in the mainstream print and electronic media, and evaluate how these articles present the potential benefits and health risks of this new technology.
4. What factors do you see as barriers to a more precautionary approach in the development and use of new technologies in the United States?
5. In your view, do the industrialized nations have any special responsibility in the international trade in hazardous wastes?

References

1. US Department of Labor, Bureau of Labor Statistics. *Employment Situation Summary June 2006*. Available at: http://www.bls.gov/news.release/empsit.nr0.htm. Accessed July 10, 2006.
2. US Environmental Protection Agency. *Profile of the Petroleum Refining Industry, 1995*. Available at: http://www.epa.gov/oecaerth/resources/publications/assistance/sectors/notebooks/petrefsn.pdf . Accessed April 15, 2008.
3. Zogorski JS, Carter JM, Ivahnenko T, Lapham W, Moran MJ, Rowe BL, et al. *The Quality of Our Nation's Waters: Volatile Organic Compounds in the Nation's Ground Water and Drinking-Water Supply Wells, 2006*. Available at: http://pubs.usgs.gov/circ/circ1225/. Accessed April 15, 2008.
4. US Environmental Protection Agency. *Profile of the Textile Industry, 1997*. Available at: http://www.p2pays.org/ref/01/00506.pdf. Accessed April 15, 2008.

5. Levin SM, Lilis R. Organic compounds. In: Wallace RB, Doebbeling BN, eds. *Maxcy-Rosenau-Last Public Health and Preventive Medicine*. Stamford, Conn: Appleton & Lange; 1998:509–542.

6. International Agency for Research on Cancer. *Agents Reviewed by the IARC Monographs*. Available at: http://monographs.iarc.fr/ENG/Classification/Listagentsalphorder.pdf. Accessed February 4, 2007.

7. Shea KM. Pediatric exposure and potential toxicity of phthalate plasticizers. *Am Acad Pediatr*. 2003;111(6):1467–1474.

8. Schettler T. Human exposure to phthalates via consumer products. *Int J Androl*. 2006; 29:134–139.

9. US Centers for Disease Control and Prevention. *Third National Report on Human Exposure to Environmental Chemicals, 2005*. Available at: http://www.cdc.gov/exposurereport/pdf/thirdreport.pdf. Accessed April 15, 2008.

10. Sharpe RM. The "oestrogen hypothesis"—where do we stand now? *Int J Androl*. 2003;26:2–15.

11. Swan S, Main K, Liu F, Stewart S, Kruse R, Calafat A, et al. Decrease in anogenital distance among male infants with prenatal phthalate exposure. *Environ Health Perspect*. 2005;113(8):1056–1061.

12. National Institute of Environmental Health Sciences. *Endocrine Disruptors, 2006*. Available at: http://www.niehs.nih.gov/health/topics/agents/endocrine/docs/endocrine.pdf. Accessed April 15, 2008.

13. vom Saal F, Hughes C. An extensive new literature concerning low-dose effects of bisphenol A shows the need for a new risk assessment. *Environ Health Perspect*. 2005; 113(8):926–933.

14. Grun F, Watanabe H, Zamanian Z, Maeda L, Arima K, Cubacha R, et al. Endocrine-disrupting organotin compounds are potent inducers of adipogenesis in vertebrates. *Mol Endocrinol*. 2006;20(9):2141–2155.

15. Stahlhut S, van Wijngaarden E, Dye T, Cook S, Swan S. Concentrations of urinary phthalate metabolites are associated with increased waist circumferences and insulin resistance in adult US males. *Environ Health Perspect*. 2007;115(6):876–882.

16. Commoner B. *Making Peace with the Planet*. New York, NY: Pantheon Press; 1990.

17. US Agency for Toxic Substances and Disease Registry. *Toxicological Profile for Polychlorinated Biphenyls (PCBs), 2000*. Available at: http://www.atsdr.cdc.gov/toxprofiles/tp17.html. Accessed February 7, 2007.

18. Webster TF, Commoner B. Overview: the dioxin debate. In: Schecter A, Gasiewicz T, eds. *Dioxins and Health*. 2nd ed. New York, NY: John Wiley and Sons; 2003:1–53.

19. US Environmental Protection Agency. *Hudson River PCBs: Background and Site Information*. Available at: http://www.epa.gov/hudson/background.htm. Accessed February 5, 2007.

20. US Department of Veterans Affairs. *Become Familiar with Agent Orange and the Health of our Vietnam Veterans*. Available at: http://www1.va.gov/agentorange/. Accessed February 8, 2007.

21. US Environmental Protection Agency. *NPL Site Narrative for Times Beach Site.* Available at: http://www.epa.gov/superfund/sites/npl/nar833.htm. Accessed February 7, 2007.

22. Bernard A, Hermans C, Broeckaert F, De Poorter G, De Cock A, Houins G. Food contamination by PCBs and dioxins. *Nature.* 1999;401:231–232.

23. Baccarelli A, Pesatori AC, Consonni D, Mocarelli P, Patterson D, Caporaso NE, et al. Health status and plasma dioxin levels in chloracne cases 20 years after the Seveso, Italy accident. *Br J Dermatol.* 2005;152:459–465.

24. Yoshimura T. Yusho in Japan. *Ind Health.* 2003;41:139–148.

25. BBC News. *Deadly Dioxin Used on Yushchenko.* December 17, 2004. Available at: http://news.bbc.co.uk/2/hi/europe/4105035.stm. Accessed February 8, 2007.

26. US Environmental Protection Agency. *Polychlorinated Biphenyls (PCBs): Health Effects of PCBs.* Available at: http://www.epa.gov/pcb/pubs/effects.html. Accessed February 5, 2007.

27. de Wit CA. An overview of brominated flame retardants in the environment. *Chemosphere.* 2002;46:583–624.

28. Hale RC, La Guardia MJ, Harvey E, Mainor TM. Potential role of fire retardant-treated polyurethane foam as a source of brominated diphenyl ethers to the US environment. *Chemosphere.* 2002;46:729–735.

29. Alcaee M, Wenning RJ. The significance of brominated flame retardants in the environment: current understanding, issues and challenges. *Chemosphere.* 2002;46:579–582.

30. McDonald TA. A perspective on the potential health risks of PBDEs. *Chemosphere.* 2002;46:745–755.

31. Meironyte D, Noren K, Bergman A. Analysis of polybrominated diphenyl ethers in Swedish human milk. A time-related trend study, 1972–1997. *J Toxicol Environ Health.* 1999;Part A(58):329–341.

32. Calafat AM, Kuklenyik Z, Caudill SP, Reidy JA, Needham LL. Perfluorochemicals in pooled serum samples from United States residents in 2001 and 2002. *Environ Sci Technol.* 2006;40(7):2128–2134.

33. Edgerly M. *Toxic Traces.* Available at: http://news.minnesota.publicradio.org/features/2005/02/22_edgerlym_3mscience/. Accessed February 10, 2007.

34. US Environmental Protection Agency. Perfluorooctanoic Acid (PFOA), Fluorinated Telomers; Request for Comment, Solicitation of Interested Parties for Enforceable Consent Agreement Development, and Notice of Public Meeting. *Federal Register.* 2003;68(73):18626–18633.

35. Inoue K, Okada F, Ito R, Kato S, Sasaki S, Nakajima S, et al. Perfluorooctane sulfonate (PFOS) and related perfluorinated compounds in human maternal and cord blood samples: assessment of PFOS exposure in a susceptible population during pregnancy. *Environ Health Perspect.* 2004;112(11):1204–1207.

36. Giesy JP, Kannan K. Global distribution of perfluorooctane sulfonate in wildlife. *Environ Sci Technol.* 2001;35(7):1339–1342.

37. Kannan K, Koistinen J, Beckmen K, Evans T, Gorzelany JF, Hansen KJ, et al. Accumulation of perfluorooctane sulfonate in marine mammals. *Environ Sci Technol.* 2001;35(8):1593–1598.

38. Organisation for Economic Co-operation and Development. *Co-operation on Existing Chemicals: Hazard Assessment of Perfluorooctane Sulfonate (PFOS) and Its Salts: Joint Meeting of the Chemicals Committee and the Working Party on Chemicals, Pesticides and Biotechnology; 2002.* Available at: http://www.oecd.org/dataoecd/23/18/2382880.pdf. Accessed April 15, 2008.

39. Lau C, Butenhoff JL, Rogers JM. The developmental toxicity of perfluoroalkyl acids and their derivatives. *Toxicol Appl Pharmacol.* 2004;198:231–241.

40. Environmental Working Group. *Canaries in the Kitchen.* Available at: http://www.ewg.org/reports/toxicteflon. Accessed February 3, 2007.

41. DuPont. *PFOA.* Available at: http://www2.dupont.com/PFOA/en_US. Accessed February 10, 2007.

42. US Environmental Protection Agency. *Perfluorooctanoic Acid (PFOA) and Fluorinated Telomers.* Available at: http://www.epa.gov/oppt/pfoa/index.htm. Accessed February 8, 2007.

43. World Meteorological Organization. *Scientific Assessment of Ozone Depletion: 2006.* 2006. Available at: http://www.esrl.noaa.gov/csd/assessments/2006/executivesummary .html. Accessed April 15, 2008.

44. Armstrong BK, Kricker A. The epidemiology of UV induced skin cancer. *J Photochem Photobiol.* 2001;B(63):8–18.

45. American Cancer Society I. *How many People Get Nonmelanoma Skin Cancer?* Available at: http://www.cancer.org/docroot/CRI/content/CRI_2_2_1X_How_many_people_get_ nonmelanoma_skin_cancer. Accessed February 12, 2007.

46. McCarty CA. A review of the epidemiologic evidence linking ultraviolet radiation and cataracts. *Dev Ophthal.* 2002;35:21–31.

47. World Health Organization. *Health Effects of UV Radiation.* Available at: http://www .who.int/uv/health/en/. Accessed February 7, 2008.

48. Sleijffers A, Garssen J, Van Loveren H. Ultraviolet radiation, resistance to infectious diseases, and vaccination responses. *Methods.* 2002;28:111–121.

49. Gidlow DA. Lead toxicity. *Occup Med.* 2004;54(2):76–81.

50. Papanikolaou NC, Hatzidaki EG, Belivanis S, Tzanakakis GN, Tsatsakis AM. Lead toxicity update. A brief review. *Med Sci Monitor.* 2005;11(10):RA329–RA336.

51. US Agency for Toxic Substances and Disease Registry. *Toxicological Profile for Mercury, 1999.* Available at: http://www.atsdr.cdc.gov/toxprofiles/tp46.html . Accessed April 15, 2008.

52. Gwinn M, Vallyathan V. Nanoparticles: health effects—pros and cons. *Environ Health Perspect.* 2006;114(12):1818–1825.

53. Witschi, HR, Pinkerton, KE, VanWinkle, LS, Last, JA. Toxic Responses of the Respiratory System. Chapter 15 in: Klaassen, CD (ed.). *Casarett & Doull's Toxicology: The Basic Science of Poisons* (7th ed.). New York: McGraw-Hill Medical, 2008.

54. Delfino R, Sioutas C, Malik S. Potential role of ultrafine particles in associations between airborne particle mass and cardiovascular health. *Environ Health Perspect.* 2005; 113(8):934–946.

55. Ozonoff D. Failed warnings: asbestos-related disease and industrial medicine. In: Bayer R, ed. *The Health and Safety of Workers: Case Studies in the Politics of Professional Responsibility*. New York, NY: Oxford University Press; 1988.

56. Case BW. Asbestos, smoking, and lung cancer: interaction and attribution. Occup Environ Med. 2006;63(8):507–508.

57. Robinson BW, Musk AW, Lake RA. Malignant mesothelioma. *Lancet.* 2005;366:397–408.

58. US Centers for Disease Control and Prevention. *Work-Related Lung Disease Surveillance Report 2002*. 2002. Available at: http://www.cdc.gov/niosh/docs/2003-111/2003-111 .html. Accessed April 15, 2008.

59. Joshi TK, Gupta RK. Asbestos-related morbidity in India. *Int J Occup Environ Health*. 2003;9(3):249–253.

60. Joshi TK, Gupta RK. Asbestos in developing countries: magnitude of risk and its practical implications. *Int J Occup Med Environ Health*. 2004;17(1):179–185.

61. US Occupational Safety and Health Administration. *Fact Sheet: Cotton Dust*. Available at: http://www.osha.gov/pls/oshaweb/owadisp.show_document?p_id=169&p_table= FACT_SHEETS. Accessed February 7, 2008.

62. National Institute for Occupational Safety and Health. *Work-Related Lung Disease (WoRLD) Surveillance System*. Available at: http://www2.cdc.gov/drds/WorldReportData/ SectionDetails.asp?SectionTitleID=4. Accessed February 7, 2008.

63. Wang X-R, Eisen EA, Zhang H-X, Sun B-X, Dai H-L, Pan L-D, et al. Respiratory symptoms and cotton dust exposure; results of a 15 year follow up observation. *Occup Environ Med.* 2003;60:935–941.

64. Saiyed HN, Tiwari RR. Occupational health research in India. *Ind Health*. 2004; 42:141–148.

65. US Bureau of Labor Statistics. *Workplace Injuries and Illnesses in 2004*. 2005. Available at: http://www.bls.gov/news.release/archives/osh_11172005.pdf. Accessed April 15, 2008.

66. Canadian Centre for Occupational Health and Safety. *What Are the Health Effects of Hand-Arm Vibration?* Available at: http://www.ccohs.ca/oshanswers/phys_agents/ vibration/vibration_effects.html. Accessed February 21, 2007.

67. Canadian Centre for Occupational Health and Safety. *Work-Related Musculoskeletal Disorders (WMSDs)*. Available at: http://www.ccohs.ca/oshanswers/diseases/rmirsi.html ?print. Accessed February 21, 2007.

68. National Institute for Occupational Safety and Health. *Worker Health Chartbook*. Fig 2-31. Available at: http://www2.cdc.gov/NIOSH-Chartbook/imagedetail.asp?imgid=73. Accessed February 19, 2007.

69. Stansfeld SA, Matheson MP, Mark P. Noise pollution: non-auditory effects on health. *Br Med Bull.* 2003;68:243–257.

70. Matheson MP, Stansfeld SA, Haines MM. The effects of chronic aircraft noise exposure on children's cognition and health: 3 field studies. *Noise Health*. 2003;5(19):31–40.

71. Straif K, Baan R, Grosse Y, Secretan B, El Ghissassi F, Bouvard V, et al. Carcinogenicity of shift-work, painting, and fire-fighting. *Lancet: Oncol.* December 2007;8:1065–1066.

72. Mapp CE. Agents, old and new, causing occupational asthma. *Occup Environ Med.* 2001;58:354–360.

73. US Occupational Safety and Health Administration. *Safety and Health Topics: Isocyanates.* Available at: http://www.osha.gov/SLTC/isocyanates/index.html. Accessed February 20, 2007.

74. US Census Bureau. *Bituminous Coal Underground Mining: 2002.* 2002. Available at: http://www.census.gov/prod/ec02/ec0221i212112.pdf. Accessed April 15, 2008.

75. US Census Bureau. *Bituminous Coal and Lignite Surface Mining: 2002.* 2002. Available at: http://www.census.gov/prod/ec02/ec0221i212111.pdf. Accessed April 15, 2008.

76. US Census Bureau. *Anthracite Mining: 2002.* 2002. Available at: http://www.census.gov/prod/ec02/ec0221i212113.pdf. Accessed April 15, 2008.

77. Mazumdar S, Redmond C, Sollecito W, Sussman N. An epidemiological study of exposure to coal tar pitch volatiles among coke oven workers. *J Air Pollution Control Assoc.* 1975;25(4):382–389.

78. Kruvant WJ. People, energy, and pollution. In: Newmand DK, Day D, eds. *The American Energy Consumer.* Cambridge, Mass: Ballinger; 1975:125–167.

79. Zupan JM. *The Distribution of Air Quality in the New York Region.* Baltimore, Md: Johns Hopkins University Press for Resources for the Future; 1975.

80. Burch WR. The peregrine falcon and the urban poor: some sociological interrelations. In: Richerson P, McEvoy J, eds. *Human Ecology: An Environmental Approach.* Belmont, Calif: Duxbury Press; 1976.

81. Anderson SJ, Gardner BW, Moll BJ, Tribble GLI, Webster TF, Wilson KR, et al. Correlation between air pollution and socioeconomic factors in Los Angeles County. *Atmos Environ.* 1978;12:1531–1535.

82. Freeman AMI. Distribution of environmental quality. In: Kneese AV, Bower BT, eds. *Environmental Quality Analysis.* Baltimore, Md: Johns Hopkins University Press; 1972.

83. Berry BJL. *The Social Burdens of Environmental Pollution: A Comparative Metropolitan Data Source.* Cambridge, Mass: Ballinger Publishing Company; 1977.

84. Asch P, Seneca JJ. Some evidence on the distribution of air quality. *Land Econ.* 1978; 54(3):278–297.

85. Gelobter M. Toward a model of environmental discrimination. In: Bryant B, Mohai P, eds. *Race and the Incidence of Environmental Hazards: A Time for Discourse.* Boulder, Colo: Westview Press; 1992.

86. Perlin SA, Wong D, Sexton K. Residential proximity to industrial sources of air pollution: interrelationships among race, poverty, and age. *J Air Waste Man Assoc.* 2001;51:406–421.

87. US General Accounting Office. *Siting of Hazardous Waste Landfills and Their Correlation with Racial and Economic Status of Surrounding Communities.* Washington, DC: US General Accounting Office; 1983.

88. Chavis BF, Lee C. *Toxic Wastes and Race in the United States.* United Church of Christ, Commission for Racial Justice; 1987.

89. Mohai P, Bryant B. Environmental injustice: weighing race and class as factors in the distribution of environmental hazards. *Univ Colo Law Rev.* 1992;63:921–932.

90. Ringquist E. Assessing evidence of environmental inequities: a meta-analysis. *J Policy Analysis Man.* 2005;24(2):223–247.

91. Bullard R, Mohai P, Saha R, Wright B. *Toxic Wastes and Race at Twenty: 1987–2007.* United Church of Christ, Justice and Witness Ministries; 2007. Available at: http://www .ejrc.cau.edu/TWART%20Final.pdf. Accessed April 15, 2008.

92. Bailey PJ. *Discussion Paper: Is There a Decent Way to Break Up Ships?* International Labour Organization; 2000. Available at: http://www.ilo.org/public/english/dialogue/ sector/papers/shpbreak/index.htm Accessed April 15, 2008.

93. US Occupational Safety and Health Administration. *OSHA Fact Sheet: Shipbreaking.* 2001. Available at: http://www.osha.gov/OshDoc/data_MaritimeFacts/shipbreaking-fact sheet.pdf. Accessed April 15, 2008.

94. Testimony of Sheila Davis, Executive Director, Silicon Valley Toxics Coalition to the Senate Subcommittee on Superfund and Waste Management, Environment and Public Works Committee, July 26, 2005.

95. US Environmental Protection Agency. *National Priorities List: NPL Site Totals by Status and Milestone as of January 14, 2007.* Available at: http://www.epa.gov/ superfund/sites/npl/index.htm. Accessed February 20, 2007.

96. US Occupational Safety and Health Administration. *OSH Act of 1970.* Available at: http://www.osha.gov/pls/oshaweb/owadisp.show_document?p_table=OSHACT&p_ id=3359. Accessed February 7, 2008.

97. Lippman, M, Cohen, BS, Schlesinger, RB. *Environmental Health Science: Recognition, Evaluation, and Control of Chemical and Physical Health Hazards.* Oxford: Oxford University Press, 2003.

98. US General Accounting Office. *Actions Are Needed to Improve the Effectiveness of EPA's Chemical Review Program.* [Statement of John B. Stephenson]. 2006. Available at: http://www.gao.gov/new.items/d061032t.pdf. Accessed April 15, 2008.

99. California Air Resources Board. *Greenhouse Gas Emissions Inventory and Mandatory Reporting.* Available at: http://www.arb.ca.gov/cc/ccei.htm. Accessed February 22, 2007.

100. California Office of Environmental Health Hazard Assessment. *Proposition 65.* Available at: http://222.oehha.ca.gov/prop65/p65faq.html. Accessed February 22, 2007.

101. Massachusetts Toxics Use Reduction Institute. *An Overview of TURA.* Available at: http://turadata.turi.org/WhatIsTURA/OverviewOfTURA.html. Accessed February 21, 2007.

Producing Food

Learning Objectives

After studying this chapter, the reader will be able to:

- Define or explain the key terms throughout the chapter

- Describe typical crop production practices in the United States, including the use of chemical pesticides, and their environmental and human health impacts

- Discuss integrated pest management as an alternative to pesticide use

- Discuss the benefits and potential health risks of genetically modified crop plants

- Describe typical livestock production practices in the United States and their implications for human health

- Explain the rendering process and its link to bovine spongiform encephalopathy and variant Creutzfeldt-Jakob disease

- Describe the contribution of agriculture to global climate change

- Describe modern fishing practices, risks to workers, and the future of fishing

- Characterize the modern food supply system and contrast it with the movement toward organic farming and locally grown food

- Describe key approaches to managing the public health risks associated with modern methods of food production

- Describe the US regulatory framework for managing the public health risks associated with food production

US agriculture has seen sweeping changes over the past half century. Farms have become fewer and larger, and many large farms are now owned by institutional entities (including family-held corporations), as shown in **Table 6.1**. From 1950 to 2002, the number of farms in the United States declined from 5.4 million to 2.1 million; over the same period, the average size doubled from 216 acres to 441 acres.[1,2] Still, almost 90% of farms, and two-thirds of farm acreage, are owned by individuals or families.

In the past, most farmers both grew crops and kept animals, and these two aspects of farming were integrated. Crop wastes were fed to cows or pigs, for example, and the animals' manure was used as fertilizer on crops. Today, especially on larger farms, the production of crops and the production of animals are essentially segregated processes. Fields are treated with synthetic chemicals, and animals grown for meat are fed a modified diet to speed their growth and shorten the period before they are slaughtered. For the same reason, and also for the sake of efficiency in meat production, cattle, swine, and chickens spend much of their lives in confinement at specialized facilities, sometimes called factory farms.

Fishing, too, has changed—the fishing industry now runs on diesel and uses sophisticated electronic methods to locate fish and sophisticated mechanical means to catch them. A substantial share of the catch is now processed on factory ships at sea.

Table 6.1   Key Characteristics of US Farms, 2002

Owned By	Percentage of Farms	Percentage of Total Farm Acreage	Average Size (acres)
Individual or family	89.7	66.3	326
Partnership	6.1	15.6	1130
Family-held corporation	3.1	10.6	1485
Other corporation	0.3	1.0	1315
Other entity*	0.8	6.6	3845

*Other cooperative, estate or trust, institutional, etc.

Data from: US Department of Agriculture, National Agricultural Statistics Service. *Census of Agriculture*. 2002:Table 58. Available at: http://www.nass.usda.gov/census/census02/volume1/us/index1.htm. Accessed April 19, 2008.

This chapter describes in some depth the environmental health impacts of modern practices for the production of crops (Section 6.1) and livestock rearing (Section 6.2), including their impacts on global climate (Section 6.3). The chapter presents more briefly the modern fishing industry (Section 6.4) and then touches on some of the complexities of the modern food supply (Section 6.5) and the contrasting movement toward organic farming (Section 6.6). The chapter closes with a description of how we regulate food and the activities that produce it (Section 6.7).

6.1 Modern Crop Production Practices

The landscape of US agriculture has changed dramatically since the mid-20th century. There is little variety in the crops grown—a relatively small number of varieties of wheat, for example, are now planted on a very large scale. Similarly, crops are grown mostly in monoculture: immense swaths of land planted in wheat, for example, rather than the traditional checkerboard of smaller fields planted with different crops, or even two crops interspersed in the same field. The production process relies heavily on chemical inputs, such as pesticides and fertilizers, and on the use of heavy machinery.

Today, agricultural production in the breadbasket is also subsidized by the use of fossil fuels to power machinery: An estimated 90 liters of diesel fuel and 56 liters of gasoline were used in the production of a hectare of corn (about 2.5 acres) in the United States in 2000.[3] The same hectare of corn also required 2.1 kilograms of herbicides and 0.15 kilograms of insecticides,[3] mostly derived from petroleum.

Finally, in the Great Plains, agriculture has been increasingly subsidized by tapping the fossil groundwater of the deep Ogallala Aquifer that underlies the region. This confined aquifer is sandwiched between impermeable layers of rock and is no longer being replenished by precipitation. During the 19th century, westward-moving settlers of European origin gradually displaced the native inhabitants of the Great Plains, and in fact an entire ecosystem, converting grassland into farms. This massive disturbance of the plains ecosystem, in combination with a cyclical drought, led to the dust bowl conditions of the 1930s. To a great extent, it was deep wells into the Ogallala Aquifer that later converted the dustbowl into a breadbasket. Unfortunately, this deep groundwater is not a renewable resource on the time scale of human planning.

This section describes key aspects of crop production as practiced in the United States today:

- The use of chemical fertilizers, partly a consequence of the separation of crop cultivation and livestock rearing
- The use of synthetic chemical pesticides to kill insects and weeds, and the effects of these chemicals on human health
- Integrated pest management, an alternative approach to pest control that has a modest presence in US agriculture

- The use of crop plants that have been genetically modified in various ways, a practice that has shown some clear short-term benefits but whose broader ecological consequences are largely unknown
- The consumption of water for irrigation to a degree that is not environmentally sustainable
- Physical injuries to farmers and farmworkers from the highly mechanized production of field crops

Nitrate Contamination from the Intensive Use of Fertilizers

Nitrogen is an essential nutrient for plants, and nitrogen-containing fertilizers are widely used in agriculture. The nitrogen in fertilizers is in the form of nitrates (NO_3^-), which are highly soluble in groundwater and are readily taken up by plants. However, more fertilizer is applied than can be used by crops, and the result is elevated nitrate concentrations in groundwater. This ultimately contributes to global climate change (see Section 6.3); more immediately, if this groundwater is used as a source of drinking water, the elevated nitrate concentrations can have a direct human health impact.

Young infants who consume well water contaminated with nitrates may be made ill, usually when the well water is used to make infant formula. Nitrates, converted to nitrites either before or after ingestion, change hemoglobin in the bloodstream into a form that cannot carry oxygen. The resulting condition is called **methemoglobinemia**; with inadequate oxygen in the blood, the child takes on a bluish color. The condition, also called **blue baby syndrome**, can be fatal.

Methemoglobinemia affects hundreds of infants in the United States each year.[4] In the mid-1990s, it was estimated that 40,000 infants under 6 months of age in the United States were living in homes with private well water contaminated by nitrates,[5] mostly in rural areas. To date, epidemiologic studies do not indicate that maternal exposure to nitrates during pregnancy causes increased risk of spontaneous abortion, low birthweight, or birth defects.[6]

Use of Chemical Pesticides

A **pesticide** is a chemical used to kill pests. But what is a pest? "Pest" is not a biological grouping, but rather a cultural one. Essentially, a **pest** is any animal or plant that interferes with human well-being or interests—by causing disease or discomfort in people, or in the animals that we care about; or by competing with people for resources (for example, locusts that eat crops, or weeds that steal nutrients from them); or by destroying property (for example, termites or mold); or even simply by being where it is not wanted (for example, a dandelion in a manicured lawn).

Many of these problems are important, and so we try to kill pests, or at least control them, using chemical poisons. Some pesticides are naturally occurring substances, but most are synthetic chemicals. These synthetic pesticides are unique among environmental health hazards in that they are developed specifically to be toxic, and then are deliberately spread widely and repeatedly in the environment. When we think of the beneficial effects or health hazards of pesticides, we generally think about the effects of the **active ingredient**—the chemical that is intended to kill a pest. However, other chemicals are also present in pesticides, as agents to help disperse the active ingredient, for example. In the United States in 2001, some 888 billion pounds of pesticides (that is, active ingredient) were used, about three-quarters of this amount in agriculture.[7]* Agricultural fields are nonpoint sources of environmental pollution: Agricultural chemicals are spread across fields, and thus enter the environment over a large area.

Types of Pesticides

Within the broad group of chemical pesticides, subgroups are defined according to the type of pest they are intended to kill: **insecticides** (used against not only insects, but also arachnids), **herbicides** (used against plant pests, commonly called **weeds**), **fungicides** (used to control fungi), and **rodenticides** (used to kill rodents). In 2001, herbicides made up 46% by weight of pesticide active ingredient used in the United States; insecticides, 9%; and fungicides, 6%.[7] The remaining 39% comprises a number of smaller uses, including rodenticides, nematicides (used against worms), molluscicides, soil fumigants, and poisons used against fish and birds.

Insecticides

Many insecticides are used against vectors of human or animal disease—most important, mosquitoes, but also flies, fleas, ticks, or lice, for example. In recent years, a pest that is merely a nuisance—the bedbug—has been experiencing a resurgence in urban apartment buildings in Boston, New York, and other US cities. Although bedbugs do not cause disease, they cause enough discomfort and annoyance to be disruptive. Insecticides are also widely used in agriculture, to keep pests from consuming crops intended as food for people or farm animals. Some insecticides poison a pest when it eats the poison; others poison on contact.

In the 19th century, inorganic compounds containing toxic metals were widely used as insecticides, and some are still used today. This group includes lead arsenate, in which arsenic is the active ingredient and lead reduces the burning of foliage; Bordeaux mixture (copper sulfate and lime), in which copper is the active ingredient; and Paris Green (copper and arsenic) in which both ingredients are toxic. Kerosene and oil have also been used as insecticides—when poured into standing water, they form a film on the water's surface that suffocates insect larvae.

Natural botanical pesticides have also been used for many years, along with inorganic pesticides. For example, **pyrethrum** is a pesticide extracted from chrysanthemums, and rotenone is extracted from the roots and stems of certain woody shrubs and vines.

The first generation of synthetic organic insecticides were the **organochlorine insecticides**, also known as **chlorinated hydrocarbon insecticides**. The best-known chemical in this group is DDT (**dichloro-diphenyl-trichloroethane**), whose insecticidal properties were discovered in 1939 by a

---

*Although pesticides are the most familiar agricultural chemicals, they are not the only ones. A number of chemicals, some of which are also used as pesticides, are used as plant growth regulators. The basic purpose of these chemicals is to produce a crop that is amenable to mechanical harvesting. Thus, for example, chemicals may be used to slow down or speed up growth; to dry out leaves or even defoliate plants; to open cotton bolls; or to keep the straw of a grain crop short and strong (Sorensen M, Danielsen V. Effects of the plant growth regulator, chlormequat, on mammalian fertility. *Int J Androl.* 2006;29:129–133. Ball S, Glover C. *Defoliants, Dessicants, and Growth Regulators Used on New Mexico Cotton.* Las Cruces: New Mexico State University; 1999).

Swiss research chemist, Paul Müller, who was awarded the Nobel Prize for this discovery in 1948. At the time, Müller considered DDT's chemical stability in the environment to be a positive feature in an insecticide.[8] DDT was used extensively by the US military during World War II to protect troops against disease (**Figure 6.1**). After the war, DDT—widely viewed as a wonder chemical—was sprayed in communities to control disease and sprayed in fields to kill agricultural pests. By the mid-1950s, more than 25 organochlorine pesticides were in use in the United States (see **Figure 6.2**), including chlordane, aldrin, dieldrin, and heptachlor.

The organochlorine pesticides are nerve toxins: They disrupt the central nervous system, causing convulsions and death. However, their acute toxicity to people is very low, and for this reason it was many years before they were considered a human health problem. These chemicals are very persistent in the environment, are lipophilic, bioaccumulate in fatty tissue, and biomagnify in the food chain. In fact, it was their toxicity in wildlife that was ultimately brought to light, largely through the efforts of Rachel Carson, a naturalist and author of the famous 1962 book, *Silent Spring*. Among other effects, Carson described how DDT softened the shells of bald eagles' eggs, preventing these birds from breeding successfully. The bald eagle is a carnivorous bird at the top of

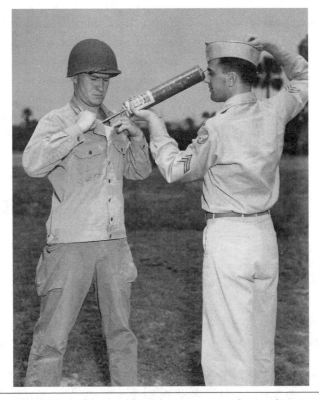

FIGURE 6.1   A World War II–era soldier demonstrates the application of DDT to US Army personnel. *Source*: Reprinted courtesy of CDC Public Health Image Library. ID 7384. Content provider: CDC. Available at: http://phil.cdc.gov/phil/details.asp. Accessed August 21, 2007.

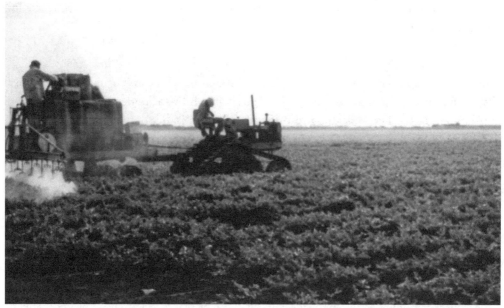

FIGURE 6.2   Agricultural workers use a tractor and sprayer to apply pesticides to crops in the 1950s. *Source*: Reprinted courtesy of CDC Public Health Image Library. ID 8982. Content provider: CDC/Barbara Jenkins (NIOSH)/Dick Robbins. Available at: http://phil.cdc.gov/phil/details.asp. Accessed August 21, 2007.

the food chain, and also a national symbol of the United States. The effects of DDT on the bald eagle caused a national outcry, and the pesticide was banned in the United States in 1972.

DDT and several other organochlorine pesticides are now banned in the United States and other industrialized nations; as noted in Chapter 5, the Stockholm Convention also restricts these chemicals. But DDT is still used for mosquito control in some lower-income countries. This practice reflects the very different view of DDT's risks and benefits in countries that are burdened with high rates of malaria and cannot afford newer, more expensive pesticides. In 2006, the World Health Organization approved the use of DDT for targeted indoor spraying of walls and roofs—killing mosquitoes that land there—both in houses and in shelters for domestic animals.[9] As of 2006, 14 countries in sub-Saharan Africa were using DDT in this targeted way.[9]

The second generation of synthetic organic insecticides were the **organophosphates**, originally developed as nerve gases to be used in war. Like the organochlorines, the organophosphates disrupt the central nervous system, causing convulsions and death at high doses. However, these chemicals are not persistent in the environment. Their acute toxicity to people varies widely: For example, parathion is highly toxic to humans, whereas malathion, familiar as a home garden pesticide, is much less toxic. The organophosphates were quickly followed by the **carbamates**, which have a similar chemical action, but low short-term toxicity in people. Sevin is an example of a carbamate pesticide widely used for gardens and mosquito control.

Most recently, synthetic insecticides called **pyrethroids** (that is, pyrethrum-like chemicals) have been developed; this group includes permethrin and resmethrin. These pesticides have low acute toxicity to people and are used in some household pesticides, mosquito repellents, and head lice treatments.

Herbicides

Synthetic herbicides have a wide range of chemical structures with considerable overlap in toxic effects, and thus it is simpler to distinguish these chemicals by their effects on different classes of plants. A **selective herbicide** kills broad-leaved plant species, but not plants in the grass family. In agriculture, this distinction means that a selective herbicide applied to a field of grain kills weeds, but not the crop; similarly, a selective herbicide applied to a lawn kills only the weeds. Atrazine is the most widely used selective herbicide in US agriculture.[7]

The first synthetic herbicide was 2,4-D, a selective herbicide introduced shortly after World War II and still used in many over-the-counter weed killers. As described in Chapter 5, 2,4-D was one of two major ingredients in the defoliant Agent Orange, used by US forces in the Vietnam War (the other, 2,4,5-T, was contaminated with dioxin). In this context, a selective herbicide was used to kill larger plants—trees and bushes—that provided cover to combatants on the ground, without wiping out all plant life.

In contrast, a **nonselective herbicide** kills all types of plants. Such an herbicide might be broadly applied, for example, in a railroad yard, to prevent workers from slipping on weeds. Or a nonselective herbicide can be applied in a targeted fashion to individual weeds in a lawn—Roundup is a nonselective herbicide used in this way. Before the 1950s, waste oils, salt, and arsenicals were used to kill plants nonselectively.

In the modern context, some genetically modified crop plants (discussed later) have been designed to be resistant to particular nonselective herbicides—specifically so that nonselective herbicides can be used in agriculture. For example, Monsanto Corporation, which produces the nonselective herbicide Roundup, has also developed Roundup-Ready genetically engineered soybeans, designed and marketed to be planted in fields treated with Roundup.

Other Pesticides

Fungicides can be critical in the protection of fruits and also of crops grown in wet conditions. Various inorganic compounds were widely used as fungicides before the era of synthetic organic compounds, and indeed Bordeaux mixture is still in use. However, today there are many synthetic organic fungicides, of different chemical types, often used in combination. For example, fungicides are commonly used in both cranberry bogs and apple orchards.

Most rodenticides are baits containing a synthetic anticoagulant; warfarin is the most commonly used active ingredient. When a rodent consumes the bait, the poison causes massive internal bleeding, resulting in death.

Limitations of Pesticides

In simple terms, pesticides are effective at killing their targets. However, their broader effectiveness is limited in two key ways, both reflecting the fact that communities of plants and pests are not static, but rather dynamic.

First, just as some bacteria are resistant to a specific antibiotic, some pests may have a genetic makeup that confers resistance to a specific pesticide. At the first application of the pesticide, the resistant organisms survive; most susceptible individuals die, though some may escape exposure somehow and survive. As a result of this differential mortality in the two groups, the resistant organisms make up a larger proportion of the population *after* the pesticide application than they did beforehand. Thus, as the population continues to multiply, its makeup changes: The selection effect is magnified through repeated pesticide applications until most or all of the surviving population carries the genetic trait that confers resistance to the pesticide. Because many pests have life spans much shorter than our own, the development of such pesticide resistance can occur rather quickly in response to this sudden change in the pests' environment— a speeded-up version of evolutionary survival of the fittest.

A second limitation on the effectiveness of pesticides is that the crop and the target pest— the pest that eats the crop and which the farmer wishes to eliminate using pesticides—do not exist in isolation (as in **Figure 6.3a**). Rather, they are part of an ecosystem in which the pest species eats—or is eaten by—other species (as in **Figure 6.3b**).

These connections cause ripple effects from the use of pesticides. For example, the pesticide may kill not only the target pest, but also another species (such as species X in Figure 6.3b)—a bystander in the war between the farmer and the target pest—which happens to serve the beneficial purpose of eating the target pest. If the population of species X is suddenly reduced, the target pest population can rebound dramatically for a time in the absence of its natural predator, a phenomenon called **target pest resurgence**.[10] Similarly, the target pest itself may not only eat the crop, but also serve the beneficial purpose of eating yet another insect (species Y in Figure 6.3b), a pest that also eats the crop. In this situation, wiping out the target pest population allows the population of the pest species Y to explode—and the crop still gets eaten. This phenomenon, in which there is surge in the population of the secondary pest, is known as a **secondary pest outbreak**.[10]

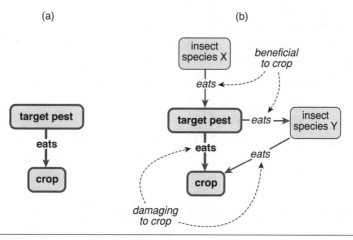

FIGURE 6.3 Unintended effects of the use of pesticides.

Human Health Effects of Pesticides

It is particularly difficult to study the chronic health effects of specific pesticides in people, mostly because it is difficult to assess exposure accurately. Many people who work with pesticides—such as farmers or pesticide applicators—are exposed to a changing mix of chemicals, and they may not know what chemicals they are using. (Organochlorines have generally been phased out in industrialized nations but are still in use in some lower-income countries.) There is great variation in pesticide application methods, training, and work practices, including the use of protective gear. Finally, the longer-term effects of a prior acute exposure may be difficult to disentangle from the effects of chronic exposure. In light of these complications, many epidemiologic studies have simply used farming occupation or agricultural work experience as a surrogate for pesticide exposure. Exposure to pesticides has been linked most clearly to neurologic effects, cancer, and reproductive and developmental outcomes.

The neurologic effects of acute pesticide exposure are well known and include headache, dizziness, nausea and vomiting, muscle weakness, and even convulsions and coma at high exposures.[11,12] In a number of studies, chronic exposure to pesticides has been associated with deficits in cognitive function (for example, memory, attention, and visual-spatial processing) and also in psychomotor function (for example, reaction time).[11,12] There is considerable support in the literature for a link between pesticide exposure and Parkinson's disease, and some evidence of an association with amyotrophic lateral sclerosis (ALS, also known as Lou Gehrig's disease).[11,12]

Among the organochlorine pesticides, DDT, aldrin, dieldrin, chlordane, and others have been shown to cause cancer in animals.[12] Risk of non-Hodgkin's lymphoma is associated with exposure to some herbicides, as well as to organochlorine and organophosphate pesticides.[12] The farming occupation has been linked to increased risk of several cancers, including leukemia, multiple myeloma, soft tissue sarcoma, and cancers of the brain, stomach, and prostate.[12–16]

Reproductive effects have been associataed with chronic exposure to some pesticides. In various studies, a woman's history of agricultural work has been linked to increased risk of spontaneous abortion and stillbirth, fetal death, and prematurity;[17] in the 1970s, the now-banned pesticide dibromochloropropane (DBCP), used to kill worms, was found to affect the fertility of male workers in a production plant.[17,18] Prenatal pesticide exposure has been linked to some birth defects, including oral clefts.[18] There is some evidence that childhood exposure to pesticides may increase the risk of leukemia and certain brain cancers and may alter thyroid function or have other endocrine-disrupting effects.[19]

The health burdens of pesticide exposures weigh more heavily on certain populations, among them pesticide production workers, farmers and their families, and hired farmworkers. In the United States, more than 80% of these farmworkers are men, about 60% are Hispanic, about 40% are foreign-born and not US citizens, and almost half lack a high school education.[20,21]

Migrant farmworkers are often at special risk from pesticide exposures because they may work with inadequate protection, live in close proximity to agricultural land, lack adequate facilities to wash, be unable to understand hazard warnings in English, whether spoken or printed, and lack health insurance and access to health care. A study of farmworkers in Oregon found that most wore no protective clothing on the job, yet wore their work clothes and boots home, and did not change their clothes within 30 minutes of arriving home,[22] suggesting that they did not appreciate the potential risk to their families.

Many agricultural workers in lower-income countries have similar vulnerabilities, compounded by the continued use of pesticides now banned in the industrialized nations. Female agricultural workers in lower-income countries may be particularly highly exposed because they are often casual workers doing low-skill, high-exposure jobs without protection or training.[23]

Integrated Pest Management as an Alternative to Pesticide Use in Agriculture

Although the concept of **integrated pest management** (IPM) predates modern synthetic pesticides, it has been expanded and elaborated in response to the obvious problems stemming from the indiscriminate use of these chemicals. These problems include the development of resistance among pests, rebound effects such as target pest resurgence and secondary pest outbreaks, and widespread environmental contamination with its impacts on wildlife and people.

The *integrated* in integrated pest management refers to the use of multiple tactics (for example, biological and chemical) to manage multiple pests in a manner consistent with ecological principles.[10] For example, a vertically integrated approach recognizes the problem of target pest resurgence, and a horizontally integrated approach recognizes the problem of secondary pest outbreaks (see Figure 6.3). The term *management* acknowledges that the goal is to suppress pests rather than to wipe them out. Integrated pest management also incorporates the notion that populations of target pests (and their predators and competitors) should be monitored, and that pest control measures should be undertaken when some predefined threshold is met, rather than on a regular schedule.[10] IPM tactics range from introducing beneficial insects (for example, predators or parasites of the pest), to using synthetic pheromones (chemicals that female insects use to attract males) that confuse male insects and reduce mating, and can also include changes to irrigation or crop rotation practices.

There is disagreement over the degree to which IPM techniques have become a part of US farming. Survey data from the US Department of Agriculture suggest widespread adoption of some IPM techniques.[24] However, critics suggest that much of what passes for IPM is simply monitoring pest populations as a way to decide when to begin treatment with pesticides.[25] In fact, the challenges of integrating the flexible and nuanced IPM approach into large-scale, mechanized agriculture are substantial.

Genetically Modified Crop Plants

The fundamental rationale for developing **genetically modified** (GM) plants is to augment the world's food supply. The global population was estimated at 6.6 billion in 2007 and is expected to increase to 8.3 billion by 2030 and 9.4 billion by 2050.[26] Because most of the world's arable land is already under cultivation, the only way to increase total production is to increase crop yield per acre. Genetically modified (or **genetically engineered**) crops are seen by many as the only plausible means to achieve this goal. For example, it would be advantageous to create plants that are not susceptible to disease, that repel pests (yet another approach to pest control), or that ripen more quickly. Crop plants might also be genetically modified to improve their nutritional value—for example, to be richer in essential vitamins.

Of course, people have been modifying plants through selective breeding for centuries. But the new technologies work at the level of DNA rather than at the level of the individual plant—in fact, such techniques are sometimes called "molecular breeding."[27] The basic approach is to first isolate a gene that codes for the desired characteristic—it might come from any species—and then transfer this DNA to the species of interest, for example, corn. Specifically, the gene being transferred (called the **transgene**, or **biotech gene**) is inserted into a simple loop of bacterial DNA, which is used to make the transfer. The processes by which the gene is integrated into the corn DNA—so that it causes the corn to take on the desired characteristic—and appears in seed are far too complex to describe here. But if these steps are successful, then subsequent generations of the **transgenic** corn (the corn into whose DNA the transgene has been imported) will have the characteristic coded by the imported DNA. For example, plants of one variety of transgenic corn produce a protein that is toxic to certain insect pests, thus protecting the plants from the pests; the gene that produces this effect comes from a soil bacterium called *Bacillus thuringiensis*, and the corn is referred to as Bt corn. This corn has, in effect, a built-in pesticide.

The cultivation of genetically modified crop plants, and the consumption of foods made from these plants, raise two distinct public health concerns: The first arises directly from the foreign genes present in transgenic plants; the second arises from the techniques used to transfer genes from one species to another.

Allergic Reactions to Genetically Modified Foods

The core human health concern related to genetically modified foods is that they may cause allergic reactions in susceptible individuals. Allergens—the biological substances that induce allergic reactions—are proteins, and the proteins in a plant species (for example, peanuts) have characteristic chemical structures determined by the genes of that species. Thus, if a peanut gene is transferred into a soybean plant, for example, peanut proteins will be present in the genetically modified soybeans. If any of the peanut proteins is an allergen, a person with a peanut allergy who eats these soybeans will have an allergic reaction to it. And because the modified soybeans don't look different or taste different, the allergic individual has no way to avoid them. Before candidate biotech genes are transferred to a different species, they are studied to see if any of the proteins they encode are considered likely to be allergenic—for example, whether a sequence of amino acids in the protein is similar to a sequence in a known allergen.[27] However, some concern remains about allergic reactions to genetically modified foods.

The safety of specific transgenic plants is a critical question because the practical challenges of limiting the spread of genetic material in the environment are truly intractable. For example, fields planted in genetically modified corn are not physically segregated from fields of traditional corn, and thus pollen from genetically modified corn can easily be carried on the wind to traditional corn plants. As a result, the ecological impacts of planting genetically modified food plants cannot be predicted at this time. Equally daunting is the task of keeping track of biotech ingredients as they wend their way through the labyrinth of the modern food supply (see Section 6.5).

Genetically Modified Foods and the Spread of Antibiotic Resistance

As described in Chapter 3, bacterial populations can become resistant to an antibiotic over time, much as pests develop resistance to pesticides. Such antibiotic resistance among pathogens is a major challenge in the battle against infectious disease because it makes certain antibiotics ineffective. There has been some concern that transgenic plants could contribute to the problem of antibiotic resistance through a somewhat convoluted series of events.

When a culture of plant cells is exposed to a foreign gene in the laboratory, in hopes that the cells will take up the transgene and integrate it into their DNA, only a small percentage of the cells actually do so. Thus it is a practical challenge to locate those cells that have been modified and which can be used to start the new genetic line—of transgenic corn, for example. This has usually been done by coupling a gene for antibiotic resistance to the gene being transferred— then, when the plant cells are exposed to the appropriate antibiotic, those few that survive are identifiable as those carrying the transgene.

But these survivors, of course, also carry the antibiotic resistance gene. Thus, the concern is that, in the broader environment, the antibiotic resistance genes might somehow be transferred from transgenic plants to bacteria. The two settings in which this is most likely to occur may seem rather different, but they share an important bacterial process. One is silos on farms (**Figure 6.4**)—storage cylinders where resident bacteria digest crop wastes, producing a moist material called silage, which is used as animal feed. The other is the gut of humans or other an-

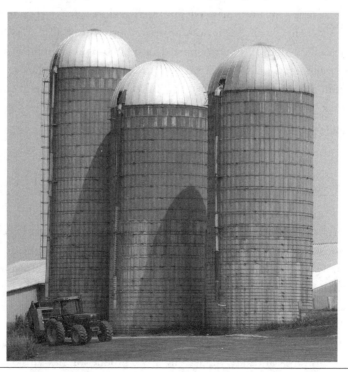

FIGURE 6.4   Bacteria digest crop wastes in silos like these.

imals, where resident bacteria help to digest plant matter in food.[28] No one knows how likely it is that antibiotic resistance genes might be transferred from transgenic plants to bacteria in the environment; the FDA's stance is that it is a remote possibility, but not all scientists agree.[29]

Use of Water for Irrigation

The irrigation of crops accounted for 34% of US water consumption in 2000, and some 42% of these withdrawals of water for irrigation came from groundwater.[30] In all, about 137 billion gallons per day was used for irrigation during the year, or almost 500 gallons per person per day. California alone accounted for 22% of water used for irrigation; other leading states were Idaho, Colorado, Nebraska, Texas, and Montana. Depending on the method of irrigation used, water losses to evaporation can be substantial—for example, much more water is lost when large sprinkling systems are used than when water is dripped slowly into the soil.

Even in 1995, the United States Geological Survey had identified the region of the Lower Colorado River as an area where the consumptive use of water exceeded its renewable water supply;[31] in 2006, the World Health Organization named parts of the Central Plains and the Southwest as areas where water use exceeds the natural supply.[32] Thus, current irrigation practices are not sustainable over the long term.

Mechanical Hazards to Workers

In addition to exposures to chemicals in crop production, farmers and farmworkers face mechanical hazards. In the period 2003–2005, there were 1006 fatal injuries in crop production in the United States. Three percent of these fatalities were children under 16, and 41% were persons aged 65 or older; nearly all (96%) were males. Nearly half of all deaths (45%) involved tractors.[33] In the same period, there were more than 63,000 nonfatal injuries in crop production, reflecting an annual incidence that runs 15% to 20% higher than the overall incidence of nonfatal injuries in private industry as a whole.[33] In epidemiologic studies, farmers commonly report being struck by objects or equipment, with injuries to fingers and feet, and they cite human error and hurry as important sources of injury.[34]

6.2 Modern Livestock Production Practices

In energy terms, eating meat is a luxury. Only a small part of the energy stored in a plant's tissues ends up stored in the tissues of an herbivore that eats the plant. Similarly, only a small part of the energy stored in the tissues of an herbivore ends up stored in the tissues of a carnivore that eats the herbivore. This is because animals—whether herbivore or carnivore—use most of the energy they take in to stay warm, move around, reproduce, and so forth. People, of course, can be either vegetarians (herbivores) or meat eaters (carnivores). For example, people can either eat the corn grown on 100 acres of land or eat the beef from the cows supported by the 100 acres of corn—but they will derive much more energy if they simply eat the corn.

In the face of this physical reality, modern livestock production has subsidized the growing of feed crops with fossil fuels and synthetic chemicals, has emphasized mechanization and economies of scale, and has introduced new feeding and veterinary practices for livestock. This section presents key elements of modern livestock production:

- Concentrated animal feeding operations where cattle, pigs, and poultry are brought to market weight
- The processes of slaughter and meat processing
- The rendering of animal carcasses, a recycling process implicated in the spread of bovine and human diseases caused by prions
- Consolidation in dairy farming
- The use of hormones to increase the productivity of both beef and dairy cattle

Concentrated Animal Feeding Operations

Some people in the United States—and many more worldwide—are vegetarians, either by economic necessity or by preference. In nature, however, human beings are omnivorous, eating both plants and animals, and animal husbandry is an integral part of traditional agriculture. In this tradition, there is a sort of contract between farmer and animal: In return for his food supply, the farmer cares for his animals so that they thrive; and the farmer's own productivity is tied to the welfare of his animals.[35]

In contrast, modern industrial agriculture in the United States is not driven by the farmer's need to survive but by the corporate objective to produce food more cheaply to increase profits. And on the scale of industrial agriculture, productivity no longer reflects the welfare of individual animals. For example, "crowding hens results in less egg laying per hen, but also in high productivity for the whole operation, since hens are cheap and cages are expensive."[35] Thus, what has been lost in industrial agriculture is the element of *husbandry*: caring for animals in a way that allows them not just to survive, but to thrive in a natural way.

In the United States today, most animals raised for their meat are brought to market weight in **concentrated animal feeding operations**, or CAFOs ("kay-foes"), after weaning. Animals are transported from CAFOs to slaughtering and meatpacking facilities, from which meat enters the marketplace and carcasses become a waste stream, undergoing a process called rendering.

A Profile of CAFOs in the United States

In the United States in 2002, some 35.7 million cattle, 100 million hogs, and 8.7 billion chickens were slaughtered for meat.[36,37] Most of these animals were raised in confinement—cattle in outdoor pens, and swine and chickens in enclosed housing.

About two-thirds of US beef cattle are to be found in very large CAFOs—those confining more than 16,000 animals (**Table 6.2**), and nearly half are in operations of more than 32,000. More than half of these very large operations are concentrated in two states: 27% of operations in the largest category are in Texas, and 26% are in Kansas; in the second size tier, the same two states dominate, though their positions are reversed.[38]

Overall, US swine CAFOs have fewer animals than cattle feedlots, but the profile of the industry is strikingly similar (Table 6.2). More than half of US hogs are in the largest facilities, and about half of the larger facilities are in just two states. Of facilities in the largest category,

Table 6.2 Distribution of US Beef Cattle and Swine Inventories, by Capacity of Feedlot, 2002

Beef cattle		Swine	
Capacity (no. animals)	Percentage of Total Inventory	Capacity (no. animals)	Percentage of Total Inventory
1000–1999	4	1 to 99	1
2000–3999	7	100–499	5
4000–7999	9	500–999	7
8000–15,999	11	1000–1999	12
16,000–31,999	20	2000–4999	23
≥ 32,000	48	≥5000	53

Data from: US Department of Agriculture, National Agricultural Statistics Service. *Cattle: Final Estimates 1999–2003.* 2004. Available at: http://usda.mannlib.cornell.edu/usda/reports/general/sb/sb989.pdf. US Department of Agriculture, National Agricultural Statistics Service. *Livestock Operations: Final Estimates 1998–2002.* 2004. Available at: http://usda.mannlib.cornell.edu/usda/reports/general/sb/sb1002.pdf. Accessed April 19, 2008.

27% are in North Carolina, and 22% are in Iowa; in the second size tier, the same two states dominate, but in reverse order.[39]

Some 98% of commercially produced chickens are **broilers**—that is, chickens under 13 weeks old, raised for meat;[37] chickens raised for their eggs (layers) are produced separately. The production of broilers is somewhat more dispersed geographically than cattle and swine production (see Table 6.3), but all the leading states are in the south. North Carolina, the leading

Table 6.3 Leading US States in Production of Broilers, 2002

State	Percentage of Broilers Produced
Georgia	15
Arkansas	14
Alabama	12
Mississippi	9
North Carolina	9
Other states	41
Total	100

Data from: US Department of Agriculture, National Agricultural Statistics Service. *Poultry Production and Value: Final Estimates 1998–2002.* 2004. Available at: http://usda.mannlib.cornell.edu/usda/reports/general/sb/sb994.pdf. Accessed April 19, 2008.

state in swine CAFOs, also hosts 9% of broiler production. The production of broilers increased 21-fold in the United States between 1950 and 1999,[1] transforming chicken from something of a luxury into a relatively inexpensive and accessible food.

Conditions of Animal Confinement

The US EPA has provided a description of conditions in confined feeding operations,[40] which are summarized here. Beef cattle are generally held in open feedlots (**Figure 6.5**), which may be unpaved, paved in the areas where food and water are provided, or fully paved. Urine and manure accumulate and are removed periodically. Cattle in CAFOs are fed grain, although they are grazing animals whose natural diet is grass.

Swine are raised in enclosed housing (**Figure 6.6**), usually with slotted floors so that urine and manure can drop into a collection area below. Beef cattle and swine produce manure equal to their own body weight about every 16 days. Wastes from feedlots are generally removed by scraping; swine houses are flushed with water to move wastes into the receptacle below the pens. In hog CAFOs like the one sketched in Figure 6.6, about a thousand animals are held in pens in each of the long, narrow buildings, and manure is held in a manmade lagoon nearby.

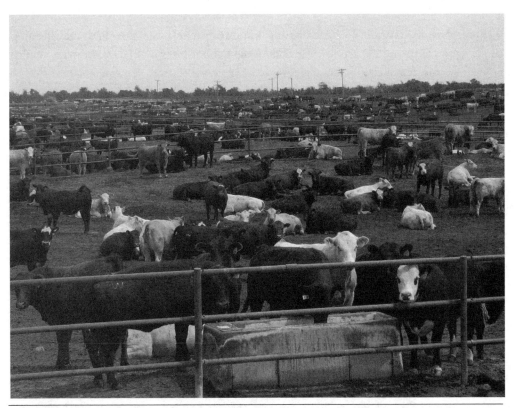

FIGURE 6.5   Cows study the photographer from the fringes of a mass of cattle in this CAFO. © 2008 Cathryn Dowd. Used with permission.

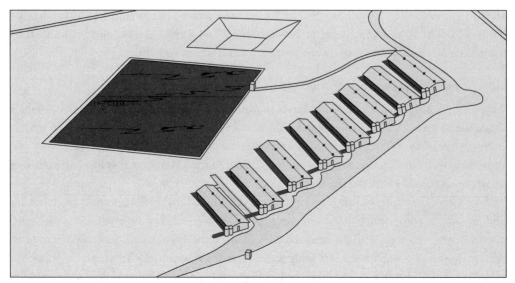

FIGURE 6.6 This sketch shows a typical layout for a hog CAFO, with a series of barns and an associated manure lagoon. A large operation might consist of several such units.

Broilers are also raised in enclosed housing, but usually with a solid floor and straw bedding. Broilers produce manure equal to their body weight about every $12^{1}/_{2}$ days. In many poultry houses, the top few inches of litter is removed five or six times a year when a new flock is brought in, and the building is fully cleaned just once a year.

In all confined animal feeding operations, feed is ground and pelletized to increase its digestibility, and is provided in troughs or by mechanical feeding devices. Pesticides may be applied both to the buildings and directly to the animals.

Animal wastes release two toxic gases: ammonia, created as nitrogen from urine moves into the air; and hydrogen sulfide, produced as manure is broken down by bacteria in the absence of oxygen. Mechanical ventilation systems run constantly in swine and poultry houses to protect both workers and animals from inhaling toxic gases and dusts at high concentrations, but the fans cannot dispel the odors or eliminate respiratory effects.

Most beef cattle in the United States are slaughtered at age 15 to 18 months[41] and may change hands several times during this period. In 2005, approximately 2% of cattle over 500 pounds (that is, excluding calves) died before slaughter; the most common single cause of death was respiratory problems (24% of deaths).[42] Most hogs in the United States are slaughtered at about 6 months of age and are brought to slaughter weight in one location.[43] In 2000, the mortality rate among postnursery swine was 2.9%; respiratory problems accounted for 39% of deaths.[44]

Environmental Impacts of CAFOs

The environmental and human health impacts of the industrialized rearing of beef cattle, swine, and broilers falls most heavily on the South and Midwest (see **Figure 6.7**). Animal wastes

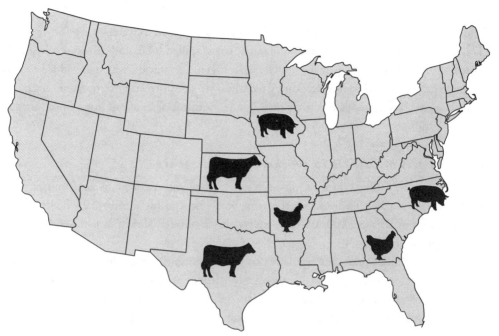

FIGURE 6.7   Concentration of beef cattle, swine, and broiler production in states in the Midwest and the South. *Data from*: US Department of Agriculture, National Agricultural Statistics Service. *Cattle: Final Estimates 1999–2003*, 2004. Available at: http://usda.mannlib.cornell.edu/usda/reports/general/sb/sb989.pdf; US Department of Agriculture, National Agricultural Statistics Service. *Livestock Operations: Final Estimates 1998–2002*, 2004. Available at: http://usda.mannlib.cornell.edu/usda/reports/general/sb/sb1002.pdf; US Department of Agriculture, National Agricultural Statistics Service. *Poultry Production and Value: Final Estimates 1998–2002*, 2004. Available at: http://usda.mannlib.cornell.edu/usda/reports/general/sb/sb994.pdf. All accessed April 19, 2008.

from cattle and hog CAFOs are stored in lagoons, or sprayed on fields, or released to bodies of water. Flooding associated with heavy rains contributes to broader releases of animal wastes. Wastes placed on land contribute heavy nitrogen loads to soil, where bacteria convert nitrogen to nitrates. Thus, like fertilizers used on crops, animal wastes contribute highly soluble nitrates to local groundwater, with the potential to cause methemoglobinemia in infants.[45] CAFO wastes also contribute to global climate change (see Section 6.3).

When CAFO wastes are released in large quantities to surface waters, they cause a different problem: a dramatic reduction in the dissolved oxygen in the water. This decline occurs through two natural processes. First, organic wastes like manure are decomposed by bacteria in the water, a process that consumes oxygen—and when large amounts of organic waste reach a river or lake, the level of dissolved oxygen in the water can fall dramatically as the decomposers do their work. Second, the overload of the nutrients phosphorus and nitrogen to the aquatic system supports an overgrowth of algae (called **eutrophication**); and as the algae die off and are decomposed by bacteria, more dissolved oxygen is consumed. Thus heavy inputs of waste may cause the receiving water to become anaerobic or nearly so, resulting in wholesale die-offs of fish and other aquatic organisms that depend on oxygen dissolved in water.

Poultry house waste, which is a mix of manure, straw, spilled food, and carcasses, is typically disposed of on land. There is growing concern that organic arsenicals, which are added to feed to promote growth and prevent infection by parasites, are transformed into inorganic arsenic in soil, in the waste, and perhaps in the chicken.[46] The inorganic arsenic can leach from waste or soil into groundwater.[46]

Health Impacts of CAFOs to Workers and Neighbors

In 2004, there were 10 fatal injuries to workers at US hog and pig feedlots, and four fatal injuries to workers at cattle feedlots. For the same year, hog and pig farmworkers had a rate of nonfatal injuries of 16.5 per 100 full-time-equivalent employees, almost four times the overall average for private industry.[33]*

Both neighbors and workers are regularly exposed to ammonia emanating from CAFOs; ammonia is a respiratory irritant, as is the organic dust from CAFOs, which may contain a wide range of irritants and allergens including fecal matter, antigenic urinary proteins, animal dander, pollens, antibiotics, and pesticides.[45] Asthmatics may be particularly vulnerable to the respiratory effects of CAFO dust.[47] Workers also face the risk of death by respiratory arrest from exposure to high concentrations of hydrogen sulfide—for example, when pumping manure out of storage lagoons.[18] Concentrations of hydrogen sulfide, ammonia, carbon dioxide, and methane may rise to dangerous levels in manure pits at CAFOs.[48] Even family members may be at risk: Manure pits have repeatedly claimed multiple lives when family members jump into the pit in a vain attempt to rescue a relative.[48,49]

The putrid odors associated with CAFOs—manure, dead fish, ammonia, the rotten-egg smell of hydrogen sulfide—are very disturbing to those who live nearby, often profoundly affecting their quality of life. At least one study suggests that residential exposure to odors from a hog CAFO is associated with increased feelings of stress, depression, fatigue, and confusion.[50]

In North Carolina, where hogs now outnumber people, poor nonwhite communities bear a heavier burden of CAFOs and their impacts.[51] Although the state has a long history of hog farming, recent decades have seen a shift from family-owned hog farms to a new way of doing business, in which a large corporation owns the animals and provides feed and transport; and the local farm operator owns the land, the buildings, and the wastes.[51]

Routine Administration of Antibiotics to Food Animals

Antibiotics are given to livestock in CAFOs to promote growth, thus bringing animals to market weight more quickly on less feed. Antibiotics used for this purpose are administered to poultry, beef cattle, and swine at low doses through much of the animals' lifetime. An antibiotic is even injected into the eggs that will hatch into broilers.[52]

---

*Data on nonfatal injuries in 2004 were not available for workers in cattle feedlots.

As previously described, the routine use of an antibiotic shapes populations of bacteria, over time increasing the share of the population that is resistant to the drug. A number of the same antibiotics are used to treat illness in people, to treat illness in farm animals and pets, and to promote growth in food animals. Estimates of the share of US antibiotic use attributable to growth promotion in food animals range from 32% (as estimated by the Institute of Medicine) to 78% (as estimated by a national public interest organization)—but in any event, it amounts to more than 15 million pounds of antimicrobials every year.[53]

Antibiotic resistance among bacterial populations in livestock has a direct effect on human health. During the process of slaughtering, it is not uncommon for the flesh of an animal to be contaminated by fecal matter from its intestine, in which certain bacteria are naturally present. For example, as described in Chapter 3, *Campylobacter* and *Salmonella* bacteria are often present on poultry products when they are purchased and are common causes of foodborne illness. If these organisms are resistant to certain antibiotics, then the antibiotics are ineffective in treating human illness.

But the ineffectiveness of antibiotics in treating foodborne illness is merely the tip of the iceberg. Whether in an animal's gut or in the broader environment, bacteria routinely swap genes, including genes for antibiotic resistance. Resistant organisms that enter the environment in CAFO wastes or slaughterhouse wastes or human sewage circulate through many ecological niches, trading in what has been called a "global web of bacterial genetics."[54] Thus, antibiotic resistance—including multidrug resistance—poses a very broad public health challenge, and the overuse of antibiotics in livestock rearing is a key part of this problem.

Slaughter and Meat Processing

Slaughter and meat processing are the conjoined industries that together convert animals on the hoof into meat on the table. These processes are largely invisible in many parts of the United States, but they are well known for their difficult and hazardous working conditions. In fact, dangers faced by slaughterhouse workers were first brought to light in the early 20th century in Upton Sinclair's famous novel *The Jungle*, about Chicago's meatpacking industry. Much has changed since that time, but even today meatpacking and poultry processing are hazardous trades.

Processing of larger animals, such as cattle and swine, begins with the animals being herded single file through a chute, stunned with a bolt to the brain, hung by the hind legs, and bled.[55] The carcasses then move down a production line at a set pace; they are cut open, eviscerated, cleaned, split in half, and then placed in walk-in coolers overnight. Each task on the production line is allotted about 5 seconds per carcass. Workers stand on elevated grated platforms (the floor is slippery) and wear protective gear. The line is noisy, and temperatures range from about 75°F to 100°F, depending on the season. Later, the refrigerated carcass is cut up in a cold room; with temperatures hovering around 40°F, these workers use power saws, power knives, and manual knives to produce chops, loins, and so forth.[55]

Chickens, because they are much smaller animals, are electrically stunned, bled, scalded to facilitate defeathering, eviscerated, cut into parts, deboned, and packed in a continuous process before being refrigerated. The division of labor in poultry processing is extreme—the

Occupational Safety and Health Administration (OSHA) defines 13 steps in evisceration, nine in cutting, and six in deboning[56]—and the production line moves rapidly.[57]

Workers who process meat or poultry face an array of occupational hazards, with overall injury and especially illness rates higher than the overall average for private industry (see **Table 6.4**). Acute injuries, including lacerations from knives, are common; in slaughterhouses, slips and falls, strains and sprains are also common.[55] Meat and poultry workers also suffer repetitive strain injuries, including carpal tunnel syndrome, from doing the same task over and over.[57] Noise is a hazard, especially in meatpacking.

In addition, workers are potentially exposed to zoonotic diseases through contact with infected animals. Preventive measures vary; for example, prevention of brucellosis (a flu-like disease that can lead to severe infections or cause chronic symptoms) has focused on eliminating the disease in US animals; whereas risks of *Salmonella* and *Campylobacter* are managed through measures to prevent workers from contacting fecal matter.[58] Respiratory irritation is common because pathogens, animal dander, or bits of feathers are likely to be present in the air of the workplace.[58] There is some evidence of elevated risk of lung cancer, oral cancer, and stomach cancer among meatpackers and butchers, but it is not known what specific exposures might be responsible.[59–61]

Finally, the origin of some foodborne illness is in the processes of slaughter and meat processing. Given the rapid pace of production lines, meat or chicken products can easily be contaminated with an animal's fecal matter. Contamination by *Salmonella* and *Campylobacter*—two very common but rarely fatal illnesses—originates in this way. As described in Chapter 3, undercooked hamburgers are the most common vehicle for exposure to the potentially fatal bacterial strain *E. coli* O157:H7, and as few as 10 organisms can cause illness. Two features of the production of ground beef make it more susceptible to contamination than solid cuts of beef, such as steaks. First, in a major meatpacking plant, many cows contribute to a single well-mixed batch of ground beef, increasing the chance of contamination.

Table 6.4   Occupational Injuries and Illnesses in Slaughtering and Meat Processing, 2004

NAICS*	Industry	Fatal Injuries (n)	Nonfatal Injuries per 100 FTE Employees	Illnesses per 10,000 FTE Employees
	Private industry (overall)	4257	4.5	27.9
311611	Slaughtering (except poultry)	4	8.3	504.2
311612	Meatpacking	9	7.8	148.7
311615	Poultry processing	10	5.5	226

*North American Industry Classification System code.

Data from: US Department of Labor, Bureau of Labor Statistics. *Occupational Injuries and Illnesses and Fatal Injuries Profiles*. Available at: http://data.bls.gov/GQT/servlet/InitialPage. Accessed March 12, 2007.

And second, grinding the meat aerates it and increases the surface area available for bacterial growth.

Rendering of Animal Carcasses

In industrialized livestock operations, the disposal of carcasses after the meat has been removed at slaughter is an enormous logistic challenge. In the United States today, for example, more than 30 million cattle are slaughtered commercially each year,[62] leaving the same number of carcasses to be disposed of. These animal carcasses are reprocessed into animal feed and other products through a process called rendering, as shown in **Figure 6.8**. Dead animals from feedlots, veterinary practices, shelters, and zoos also enter the rendering stream.

Rendering is essentially the heating of animal remains in a large vat. Fat is separated and removed—this rendered fat is **tallow**, used as an ingredient in various products, including candles, soap, and some cosmetics. The remaining slurry is dried and then ground, producing what is called **meat and bone meal**. This meal is fed to farm animals as a high-protein dietary supplement, shortening the time needed to bring the animals to market. It is also an ingredient in many pet foods.

The rendering cycle has been used, with variations, since the early 20th century, when slaughterhouse wastes became a problem. In the 1960s and 1970s, as cattle were increasingly moved from grass pastures to feedlots, meat and bone meal began to be widely used in feed. Thus, within the livestock industry, rendering has long been seen as a form of recycling—a process that turns a waste product into something useful.

But everything changed in the 1980s and 1990s, when a novel and frightening disease of cattle morphed into a novel and frightening disease of humans—both ultimately shown to be caused by prions distributed through the rendering cycle. In the United Kingdom, where these diseases emerged, about 4 million cattle were slaughtered, most of them as a precau-

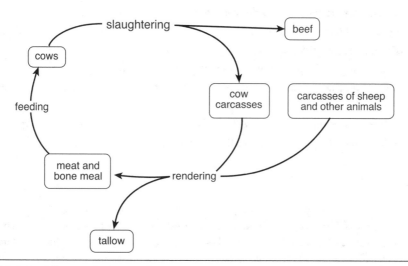

FIGURE 6.8   The rendering cycle.

tionary measure,[63] and more than 150 people have died to date from the newly identified human illness.

Familiar Prion Diseases

As described previously, abnormal prion proteins cause a set of degenerative brain diseases known as transmissible spongiform encephalopathies, which are uniformly fatal. The prions form plaques in the brain, creating gaps that create the sponge-like texture visible at autopsy— the hallmark of these illnesses. One such disease is **Creutzfeldt-Jakob disease (CJD)**, a rare human disease that has been known since the 1920s. It typically occurs in older people, causing neurological symptoms: dementia, loss of speech and coordination, and ultimately death. Cases of CJD occur sporadically, and no environmental risk factors are known for the disease, though iatrogenic transmission (that is, caused by medical treatment) can occur.*

Several transmissible spongiform encephalopathies affecting animals have also been known for some time, including **scrapie**, a familiar disease of sheep in the United Kingdom. Scrapie has never been known to pose a hazard to people who have contact with infected animals. Several prion diseases are known in other **ruminants** (animals which, like sheep and cattle, have multichambered stomachs and regurgitate and rechew food that they have previously swallowed). A chronic wasting disease that affects deer and elk, for example, is a prion disease.

Two Novel Prion Diseases

The two prion diseases that emerged in the United Kingdom late in the 20th century were new to scientists. The disease that affected cattle was given the name **bovine spongiform encephalopathy (BSE)**, though it was commonly called **mad cow disease** in reference to the dementia suffered by the animals. Affected cows also experienced a loss of coordination, and many became downer cows—cows too ill to stand (**Figure 6.9**). The human disease, like Creutzfeldt-Jakob disease, was a fatal degenerative neurological disease, but it affected mostly younger people and had a somewhat different constellation of symptoms. The new illness was designated **variant Creutzfeldt-Jakob disease (vCJD)**. The first case of BSE appeared in 1986; the first case of vCJD was diagnosed in 1993. BSE cases were also reported in several other European countries in the 1990s.

In the United Kingdom, epidemiologic evidence indicated that eating beef was a risk factor for vCJD, suggesting that prions from diseased cattle were being transmitted to people. A UK government inquiry showed that neural matter from a cow's brain or spinal cord could in fact contaminate beef at the time of slaughter.[64] As in the United States, processing of beef in the United Kingdom was a fast-moving, partially mechanized process. The UK investigation docu-

---

*For example, CJD can be transmitted through transplants of dura mater (the membrane that sheaths the spinal cord), taken from cadavers. It is estimated that 267 cases of iatrogenic CJD (that is, cases caused by medical treatment) may have occurred worldwide in the year 2000 (S-Juan P, Ward H, De Silva R, Knight R, Will R. Ophthalmic surgery and Creutzfeldt-Jakob disease. *Br J Ophthalmol.* 2004;88:446–449).

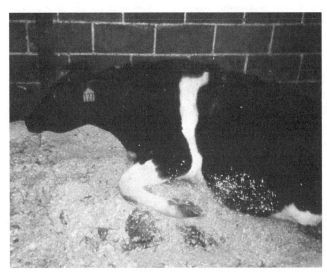

FIGURE 6.9 A cow afflicted with BSE struggles to stand up. *Source*: Reprinted courtesy of CDC Public Health Image Library. ID 5438. Content Providers: CDC/Dr. Art Davis. Available at: http://phil.cdc.gov/phil/details.asp. Accessed September 13, 2007.

mented that the carcass was split in half lengthwise using saws or cleavers, and the spinal cord was scraped out with a tool or sometimes by hand.[64] The head was removed for separate processing, and some low-quality meat was obtained from the head. All these processes created opportunities for prions to contaminate meat products intended for human consumption.

Thus, a complete transmission cycle was documented, made possible by prions' capacity to survive heat, freezing, and drying. Prions present in cattle carcasses survived the process of rendering, causing illness in cows that ate meat and bone meal; and prions present in beef survived the processes of food preparation, causing illness in people.

The Origins of the BSE Epidemic

The question remains: How did the first cow get BSE? The answer to this question is not known, but there are two likely possibilities. One is that a sporadic case of BSE occurred in a cow, much as sporadic CJD occurs in humans, and that this cow's remains were rendered, beginning the cycle of amplification. The other possibility is that prions from a sheep with scrapie, which were present in meat and bone meal, crossed the species boundary, becoming able to infect cattle.

In either case, the factor that transformed this rare event into an epidemic among cattle was the amplification of exposure through the rendering cycle—in which the remains of many animals are mixed together, and then fed to many more animals, whose carcasses ultimately also enter the rendering cycle. In contrast, if a cow on a farm in 1930 had spontaneously developed BSE, the consequences would have been limited to the circle of people who ate beef from this animal. Thus, it seems fair to say that the epidemics of BSE and vCJD resulted from breaking another "biological taboo" by turning cows into carnivores (and, in effect, cannibals).

In fact, the only other setting in which a prion disease is known to have been transmitted and amplified in this way was in a remote tribal group in New Guinea, where transmission occurred through the ritual eating of certain body parts, including the brain, of deceased family members.[65] The disease, known locally as **kuru**, was a fatal degenerative neurological condition. By the late 1960s, it had been demonstrated that kuru was transmitted by the eating of body parts,[65] and the practice came to an end. But the infectious agent remained a mystery for more than a decade as scientists painstakingly documented the existence of infectious proteins, which came to be called prions. The kuru epidemic is believed to have begun with a case of sporadic CJD in the population.[66]

Human Illness in the United Kingdom

In the United Kingdom, at the close of 2005, a total of 153 deaths from variant Creutzfeldt-Jakob disease had occurred, and nine living persons were believed to be afflicted with the disease.[67] The time pattern suggests that the episode is drawing to a close (**Figure 6.10**). However, there is some concern that it will not be so simple. There is variation in the normal prions that people carry, reflecting differences in people's genetic makeup, and individuals with certain variants of the normal prion are more susceptible to prion diseases. For example, people with a certain

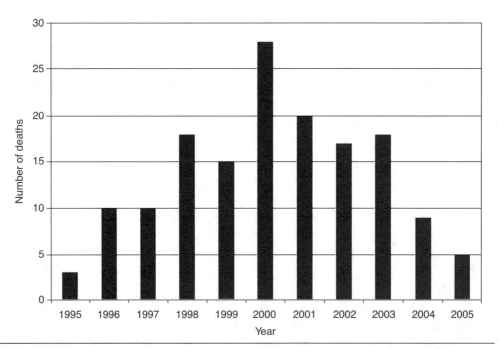

FIGURE 6.10   Deaths from variant Creutzfeldt-Jakob disease in the United Kingdom, 1995–2005. *Data from*: UK Department of Health. *Communications Summary September 2006: Creutzfeldt-Jakob Disease in the UK*. Available at: http://www.dh.gov.uk/en/ Publicationsandstatistics/Publications/CommunicationsSummary/DH_4138939. Accessed March 7, 2007.

genotype are known to be at higher risk of CJD; and all the victims of vCJD whose genetic makeup was analyzed showed this same trait.[66] Thus, if the vCJD cases to date represent a susceptible subgroup, there may be another wave of cases at some point in the future. Evidence from the waning kuru epidemic suggests that the incubation period for that illness was up to 40 years.[66] It is also possible for iatrogenic transmission of vCJD to occur if tissue from donors afflicted with the disease is unwittingly used.

Dairy Farming

Like the production of food crops and meat, the production of dairy goods is being consolidated into larger operations. From 2000 to 2006, the proportion of US dairy cows found in operations of more than 2000 animals more than doubled (to 22%), as did the proportion of dairy production found in these large operations (to 23%).[68] These large operations are less likely than small ones to be family-owned, or to be integrated into a broader farming operation—and thus they are more likely to purchase feed and young cows, rather than growing their own feed and raising their own heifers.[68] With the increasing size in dairy operations has come a geographic shift: While production in the traditional dairy regions of the Midwest and Northeast has held about steady, production in the western states has grown by about 60%.[68] Like CAFOs, large dairy operations produce large quantities of manure, with similar environmental and human health impacts.

Use of Hormones in Beef and Dairy Cattle

The administration of steroid hormones to beef cattle increases their growth rate and produces meat with less fat and more lean mass.[69] The hormones are released slowly from pellets implanted under the skin of the ear; the concentrations of the hormones in meat remain within the normal range of untreated animals.[70]

Synthetic hormones are also used in dairy cows. **Bovine growth hormone** (also called **bovine somatotropin**) is a natural hormone in cows that, among other things, regulates milk production. A genetically engineered version of this hormone, **recombinant bovine growth hormone** (**rBGH**) has been developed by Monsanto Corporation under the name Posilac.

Regular injection of slow-release rBGH to dairy cows (every 2 to 4 weeks) increases their milk production substantially and makes them convert feed to milk more efficiently.[71] There has been some concern that rBGH may increase the frequency of udder infections and may cause stress in cows. Although potential human health concerns have been raised—mainly related to possible antibiotic residues in milk from treatment of udder infections—no human health effects have been documented.

rBGH was approved in 1994 for use in the United States, though it has been banned in the European Union and in Canada. The economics of using rBGH favor larger dairy operations. In a 2002 study of US dairy farmers in 21 states, rBGH was being used in 15% of herds overall—but in 54% of large herds (500 or more cows), 32% of medium-sized herds (100 to 499 cows), and only 9% of small herds (fewer than 100 cows).[72] Farmers not using rBGH most often cited its cost and their animals' health, but some cited personal beliefs or the wish to maintain their organic status.

6.3 Impacts of Modern Agricultural Practices on Global Climate

Agriculture makes a substantial contribution to global climate change. As described in Chapter 4, both nitrous oxide and methane are greenhouse gases—nitrous oxide is estimated to account for 5.4%, and methane 16.3%, of the earth's net gain in radiation energy from the five major anthropogenic greenhouse gases (see Table 4.5). In fact, both nitrous oxide and methane are more potent greenhouse gases, molecule for molecule, than the gas with the greatest overall impact, carbon dioxide.

As described earlier in this chapter, both wastes from CAFOs and the intensive use of fertilizers on crops contribute to contamination of groundwater with nitrates. Bacteria in soil convert nitrates to either nitrogen gas (N_2) or nitrous oxide (N_2O), which are released to the atmosphere. In 2003, nitrate fertilizers accounted for more than half (56%) of US nitrous oxide emissions.[73]

Methane (CH_4) is produced by agricultural activities in which organic matter is digested or decomposes under anaerobic conditions. For example, a single cow releases 250 to 500 liters of methane per day, mainly by belching.[74] Manure from CAFOs, if allowed to accumulate in lagoons, produces methane as it decomposes. And the cultivation of rice in paddies also releases methane as crop residues decompose under flooded conditions. In the United States, cattle and rice cultivation together are estimated to account for almost one-third (29%) of US emissions of methane, though this gas is released in greater quantities through the fossil fuel cycle and by landfills.

6.4 Modern Fishing Practices

In recent decades, human capacity to catch marine fish has increased dramatically as a result of mechanized methods to take fish from the water, as well as the use of high-tech means, such as sonar, to locate fish. Large nets dragged across the sea floor—a sort of mechanized underwater harvest—disrupt or even destroy ecosystems. And, like farming, fishing is powered by fossil fuels: A recent analysis found that about 500 liters of diesel fuel was expended for every metric ton of deep sea fish caught.[75]

Declining Wild Stocks and Growth of Fish Farms

For a given fishery (the population of a species of fish in a particular location), the volume caught follows a typical time course, increasing to a peak level of production and then falling off, as shown schematically in **Figure 6.11** using hypothetical data. Marine scientists define a fishery as *fully exploited* during the period around its peak production, when yearly production is more than 50% of the peak year's production. This fully exploited period is bracketed by periods defined as *developing* and *overfished* (during which production is at 10% to 50% of peak production); and these periods in turn are bracketed by periods labeled *undeveloped* and *collapsed or closed* (during which production is at less than 10% of the peak).[76]

In 1950, more than 90% of the world's fisheries were classified as either undeveloped or developing. By 2000, fewer than 10% were classified as undeveloped or developing, and nearly 20% had collapsed.[76] To date, the challenges of protecting this resource—from gaining the

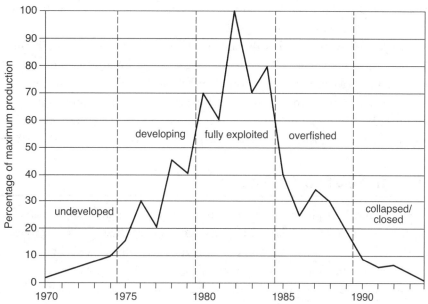

FIGURE 6.11 The typical time course of a hypothetical marine fishery. *Data from*: Froese R, Kesner-Reyes K. Impact of fishing on the abundance of marine species. Presented at: International Council for the Exploration of the Sea Annual Science Conference; 2002; Copenhagen.

compliance of fishing crews to ceding some national authority to international commissions—have largely stymied efforts to do so.[77]

In the context of declining stocks of wild fish, along with the current recommendation to eat fish as a healthy alternative to red meat, the farming of fish inside enclosures placed in natural waters has become widespread. The most commonly farmed species is salmon; the global production of farmed salmon has increased more than 40-fold over the past two decades.[78] Farmed fish are fed an intensive diet consisting mainly of fish meal and oils derived from small ocean fish. Research has shown that concentrations of PCBs and dioxins, as well as DDT and other organochlorine pesticides, are higher—sometimes up to 10 times higher—in farmed salmon than in wild-caught salmon.[78]

Occupational Hazards of Fishing

Fishing is one of the most dangerous of occupations for US workers, as documented in a recent study of death and injury in the Alaskan commercial fishing fleet.[79]* Over an 8-year period (1991–1998), a total of 167 fishermen of the Alaskan fleet died on the job, yielding an overall

---

*Even more than for farming, national data on deaths and injuries among fishermen are incomplete because many fishermen are self-employed and the number of workers on individual vessels is small. For this reason, research data on one region's fishermen are presented here.

annual fatality rate of 119 per 100,000 full-time-equivalent workers. Nearly all those who died were males, ranging in age from 10 to 67 years.

Of the fatalities, 107 were caused by the sinking or capsizing of a vessel; of the 60 deaths *not* caused by the loss of the vessel, 42 were nevertheless caused by drowning or hypothermia, mostly because a man went overboard. More than half of these fishermen were washed overboard by a wave or dragged overboard after becoming entangled in equipment; more than 20% of man-overboard events were unobserved. Other than being washed overboard, the most frequent cause of death among Alaskan fishermen was crushing by machinery or equipment.

6.5 From Source to Table

Previous sections of this chapter describe methods used to cultivate crops, to raise and slaughter food animals, and to capture or farm fish. Although some of these activities produce items ready for the table, more often they produce inputs to a complex web of manufacturing processes. This section first touches on a few specific issues related to the quality of food as it is processed, and then takes up a broader issue: the capacity to trace foods backward through the systems of production and distribution.

Food Defects, Food Additives, and the Irradiation of Food

Food products may become contaminated—on the farm or during storage or processing—by foreign substances such as mold, fruitfly eggs, insect fragments, rodent hairs, or grit. Although these things are unappetizing, at low levels they do not make people sick, and they are unavoidable at acceptable levels of pesticide use. The regulatory term for such contaminants is **food defects**, and acceptable levels of these substances in food have been established.

In contrast to these accidental additions to food products, various substances are deliberately added to foods during processing to achieve specific purposes. Such **food additives** are used as preservatives (for example, BHA), sweeteners (for example, aspartame), flavor enhancers (for example, MSG), fat replacers (for example, Olestra), nutrients (for example, vitamin C), thickeners, leavening agents, anti-caking agents, and so forth. The additives that can be used, and the amounts that can be present in food, are regulated.

Finally, foods can be irradiated during processing to kill microbes and prevent foodborne illness. Irradiation of food, though not widely used in the United States, has been technically feasible for decades. Food is irradiated relatively late in the production process to minimize the opportunity for later microbial contamination—for example, a piece of beef might be irradiated after being wrapped for sale. Typically, cobalt-60 is used as a source of gamma radiation. Food is irradiated by passing it through a machine on a conveyor belt; the speed of the conveyor belt determines the dose. This technique kills by fragmenting DNA; it is effective against insects, parasites, and bacteria, but it is not effective against viruses, prions, bacterial spores, or toxins previously produced by bacteria.[80] Similar techniques are used to sterilize instruments and materials in medical settings.

Irradiation does *not* leave food radioactive. Rather, the immediate health concerns revolve mainly around the destruction of vitamins and micronutrients in food and the potential toxicity of chemicals created by irradiation (called **radiolytic chemicals**).[80,81] Taking a broader view, irradiation substitutes a late process for preventive strategies farther upstream—for example, changes in feedlots to reduce the prevalence of *E. coli* in cattle; in addition, there is some concern over the use of nuclear technologies in a large number of local food processing facilities.[82] Radiation is not unique in creating new chemicals in food—other types of food processing (for example, broiling steak) also do so.

Although the technology for irradiating food is not new, controversy remains over its potential human health effects. Numerous studies of the health effects of radiolytic chemicals have been conducted in animals, with inconsistent results.[80] Two studies in humans, one conducted in India in the 1970s and one in China in the 1980s, showed evidence of chromosomal breaks in subjects given irradiated foods, but this evidence is considered weak because of methodological limitations.[81]

"Traceability" in the Modern Food Supply System

The modern food system is marked by the complexity and scale of its operations and the rapid distribution of foods. Taken together, these factors make it challenging to trace food products backward through the system—but events have shown that this can be important.

For example, tracing meat to its origins has been critical in containing outbreaks of illness from the virulent pathogen *E. coli* O157:H7. Just four major companies slaughter about 84% of US cattle, and 13 large meatpacking facilities produce most US beef.[83] Ground beef from these large facilities—some in the form of ready-made hamburger patties—is promptly shipped to locations around the country. For reasons detailed previously, ground beef is particularly susceptible to contamination with *E. coli* O157:H7.

Fast-food restaurants further promote the rapid distribution of pathogens. In 1993, more than 200 people were made ill, and four died, from an *E. coli* O157:H7 outbreak traced to hamburgers served by the Jack-in-the-Box fast-food chain.[83] Although recalls of meat can prevent some illness, their effectiveness is limited in the context of a rapid-distribution food system. For example, the source of an *E. coli* O157:H7 outbreak in Colorado in 1997 was traced to ground beef, sold as hamburger patties in grocery stores, from a large meatpacking plant in Nebraska. The company voluntarily recalled about 35 million pounds of ground beef—but 25 million pounds had already been eaten.[83]

Although corn is not transformed into grain products as rapidly as livestock is transformed into meat, it has proved extremely difficult to trace or recall grain from genetically modified crop plants. This became clear in 1998, when the US EPA took the highly unusual step of restricting the use of a specific genetically engineered corn to animal feed. A Bt corn named StarLink was not to be used in foods for human consumption because proteins of this transgenic corn had been found to be similar to known human allergens.[29]

However, it soon became clear that corn bound for human consumption was not necessarily segregated from corn bound for animal consumption. And because corn is processed and transported en masse, some mixing is likely to occur in grain elevators or elsewhere. Testing of corn products from supermarket shelves documented the presence of StarLink corn in taco shells made by Taco Bell. Ultimately, StarLink corn was found in various other products, including non–genetically modified seed corn and corn shipped to Japan.[29] Unlike cattle, kernels of corn cannot be tagged and tracked, and it does not appear realistic to segregate genetically modified grains from other grains. The StarLink saga ultimately involved about 2500 farmers and 350 grain elevators, as well as 17 corporate entities that produced or sold seed or flour or taco shells.[29]

In sum, the broad-scale industrial systems that make it possible to produce and distribute foods rapidly also make it difficult to manage certain hazards of the food supply.

6.6 Organic Farming and Locally Grown Foods

Since the 1950s, the US food industry has succeeded in making varied and nutritional foods—including high-protein meat, poultry, and fish products—available to a much broader segment of the population. These achievements are attributable mainly to economies gained through large-scale, mechanized processes, along with the use of synthetic chemicals and other technical innovations. Of course, these changes bring costs as well as benefits. As detailed earlier, various practices of modern agriculture may leave residues in foods, including low levels of pesticides, hormones, or antibiotics; and genetically modified foods can cause unexpected allergic reactions.

In addition to these concerns, some people are uncomfortable with the extent to which we have manipulated nature, or contaminated the environment, or treated animals as mere inputs to industrial processes. Others are disturbed by the homogenizing effect—not to mention the empty calories—of many fast foods and convenience foods. These concerns are evidenced in a renewed interest in organic farming, as well as in locally grown foods bought at farmers' markets or grown in community gardens (**Figure 6.12**).

The organic approach to farming is roughly the antithesis of the modern approach described in the introduction to this chapter, which characterizes most US agriculture. **Organic farming** is, at a minimum, sustainable—its practices do not degrade the soil, but rather maintain and even build it, because good soil is the foundation of successful agriculture.[84] A second defining characteristic of organic farming is that it rejects the use of synthetic pesticides and commercial fertilizers.[84]

Together, these principles yield the typical features of organic farming—for example, raising both crops and animals, feeding crops to animals and using manure to fertilize crops. Similarly, organic farmers may grow two crops together or in rotation. For example, grains may be alternated with legumes such as peas or beans, whose roots have nodules containing nitrogen-fixing bacteria. These bacteria convert organic nitrogen compounds to nitrates, which are water-soluble nutrients easily taken up by plants. Organic farming shares some features with traditional farming—that is, farming in the era before gasoline-powered tractors and synthetic organic chemicals—but unlike traditional agriculture, organic farming is explicitly sustainable. Although organic farming does not have to be small in scale, it usually is.

It was only in 1990 that organically grown produce and meats gained official regulatory standing at the federal level, though various private and regional entities had offered organic

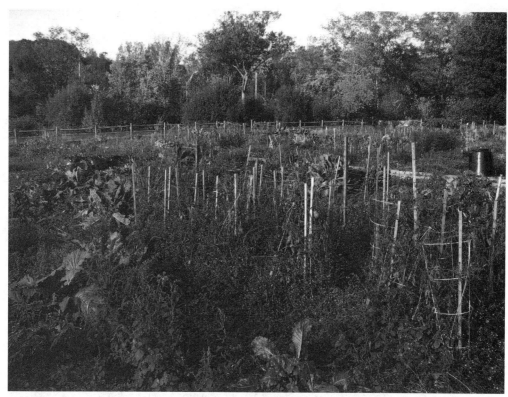

FIGURE 6.12 This urban community garden, seen here in autumn, provides homegrown vegetables for city dwellers. *Source*: Courtesy of Keith J. Maxwell.

certification for some time. In 2005, just one-half of 1% of all US cropland was certified organic.[85] In some categories, the percentage is somewhat higher—4.7% of acreage planted in vegetables, for example, and 2.5% of fruit acreage, was organic—and the acreage planted in organic crops in 2005 was nearly three times that estimated in 1995. Nearly 1% of milk cows and layers (chickens raised to produce eggs) were certified organic in 2005; only a tiny fraction of beef cattle, swine, and broilers were organically produced.[85]

6.7 Regulation of Food and the Activities That Produce It

The regulation of food, agriculture, and fisheries in the United States is complex, involving numerous laws implemented by several agencies. It also has very deep roots. The Meat Inspection Act was passed in 1906 and later amended as the Wholesome Meat Act (1967); the Poultry Products Inspection Act was passed in 1957. The original Food and Drug Act was also passed in 1906; it has been amended several times and is known today as the Federal Food, Drug, and Cosmetics Act (FFDCA). Two other laws are central to food regulation: the Federal Insecticide,

Fungicide, and Rodenticide Act (FIFRA; "fif-ra") of 1972, and the Food Quality Protection Act (FQPA) of 1996, which amended some sections of both FIFRA and the FFDCA.

Three federal agencies are most involved in the regulation of food and agriculture[86]:

- The US Department of Agriculture regulates the safety and labeling of most meat and poultry.
- The US Environmental Protection Agency is responsible for controlling the effects of pesticides on human health.
- The Food and Drug Administration is responsible for the safety, nutritional value, and labeling of most foods other than meat and poultry, and related to concerns other than pesticides.

Key elements of the US regulatory framework for food and agriculture appear in **Table 6.5**. This table is the sixth in a series of similar tables that place regulatory provisions within the traditional regulatory domains of environmental health.

Table 6.5 Overview of US Regulatory Framework for Environmental Health Hazards (6)

Environmental Health Domain	Major Laws and Key Provisions for the Control of Environmental Health Hazards
Biological hazards	Public Health Service Act (PHSA)—development of guidelines for vaccination; use of quarantine or isolation to prevent entry of infectious diseases into the United States; conduct of surveillance and investigation of outbreaks
Air pollution	Clean Air Act (CAA)—ambient standards (NAAQS) for Criteria Air Pollutants; emissions standards for Hazardous Air Pollutants, including mercury; emission allowances for SO_2 (to control acid deposition); removal of lead from gasoline; requirement to sell reformulated gasoline in high-smog areas
Ionizing radiation	Energy Reorganization Act (ERA)—safety requirements for operating nuclear power plants, including licensing, emissions limits, storage of wastes
	Nuclear Waste Policy Act (NWPA)—requirements to build and regulate a repository for radioactive wastes, including spent reactor fuel
	Uranium Mill Tailings Radiation Control Act —standards for management of abandoned mill tailings
Alternative energy sources	Energy Policy Act (EPAct)—modest supports for alternative energy sources
Hazardous wastes	Comprehensive Environmental Response Compensation and Liability Act ("Superfund") / Superfund Amendments and Reauthorization Act (CERCLA/SARA)—identify, assess health risks of, and remediate abandoned hazardous waste sites
	Resource Conservation and Recovery Act (RCRA)—"cradle-to-grave" manifest system for hazardous wastes; standards and permits for hazardous waste storage or disposal facilities; provisions to promote hazardous waste minimization (source reduction) and recycling of hazardous wastes

Table 6.5 *(Continued)*

Environmental Health Domain	Major Laws and Key Provisions for the Control of Environmental Health Hazards
Occupational health	Occupational Safety and Health Act (OSHAct)—ambient standards (Permissible Exposure Limits) for workplace air; employers must provide Materials Safety Data Sheets (MSDSs) to workers
Industrial water pollution	Clean Water Act (CWA)—ambient standards (Ambient Water Quality Criteria, or AWQC) for about 150 pollutants; technology requirements and permitting system for discharges to ambient water from industry
Toxic chemicals	Toxic Substances Control Act (TSCA)—premanufacture notice for new chemicals; EPA can restrict manufacture, distribution, or use if new chemical poses unreasonable risk
	Emergency Planning and Community Right-to-Know Act (EPCRA)—local and state emergency response commissions; yearly chemical reporting requirements for manufacturing facilities; data available as Toxics Release Inventory; facilities must provide Materials Safety Data Sheets (MSDSs) to local commissions
	Pollution Prevention Act (PPA)—support for source reduction/waste prevention as preferable to treatment or disposal of wastes
Pesticides	*Federal Insecticide, Fungicide, and Rodenticide Act (FIFRA)— registration of pesticides*
Food supply	*Federal Food, Drug, and Cosmetic Act (FFDCA)/Food Quality Protection Act (FQPA)—setting pesticide tolerances in food; setting food defect action levels; approval of food additives, including potential chemical by-products of irradiation; requirements for HACCP systems for food safety; BSE surveillance and controls on feed for ruminants*
	Humane Methods of Slaughter Act (HMSA)—standards for humane slaughter
	Wholesome Meat Act (WMA)/Poultry Products Inspection Act (PPIA)—inspection of meat and poultry
	Magnuson-Stevens Fishery Conservation and Management Act (MSFCMA)—conservation of fisheries
	Organic Foods Production Act (OFPA)—standards for labeling food as organic
Sewage wastes and community water supply	
Municipal solid waste	
Consumer products	
Environmental noise	

Note: New information appears in italics.

Pesticides

Before a pesticide can be sold or distributed in the United States, the pesticide must be registered with (licensed by) the US EPA. Pesticides are registered for a specific use or set of uses. Registration is intended to ensure that if the pesticide is used as instructed on its label, there is a "reasonable certainty of no harm to human health" (that is, to workers or others at hand when it is applied) and the pesticide will not pose "unreasonable risks to the environment."[87] For pesticides used on crops consumed by people or by food animals, EPA also sets a **pesticide tolerance**, which is the maximum pesticide residue level allowed in human food. Pesticide tolerances are to be set low enough to protect infants and children.

Genetically Modified Food Plants

There is no single federal law governing genetically modified foods or **biotechnology** more generally. (The term *biotechnology* is often used synonymously with **genetic engineering**, but also refers more broadly to applied biological science.) This fact reflects a 1986 policy judgment that biotechnology does not pose any unique risks and that its products can be regulated in the same way as conventional products, using laws that predate biotechnology.[88] As a result, at least three federal agencies are involved in the regulation of genetically modified food plants—the USDA, EPA, and FDA—and their responsibilities in this area are closely intertwined.[88,89]

The USDA regulates plant pests, and therefore also evaluates whether genetically modified plants could harm other plants—for example, a plant that incorporates a pesticide might harm insects that are beneficial to plants. Thus, the agency issues site permits for field tests of transgenic plants, with conditions intended to limit their spread, and afterward makes a determination of the new plant's potential to cause harm to agricultural plants.

The EPA registers pesticides and sets food tolerances for pesticides, and therefore does the same for pesticides produced by genetically engineered plants.

The FDA has responsibility for food safety, and therefore has this same responsibility for foods derived from transgenic plants. The FDA recommends that developers of transgenic plants consult early with the agency and that they follow certain procedures to evaluate potential harm—for example, the potential allergenicity of new proteins—but these steps are not required. FDA also does not require that transgenic foods be labeled as such. In 2001, FDA proposed that food companies be required to notify FDA 120 days before releasing a genetically modified food into the market, along with data demonstrating that the food is safe, but this proposed change is not yet law.

Humane Slaughter of Food Animals

In keeping with the 1978 Humane Methods of Slaughter Act, the USDA employs a veterinarian and slaughter line inspectors at each of the more than 900 federally inspected slaughterhouses.[90] Mandated methods for humane slaughter are incorporated into the Hazard Analysis and Critical Control Point systems (described later) in use at these plants. USDA is currently examining its requirements to strengthen them in a revised set of regulations.

Inspection and Grading of Meat

In keeping with requirements of the Wholesome Meat Act, carcasses are inspected for wholesomeness in meat processing plants and approval is stamped on the carcass.[91] For the most part, consumers do not see this stamp because they see only individual cuts of meat in the grocery store.

However, customers typically do know the grade of the meat they buy in the grocery or eat in a restaurant. Most familiar to consumers is the US Department of Agriculture's traditional grading of beef (for example, USDA Prime and USDA Choice steaks). This voluntary grading is based on the marbling of the meat—that is, higher-grade beef has more fat streaks running through the meat, making it juicier and more flavorful.[91]

In general, beef from grain-fed cattle is fattier than beef from grass-fed cattle, and the two types of beef also taste somewhat different. USDA recently established a voluntary certification process for labeling beef as grass-fed. To be labeled as grass-fed, beef must come from cows that were not fed grain, but rather ate only grass (or forage) and had ready access to pasture.[92]

US Safeguards Against BSE

The US Food and Drug Administration (FDA) is the lead agency in putting in place measures to prevent an epidemic of BSE and variant Creutzfeldt-Jakob disease in the United States, following a 1989 ban on importing animals or animal products from any country affected by BSE. In 1997, a **ruminant feed ban** was imposed—that is, a ban on feeding *ruminant protein* (meat and bone meal from rendered ruminant mammals) to ruminants. This restriction was expanded a few years later into a full **mammalian feed ban**, banning the feeding of any *mammalian protein* to ruminants (because nonruminant mammals, such as swine and horses, might have been fed rendered ruminant protein). Nonmammalian protein (from rendered poultry, for example) can still be fed to ruminants because birds are not believed to be susceptible to prion diseases.

Some exceptions to the 1997 no-mammalian-protein rule have recently been eliminated: mammalian blood and blood products from slaughter can no longer be fed to ruminants as a source of protein, for example; neither can poultry litter or plate waste from human consumption.[93] Recent regulations also address the considerable practical challenges of preventing cross-contamination between segregated rendering processes.

In addition to establishing controls on rendering, the FDA has mounted a BSE surveillance program and developed plans to respond to a US outbreak. To date, three cases of BSE have been diagnosed in US cows, though the first, in 2003, was in a cow that had been imported from Canada. The first native case, a Texas cow about 12 years old, was confirmed in 2005; the animal had been selected for sampling on arrival at a pet food plant.[94] In 2006, a 10-year-old downer cow in Alabama was determined to have BSE; this cow's herd of origin was never determined.[95]

Conservation and Management of Fisheries

The Magnuson-Stevens Fishery Conservation and Management Act, reauthorized most recently in 2006, includes provisions to address three critical issues: overfishing of the regional fisheries in ocean waters surrounding the United States; environmental degradation in these fisheries; and the incidental catching of fish other than the species being sought, often resulting in the death of these fish.[96] Regional fishery management councils are required to define what constitutes overfishing of a given fishery and to establish plans to rebuild fish stocks.

Organic Foods

The Organic Foods Production Act of 1990 set national standards for the production and handling of foods labeled as organic. It also created the National Organic Standards Board, an advisory body that includes organic farmers and retailers, scientists, and environmental and consumer advocates. The law sets criteria that qualify crops and livestock as organically grown and certifies organic growers and handlers that conform to these criteria.[97] For example, organically raised cattle must have access to pasture and fresh air and be able to exercise. Their feed must be organically produced and cannot include products from rendering. Products from certified growers can carry the organic seal shown in **Figure 6.13**. Unlike the term *organic*, the term *natural* has no regulatory meaning under US law.

Food Safety

As described in Chapter 3, individuals can do much to prevent foodborne illness by using appropriate practices at home. Upstream controls are also important; however, using institutional controls to ensure food safety is a difficult challenge because many individuals and entities may be involved in a long line of processes in food production and food service. Inspection of food products and processes has long been at the heart of regulating food safety, as evidenced in the early laws to inspect meat and poultry. Traditionally, federal food safety efforts rested on inspectors who made a physical examination of foods, such as carcasses in a meatpacking facility. Although this approach—sometimes referred to as the "poke and sniff" method—was not fully scientific, it was a direct inspection of the food itself.

Since the 1990s, the USDA and FDA have increasingly implemented a different approach to food safety, known as the **Hazard Analysis and Critical Control Point (HACCP) system**, or "has-sip," which has broad international acceptance. The HACCP approach rests on seven key actions[98]:

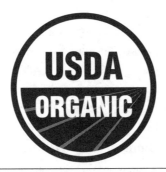

FIGURE 6.13   The USDA organic seal. *From*: US Department of Agriculture, Agricultural Marketing Service. *The National Organic Program: Production and Handling—Preamble*. Available at: http://www.ams.usda.gov/nop/NOP/standards/DefinePre.html. Accessed December 12, 2007.

- Identify the hazards that may be associated with a food (for example, microbial contamination)
- Identify **critical control points** in the production of the food—that is, points at which the hazard could be controlled or eliminated (for example, cooking); and for each critical control point establish:
  - Specific measures to prevent the hazard (for example, requirements for cooking time and temperature)
  - Procedures to monitor the preventive measures (for example, how cooking time will be monitored)
  - Corrective actions to be taken when monitoring shows a failure in preventive measures (for example, disposing of inadequately cooked food)
- Establish procedures to ensure that pieces of the system are in good working order (for example, that a cooking unit is working properly)
- Establish recordkeeping systems to document each of the preceding steps

Because HACCP systems incorporate both scientific and practical understanding of food safety, they offer the possibility of much more effective control of foodborne illness than "poke and sniff" inspections. On the other hand, HACCP systems rely on food industries, such as meatpackers and poultry processors, to police themselves. Federal inspectors no longer inspect food directly, but rather evaluate the HACCP systems that industry has created to monitor itself—a change that is of real concern to some food inspectors.[99]

The USDA and FDA have concluded that on balance the modernization offered by HACCP is an improvement over traditional food inspections. The USDA has required the meat and poultry industries to implement HACCP, and the FDA has required it of processors of seafood and seafood products, and also of processors of fruit and vegetable juice and juice products. State and local governments regulate food safety in food service and retail food establishments; however, FDA is encouraging the voluntary implementation of HACCP in these settings also.[100]

Food Defects and Additives

The FDA sets Food Defect Action Levels—maximum acceptable levels of food defects, such as insect parts, that are considered unavoidable in food. Foreign substances present in food at these levels are considered to present no health hazard to people.

Since a 1958 amendment to the FFDCA, the FDA must approve any new additive to be used in food, set limits on its use, and set labeling requirements. Two classes of additives are exempted: substances that FDA had determined to be safe before the 1958 amendment; and substances that are *generally regarded as safe* (GRAS; "grass") by scientists. This term has a regulatory meaning: Several hundred substances are on the GRAS list, which is subject to modification. No additive can be approved by the FDA if it is found to cause cancer in either humans or animals—a restriction known as the Delaney Clause.[101] (Pesticides were removed from the scope of the Delaney Clause when the Food Quality Protection Act was passed in 1996.)

The FDA has approved irradiation of meat, poultry, and some other foods, including fresh fruit and vegetables, at a specific dose for each type of food. The symbol shown in **Figure 6.14**

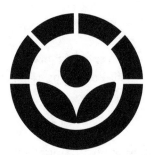

FIGURE 6.14   The radura logo, symbolizing irradiated food. *From*: Morehouse K. Food irradiation: The treatment of foods with ionizing radiation. *Food Testing Anal.* 1998;4(3):9, 32, 35.

is known as the **radura** and signifies food that has been irradiated. Under US law, irradiated food must bear the radura symbol on its label, along with the words "treated with radiation" or "treated by irradiation."[102] In regulatory terms, irradiating food without complying with these requirements amounts to using an unapproved additive.

Study Questions

1. Contrast chemical pesticides with industrial chemical pollutants as environmental health hazards.
2. Contrast the perspective of the industrialized nations of the northern hemisphere with the perspective of sub-Saharan African nations on the use of DDT.
3. Why do you think integrated pest management is not more widely used in the United States?
4. Arguments for vegetarianism have been made on grounds of ethics, equity, and sustainability. Do you find any of these arguments compelling? Why or why not?
5. What are the key lessons to be learned from the experience with bovine spongiform encephalopathy?
6. Do you think the HACCP approach to food safety is an improvement over traditional "poke and sniff" inspections? Explain.

References

1. US Department of Agriculture, National Agricultural Statistics Service. *Trends in US Agriculture*. Available at: http://www.usda.gov/nass/pubs/trends/timecapsule.htm. Accessed March 13, 2007.
2. US Department of Agriculture, National Agricultural Statistics Service. *2002 Census of Agriculture*. Available at: http://www.nass.usda.gov/census/census02/volume1/us/index1.htm. Accessed March 13, 2007.
3. Pimentel D. Industrial agriculture, energy flows in. In: Cleveland C, ed. *Encyclopedia of Energy*. Amsterdam: Elsevier, 2004:365–371.
4. Knobeloch L, Proctor M. Eight blue babies. *Wisc Med J.* 2001;100(8):43–47.

5. Greer F, Shannon M, Committee on Nutrition, Committee on Environmental Health. Infant methemoglobinemia: the role of dietary nitrate in food and water. *Pediat.* 2005;116(3):784–786.

6. Manassaram D, Backer L, Moll D. A review of nitrates in drinking water: maternal exposure and adverse reproductive and developmental outcomes. *Environ Health Perspect.* 2006;114(3):320–327.

7. US Environmental Protection Agency. *Pesticides Industry Sales and Usage: 2000 and 2001 Market Estimates.* 2004. Available at: http://www.epa.gov/oppbead1/pestsales/01pestsales/market_estimates2001.pdf. Accessed April 19, 2008.

8. Paul Hermann Muller. In: *Britannica Online Encyclopaedia*; 2007. Available at: http://www.britannica.com/eb/article-9054225/Paul-Hermann-Muller. Accessed December 9, 2007.

9. World Health Organization. *WHO Gives Indoor Use of DDT a Clean Bill of Health for Controlling Malaria.* September 15, 2006. Available at: http://www.who.int/mediacentre/news/releases/2006/pr50/en. Accessed December 9, 2007.

10. Ehler L. Integrated pest management (IPM): definition, historical development and implementation, and the other IPM. *Pest Management Sci.* 2006;62:787–789.

11. Kamel F, Hoppin J. Association of pesticide exposure with neurologic dysfunction and disease. *Environ Health Perspect.* 2004;112(9):950–958.

12. Alavanja M, Hoppin J, Kamel F. Health effects of chronic pesticide exposure: cancer and neurotoxicity. *Ann Rev Public Health.* 2004;25:155–197.

13. Blair A, Zahm S. Cancer among farmers. *Occup Med.* 1991;3:335–354.

14. Blair A, Zahm S. Patterns of pesticide use among farmers: implications for epidemiologic research. *Epidemiology.* 1993;4:55–62.

15. Blair A, Zahm S. Agricultural exposures and cancer. *Environ Health Perspect.* 1995;103:205–208.

16. Blair A, Zahm S, Pearce N, Heineman E, Fraumeni J. Clues to cancer etiology from studies of farmers. *Scand J Work Environ Health.* 1992;18:209–215.

17. Garcia A. Occupational exposure to pesticides and congenital malformations: a review of mechanisms, methods, and results. *Am J Ind Med.* 1998;33:232–240.

18. Kirkhorn S, Schenker M. Current health effects of agricultural work: respiratory disease, cancer, reproductive effects, musculoskeletal injuries, and pesticide-related illnesses. *J Agri Safety Health.* 2002;8(2):199–214.

19. Garry V. Pesticides and children. *Toxicol Appl Pharmacol.* 2004;198:152–163.

20. US Department of Agriculture, Economic Research Service. *Rural Labor and Education: Farm Labor.* Available at: http://www.ers.usda.gov/Briefing/LaborAndEducation/FarmLabor.htm#demographic. Accessed March 4, 2007.

21. Runyan J. Almost half of hired farmworkers 25 years and older earn poverty-level wages. *Rural Conditions Trends.* 2000;11(2):47–50.

22. McCauley LA, Lasarev MR, Higgins G, Rothlein JE, Muniz J, Ebbert C. Work characteristics and pesticide exposures among migrant agricultural families: a community-based research approach. *Environ Health Perspect.* 2001;109(5):533–538.

23. London L. Occupational epidemiology in agriculture: a case study in the Southern African context. *Int J Occup Environ Health.* 1998;4:245–256.

24. Brower V. Growing greener: the impact of integrated pest management. *EMBO Reports.* 2002;3(5):403–406.

25. Ehler L, Bottrell D. The illusion of integrated pest management. *Issues Science Technol.* Spring 2000. Available at: http://www.issues.org/16.3/ehler.htm. Accessed March 3, 2007.

26. US Census Bureau. *World Population Information.* Available at: http://www.census.gov/ipc/www/world.html. Accessed March 3, 2007.

27. Lehrer S, Bannon G. Risks of allergic reactions to biotech proteins in foods: perception and reality. *Allergy.* 2005;60:559–564.

28. Heritage J. Transgenes for tea? *Trends Biotechnol.* 2005;23(1):17–21.

29. Nestle M. *Safe Food: Bacteria, Biotechnology, and Bioterrorism.* Berkeley: University of California Press; 2003.

30. Hutson S, Barber N, Kenny J, Linsey K, Lumia D, Maupin M. *Estimated Use of Water in the United States in 2000.* US Geological Survey Circular 1268; 2004. Available at: http://pubs.usgs.gov/circ/2004/circ1268/. Accessed April 19, 2008.

31. US Geological Survey. *Comparisons of Average Consumptive Use and Renewable Water Supply for the 21 Water-Resources Regions of the United States, Puerto Rico, and US Virgin Islands (updated using 1995 estimates of water use).* Available at: http://water/usgs.gov/watuse/misc/consuse-renewable.html. Accessed December 17, 2007.

32. United Nations. *Water: A Shared Responsibility.* Paris: UNESCO; 2006. Report No. 92-3-104006-5. Available at: http://unesdoc.unesco.org/images/0014/001444/144409E.pdf.

33. US Department of Labor, Bureau of Labor Statistics. *Occupational Injuries and Illnesses and Fatal Injuries Profiles.* Available at: http://data.bls.gov/GQT/servlet/InitialPage. Accessed March 12, 2007.

34. Rautiainen R, Lange J, Hodne C, Schneiders S, Donham K. Injuries in the Iowa Certified Safe Farm Study. *J Agri Safety Health.* 2004;10(1):51–63.

35. Rollin BE. Animal agriculture and emerging social ethics for animals. *J Animal Sci.* 2004;82:955–964.

36. US Department of Agriculture, National Agricultural Statistics Service. *Livestock Slaughter.* 2003. Available at: http://usda.mannlib.cornell.edu/usda/nass/LiveSlau//2000s/2003/LiveSlau-01-24-2003.pdf. Accessed April 19, 2008.

37. US Department of Agriculture, National Agricultural Statistics Service. *Poultry Slaughter: 2002 Annual Summary.* 2003. Available at: http://usda.mannlib.cornell.edu/usda/nass/PoulSlauSu//2000s/2003/PoulSlauSu-03-07-2003.pdf. Accessed April 19, 2008.

38. US Department of Agriculture, National Agricultural Statistics Service. *Cattle: Final Estimates 1999–2003.* 2004. Available at: http://usda.mannlib.cornell.edu/usda/reports/general/sb/sb989.pdf. Accessed April 19, 2008.

39. US Department of Agriculture, National Agricultural Statistics Service. *Livestock Operations: Final Estimates 1998–2002.* 2004. Available at: http://usda.mannlib.cornell.edu/usda/reports/general/sb/sb1002.pdf. Accessed April 19, 2008.

40. US Environmental Protection Agency. *Profile of the Agricultural Livestock Production Industry.* 2000. Available at: http://www.epa.gov/compliance/resources/publications/ assistance/sectors/notebooks/aglivestock.pdf. Accessed April 19, 2008.

41. US Food and Drug Administration. *A Risk-Based Approach to Evaluate Animal Clones and Their Progeny (Draft); Appendix B: Overall Reproductive Efficiency and Health Statistics for US Animal Agriculture.* 2007. Available at: http://www.fda.gov/cvm/ CloningRA_AppendixB.htm. Accessed March 10, 2007.

42. US Department of Agriculture, National Agricultural Statistics Service. *Cattle Death Loss.* 2006. Available at: http://www.nass.usda.gov/Statistics_by_State/Oregon/ Publications/Livestock_Report/cattdl06.pdf. Accessed April 19, 2008.

43. US Department of Agriculture, Economic Research Service. *Hogs: Background.* Available at: http://www.ers.usda.gov/Briefing/Hogs/Background.htm. Accessed March 10, 2007.

44. US Department of Agriculture, Animal and Plant Health Inspection Service. *Swine 2000.* 2005. Available at: http://nahms.aphis.usda.gov/swine/swine2000/swine2kPt4.pdf. Accessed April 19, 2008.

45. Cole D, Todd L, Wing S. Concentrated swine feeding operations and public health: a review of occupational and community health effects. *Environ Health Perspect.* 2000;108(8):685–699.

46. Nachman K, Graham J, Price L, Silbergeld E. Arsenic: a roadblock to potential animal waste management solutions. *Environ Health Perspect.* 2005;113(9):1123–1124.

47. Sigurdarson S, O'Shaughnessy P, Watt J, Kline J. Experimental human exposure to inhaled grain dust and ammonia: towards a model of concentrated animal feeding operations. *Am J Ind Med.* 2004;46:345–348.

48. National Institute of Occupational Safety and Health. *NIOSH Warns: Manure Pits Continue to Claim Lives.* Available at: http://www.cdc.gov/Niosh/updats/93-114.htm. Accessed December 2, 2007.

49. Brubaker B. Four family members, farmhand killed by gas fumes in manure pit. *Washington Post,* July 4, 2007.

50. Schiffman S. Livestock odors: implications for human health and well-being. *J Animal Sci.* 1998;76:1343–1355.

51. Wing S, Cole D, Grant G. Environmental injustice in North Carolina's hog industry. *Environ Health Perspect.* 2000;108(3):225–231.

52. Marano N, Stamey K, Barrett T, Angulo F. High prevalence of gentamicin resistance among selected *Salmonella* serotypes in the United States: associated with heavy use of gentamicin in poultry. Infect Disease Society of America 37th Annual Meeting; Philadelphia, Pa.; 1999.

53. Shea K. Antibiotic resistance: what is the impact of agricultural uses of antibiotics on children's health? *Pediatrics.* 2003;112(1):253–258.

54. Sorum H, L'Abee-Lund T. Antibiotic resistance in food-related bacteria—a result of interfering with the global web of bacterial genetics. *Int J Food Microbiol.* 2002;78: 43–56.

55. Cai C, Perry M, Sorock G, Hauser R, Spanjer K, Mittleman M, et al. Laceration injuries among workers at meat packing plants. *Am J Ind Med.* 2005;47:403–410.

56. US Occupational Safety and Health Administration. *Poultry Processing Industry eTool.* Available at: http://www.osha.gov/SLTC/etools/poultry/index.html. Accessed March 24, 2007.

57. Quandt S, Grzywacz J, Marin A, Carrillo L, Coates M, Burke B, et al. Illnesses and injuries reported by Latino poultry workers in western North Carolina. *Am J Ind Med.* 2006;49:343–351.

58. Campbell D. Health hazards in the meatpacking industry. *Occup Med: State Art Rev.* 1999;14(2):351–372.

59. Besson H. Cancer mortality among butchers: a 24-state death certificate study. *J Occup Environ Med.* 2006;48(3):289–293.

60. McLean D, Pearce N. Cancer among meat industry workers. *Scand J Work, Environ Health.* 2004;30(6):425–437.

61. Boffetta P, Gridley G, Gustavsson P, Brennan P, Blair A, Ekstrom A, et al. Employment as butcher and cancer risk in a record-linkage study from Sweden. *Cancer Causes Control.* 2000;11(7):627–633.

62. US Department of Agriculture, National Agricultural Statistics Service. *QuickStats: Agricultural Statistics Database.* Available at: http://www.nass.usda.gov/QuickStats/. Accessed March 7, 2007.

63. BBC News. Why mad cow disease lingers on. October 29, 1999. Available at: http://news.bbc.co.uk/2/hi/uk_news/493435.stm. Accessed March 23, 2007.

64. UK Ministry of Agriculture, Fisheries and Food. *The BSE Inquiry Report: BSE Inquiry.* 2000. Available at: http://www.bseinquiry.gov.uk/. Accessed March 22, 2007.

65. Rhodes R. *Deadly Feasts.* New York, NY: Simon & Schuster; 1997.

66. Doyle E. *Bovine Spongiform Encephalopathy: An Updated Scientific Literature Review.* Madison: University of Wisconsin, Food Research Institute; 2004. Available at: http://www.wisc.edu/fri/briefs/BSE04update.pdf. Accessed April 19, 2008.

67. UK Department of Health. *Communications Summary September 2006: Creutzfeldt-Jakob Disease in the UK.* Available at: http://www.dh.gov.uk/en/Publicationsandstatistics/Publications/CommunicationsSummary/DH_4138939. Accessed March 7, 2007.

68. MacDonald J, O'Donoghue E, McBride W, Nehring R, Sandretto C, Mosheim R. *Profits, Costs, and the Changing Structure of Dairy Farming.* USDA Economic Research Report No. 47; 2007.

69. Lone K. Natural sex steroids and their xenobiotic analogs in animal production: growth, carcass quality, pharmacokinetics, metabolism, mode of action, residues, methods, and epidemiology. *Crit Rev Food Sci Nutr.* 1997;37(2):93–209.

70. US Food and Drug Administration. *The Use of Steroid Hormones for Growth Promotion in Food-Producing Animals.* Available at: http://www.fda.gov/cvm/hormones.htm. Accessed March 12, 2007.

71. Keown J, Kononoff P. *Can You Afford to Use Bovine Somatotrophin (Bovine Growth Hormone)?* University of Nebraska-Lincoln Extension, Institute of Agriculture and

Natural Resources; 2007. Available at: http://www.ianrpubs.unl.edu/epublic/live/g1664/build/g1664.pdf. Accessed April 19, 2008.

72. US Department of Agriculture, Animal and Plant Health Inspection Service. *Bovine Somatotropin*. 2003. Available at: http://www.aphis.usda.gov/vs/ceah/ncahs/nahms/dairy/dairy02/Dairy02BST.pdf. Accessed April 19, 2008.

73. US Energy Information Administration. *Emissions of Greenhouse Gases in the United States 2004*. 2005. Available at: http://www.eia.doe.gov/oiaf/1605/archive/gg05rpt/pdf/executive_summary.pdf. Accessed April 19, 2008.

74. Johnson K, Johnson D. Methane emissions from cattle. *J Anim Sci*. 1995;73:2483–2492.

75. Tyedmers P. Fisheries and energy use. In: Cleveland C, ed. *Encyclopedia of Energy*. Amsterdam, Elsevier: 2004:683–693.

76. Froese R, Kesner-Reyes K. *Impact of Fishing on the Abundance of Marine Species*. International Council for the Exploration of the Sea Annual Science Conference; Copenhagen; 2002.

77. Grainger R. *Global Trends in Fisheries and Aquaculture (National Oceanic and Atmospheric Administration's National Dialogues on Coastal Stewardship)*. 1999. Available at: http://www.oceanservice.noaa.gov/websites/retiredsites/natdia_pdf/2grainger.pdf. Accessed April 19, 2008.

78. Hites R, Foran J, Carpenter D, Hamilton M, Knuth B, Schwager S. Global assessment of organic contaminants in farmed salmon. *Science*. 2004;303:226–229.

79. Thomas T, Lincoln J, Husberg B, Conway G. Is it safe on deck? Fatal and non-fatal workplace injuries among Alaskan commercial fishermen. *Am J Ind Med*. 2001; 40:693–702.

80. Shea K, American Academy of Pediatrics, Committee on Environmental Health. Technical report: irradiation of food. *Pediatrics*. 2000;106(6):1505–1510.

81. Louria D. Counterpoint on food irradiation. *Int J Infect Dis*. 2000;4(2):67–69.

82. Epstein SS, Hauter W. Preventing pathogenic food poisoning: sanitation, not irradiation. *Int J Health Serv*. 2001;31(1):187–192.

83. Schlosser E. *Fast Food Nation*. New York, NY: Perennial; 2002.

84. Kuepper G, Gegner L. *Organic Crop Production Overview*. 2004. US Department of Agriculture, National Center for Appropriate Technology. Available at: http://attra.ncat.org/attra-pub/PDF/organiccrop.pdf. Accessed April 19, 2008.

85. US Department of Agriculture, Economic Research Service. *Organic Production*. Available at: http://www.ers.usda.gov/Data/Organic/Data/Certified%20and%20total%20US%20acreage%20selected%20crops%20livestock%2095-05.xls. Accessed March 22, 2007.

86. Congressional Research Service. *Food Biotechology in the United States: Science, Regulation, and Issues*. 2001. Available at: http://www.ncseonline.org/nle/crsreports/science/st-41.pdf. Accessed April 19, 2008.

87. US Environmental Protection Agency. *Pesticides: Regulating Pesticides*. Available at: http://www.epa.gov/pesticides/regulating/. Accessed March 22, 2007.

88. Pew Initiative on Food and Biotechnology. *Guide to US Regulation of Genetically Modified Food and Agricultural Biotechnology Products*. 2001. Available at: http://www.pewtrusts.org/uploadedFiles/wwwpewtrustsorg/Reports/Food_and_Biotechnology/hhs_biotech_0901.pdf. Accessed April 19, 2008.

89. Rawson JM and Vogt DU. CRS Report for Congress: *Food Safety Agencies and Authorities: A Primer*. 1998. Available at: http://www.ncseonline.org/NLE/CRSreports/Agriculture/ag-40.cfm. Accessed March 21, 2007.

90. US Department of Agriculture, Food Safety and Inspection Service. *Key Facts: Humane Slaughter*. Available at: http://www.fsis.usda.gov/Fact_Sheets/Key_Facts_Humane_Slaughter/index.asp. Accessed March 22, 2007.

91. US Department of Agriculture, Agricultural Marketing Service. *How to Buy Meat*. July 1995. Available at: http://www.ams.usda.gov/howtobuy/meat.htm. Accessed December 10, 2007.

92. US Department of Agriculture, Agricultural Marketing Service. *USDA Establishes Grass (Forage) Fed Marketing Claim Standard*. October 15, 2007. Available at: http://www.ams.usda.gov/news/178-07.htm. Accessed December 10, 2007.

93. US Food and Drug Administration. Statement by Lester M. Crawford before the Senate Committee on Agriculture, Nutrition, and Forestry. Available at: http://www.fda.gov/ola/2002/schoollunches430.html. Accessed March 12, 2007.

94. US Department of Agriculture. Statement by USDA Chief Veterinarian John Clifford. Available at: http://www.aphis.usda.gov/lpa/issues/bse/BSE_statement6-29-05.pdf. Accessed January 2, 2007.

95. US Centers for Disease Control and Prevention. *About BSE*. Available at: http://www.cdc.gov/ncidod/dvrd/bse/. Accessed March 12, 2007.

96. National Oceanic and Atmospheric Administration. *Sustainable Fisheries Act*. Available at: http://www.nmfs.noaa.gov/sfa/. Accessed March 14, 2007.

97. US Department of Agriculture, Agricultural Marketing Service. *The National Organic Program: Production and Handling—Preamble*. Available at: http://www.ams.usda.gov/nop/NOP/standards/DefinePre.html. Accessed December 12, 2007.

98. US Food and Drug Administration. *HACCP: A State-of the-Art Approach to Food Safety*. Available at: http://www.cfsan.fda.gov/~lrd/bghaccp.html. Accessed February 7, 2008.

99. PBS Frontline. *Modern Meat*. Available at: http://www.pbs.org/wgbh/pages/frontline/shows/meat/evaluating/haccp.html. Accessed March 22, 2007.

100. US Food and Drug Administration. *Managing Food Safety: A Manual for the Voluntary Use of HACCP Principles for Operators of Food Service and Retail Establishments*. Available at: http://www.cfsan.fda.gov/~dms/hret2toc.html. Accessed March 22, 2007.

101. US Food and Drug Administration. *Food Additives*. Available at: http://www.cfsan.fda.gov/~lrd/foodaddi.html. Accessed February 7, 2008.

102. US Food and Drug Administration. *Food Irradiation: The Treatment of Foods with Ionizing Radiation*. Available at: http://www.cfsan.fda.gov/~lrd/bghaccp.html. Accessed March 22, 2007.

Living in the World We've Made

Learning Objectives

After studying this chapter, the reader will be able to:

- Define or explain the key terms throughout the chapter

- Describe how various types of municipal waste are consolidated into waste streams that are treated

- Describe the problem that combined sewer overflows are intended to address and how they address it

- Describe the typical steps in municipal wastewater treatment, along with the objectives of each step

- Explain the key principle behind a sustainable approach to sanitation, whether in industrialized or lower-income countries

- Describe the potential hazards of land application of treated sewage sludge

- Explain how the objectives of drinking water treatment are met through the treatment processes

- Identify the four major approaches to handling municipal solid waste, and describe the challenges of managing this mundane waste stream

- Describe the US regulatory framework for managing the public health risks associated with drinking water, municipal wastewater, and municipal solid waste

- Describe the environmental health hazards of megacities in lower-income countries

- Describe the environmental health hazards of urban and suburban or exurban settings in industrialized countries, and of specific hazards of modern life

- Explain and compare the carbon footprint and the ecologic footprint and their implications for the sustainability of current development patterns

As described in earlier chapters, though human beings live among other species—and are closely connected to some of them through disease—we are unique in the extent of our deliberate modification of the natural world. Especially in the industrialized nations, we have built complex systems to generate power, manufacture goods, and produce food. These systems consume raw materials and energy, and produce wastes, in vast quantities.

This final chapter is about living in the world we have created. It begins by describing the major flows into and out of communities (Section 7.1). The following three sections describe the challenges and health concerns of each in turn: handling sewage (Section 7.2), providing safe drinking water (Section 7.3), and managing trash and other types of solid waste (Section 7.4). These sections also describe pertinent US regulatory provisions. Section 7.5 considers the environmental health concerns of urban settings in our increasingly urbanized world, and Section 7.6 considers some environmental health hazards of the modern lifestyle—from cigarettes to cosmetics to noise. The chapter—and the book—concludes with a brief discussion of the globalization of environmental health concerns and the nonsustainable nature of modern development (Section 7.7).

7.1 The "Metabolism" of Communities

If we think of a city or town as an organism, then its water supply, sewage, and trash are the inputs and outputs of a kind of "urban metabolism."[1] The metabolism of today's cities, though it incorporates some thoroughly modern features, also reflects some 19th-century decisions about infrastructure.

Urban Metabolism in the 19th Century

The development of systems to handle water and waste followed a similar pattern in most cities of the United States and Europe. Through the early years of the 19th century, urine and feces were collected in pits located below privies or in larger underground vaults known as cesspools.

These had to be emptied periodically and the contents carried away. In some cities, there were sewer pipes to carry away rainwater that collected in gutters.

By the mid-19th century, it had become possible to supply urban homes with running water from a tap. This led to the development of the water closet, in which water was used to flush waste through pipes into a privy pit or cesspool. This addition of water to the waste stream meant that a much larger volume of waste was now going to storage vaults, which suddenly seemed too small. They now had to be emptied more frequently, which was both inconvenient and expensive.

Faced with this crisis, in the latter half of the 19th century many cities opted for the same technological solution—the use of water to carry away sewage.[1] And as engineers designed sewer systems, they faced a key decision: whether to channel sewage waste and street runoff into one sewer system, or build separate systems for the two waste streams. Separate systems would have been more costly, and most communities opted for combined sewer systems, which emptied wastewater into a nearby body of water.[1]

In the coming decades, scientists showed that contamination of a downstream city's drinking water intake by an upstream city's sewage could cause disease in the downstream city. Further, filtration technologies were developed during this period that could dramatically reduce microbial contamination of water. Now cities faced another decision[1]: Was it enough for a city to treat its drinking water, or should it also treat its wastewater? Again, cities took the less expensive option, treating only drinking water. It was not until the 20th century that it became common for cities to treat their wastewater in even a limited fashion.

As will be described later, the processes used to treat sewage and drinking water have costs and side effects, and we might like to imagine different technological decisions, past or future. Nevertheless, these methods have been strikingly successful overall in holding the incidence of waterborne illness to a low level in the industrialized nations.

In contrast to sewage, trash as we know it today is largely a phenomenon of the 20th century. Before that time, material goods were scarce and were scavenged and reused as a matter of course.[2] It is only in the era of the *consumer* that ordinary people buy many new items simply because they want them and continually throw out the old to make way for the new.

Community Metabolism Today

The modern metabolism of US communities is shaped by three facts so fundamental that we rarely think about them. First, on the intake side, we have a unified water supply, not separate supplies of **potable water** (water deemed suitable for drinking) and nonpotable water. There is a strong public health rationale for this approach: It avoids cross-contamination of the potable supply and various mistakes that would lead to waterborne illness. Nevertheless, the result is that we water our lawns and wash our cars with water that has been treated to drinking water standards. The second fundamental fact derives directly from the first: On the outgoing side of community metabolism, we use potable water to carry away sewage.

The third fundamental fact of modern community metabolism is the sheer scale of its inputs and outputs. In the United States today, a typical family of four uses about 280 gallons of water indoors each day, and an additional 120 gallons outdoors.[3,4] Flushing wastes down the toilet is the single largest indoor use of water (**Figure 7.1**); other major uses are washing clothes, taking

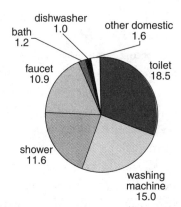

FIGURE 7.1 Estimated indoor use of water in the United States, 1999 (gallons per capita per day; excludes leaks). *Data from*: Aquacraft Inc., American Water Works Association Research Foundation. *Residential Water Use Summary from the American Water Works Association Research Foundation's End Uses of Water Study.* Available at: http://www.aquacraft.com/Publications/resident.htm. Accessed February 10, 2008.

showers, and using water from the faucet for various purposes. Four people in the United States also generate about 18 pounds of trash each day, on average,[5] as detailed below.

Thus domestic wastewater, though it is still the most basic human waste stream, is now accompanied by large quantities of trash, and in fact there is some overlap in the contents of these two waste streams. Further, once domestic wastewater enters the municipal system, it is sometimes mixed with two other waste streams: storm runoff from paved surfaces; and liquid wastes from industry. These various connections among waste streams are described here.

Municipal Wastewater and Municipal Solid Waste

The typical household produces three basic types of wastes: urine and feces; food waste; and a mixture of other wastes that includes chemical products and items made of glass, metal, plastic, paper, and other materials. As shown in **Figure** 7.2, these wastes are consolidated into two waste

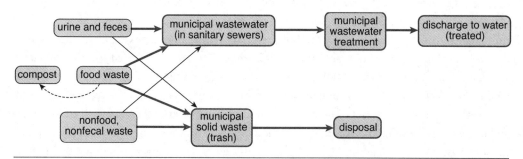

FIGURE 7.2 Contributors to municipal wastewater and municipal solid waste streams.

streams: **sewage** and **trash**.* At the community level, these two waste streams are often referred to as **municipal wastewater** and **municipal solid waste**.

Although these are separate municipal waste streams, there is some overlap in their contents, since each is simply a different mix of the same basic types of waste. Wastewater consists of anything that goes down a drain, not only from toilets but also from sinks and bathtubs, washing machines and dishwashers. Thus, in addition to urine and feces it includes paper and cotton products, soap, shampoo, other personal care products applied to the body, laundry detergents, and fabric softeners. Other items also go down the toilet—outdated medications, used condoms, dead goldfish, children's toys, jewelry, and so on. Many more of these same items are discarded as trash, along with a great variety of other household items, large and small. At the same time, a small proportion of fecal waste goes out as trash—for example, in disposable diapers, which now make up 1.5% by weight of the US municipal solid waste stream.[5]

The fate of food waste varies: Some goes down the drain, and some into the trash. If a household has a garbage disposal in the kitchen, a much greater share of its food waste enters the municipal wastewater stream. Alternatively, food waste can be composted, which is a form of recycling, and in this case food waste doesn't enter a municipal waste stream.

Municipal Wastewater and Storm Runoff

As noted earlier, many older cities channel storm runoff from gutter drains into the sanitary sewers. This urban runoff, shed mainly from streets and other impervious surfaces, is different from municipal wastewater in two important ways. First, its makeup is different. Although it may carry small quantities of animal waste, its overall burden of fecal waste and pathogens is very low. But it may include oil and grease, road salt, heavy metals, and yard chemicals, as well as a heavy load of sediment. Second, storm runoff is episodic, surging during and after storms, whereas the municipal wastewater stream is relatively constant day in and day out. This creates a problem: Treatment plants are designed to handle the steady flow of municipal wastewater, and are overwhelmed when a storm surge is added to the normal flow.

For this reason, overflow valves called **combined sewer overflows** (CSOs) are built into a combined sewer system. When the combined flow of municipal wastewater and storm runoff exceeds the treatment plant's capacity, these overflow valves open, releasing untreated wastewater directly into some body of water (see **Figure 7.3**, which zooms in on the municipal wastewater stream in Figure 7.2 and adds new elements). The treatment plant continues to operate at full capacity, but some wastewater never passes through it.

In the United States, about 46 million people live in more than 800 communities that have combined sewer overflows.[6] These overflows are found mostly in older cities, in areas of relatively dense population and high rainfall—almost no CSOs are found, for example, in the Great Plains or Rocky Mountain states, or in the arid Southwest. Modifications to such an infrastructure are difficult and expensive. In Greater Boston, for example—where the sewage sys-

---

*Some people use the term *garbage* to refer specifically to food waste; others consider it synonymous with *trash*.

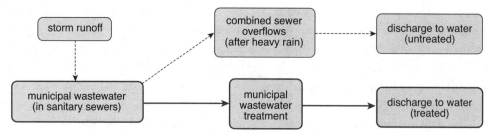

FIGURE 7.3 Use of combined sewer overflows to handle storm runoff.

tem serves 2.5 million people in 43 cities and towns, and handles 350 million gallons of sewage per day[7]—some 70 combined sewer overflows once released untreated sewage into Boston Harbor and the three rivers that flow into the harbor. Although it is not feasible to completely restructure the system, the regional water authority has taken an incremental approach. Municipal wastewater and storm water have been separated in some local areas, and in some other locations CSOs have been consolidated so that the combined waste stream can at least be screened and chlorinated before being released. And, during a rainstorm, some wastewater can be held in storage so that it can later go to the treatment plant.[8]

Municipal Wastewater and Industrial Wastes

Finally, though industrial wastes are sometimes treated and discharged separately from municipal wastewater (called a **direct discharge** of industrial wastes to the receiving body of water), they are sometimes discharged via the municipal wastewater stream (an **indirect discharge**); **Figure 7.4** adds this waste stream to the municipal sewage and storm runoff waste streams in Figure 7.3. In the case of an indirect discharge, industrial wastes are passing through a system

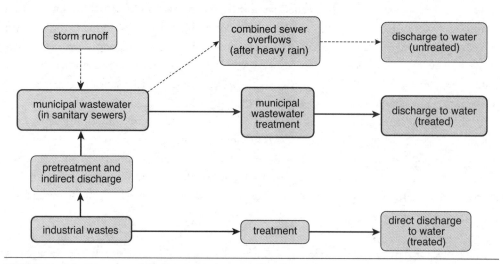

FIGURE 7.4 Direct and indirect discharge of industrial wastes.

that is not designed to treat them, and the wastes should undergo pretreatment before entering the municipal wastewater stream. Without pretreatment, acidic industrial wastes can damage sewers or the wastewater works, and pesticides or other toxic chemicals in industrial wastes may kill the bacteria that are used in wastewater treatment (described later). In addition, metals or synthetic chemicals in industrial wastes can end up in the residual material (called sludge) that remains after sewage treatment.

7.2 Management of Sewage Wastes

The biological processes involved in returning human waste safely to the environment are similar in all settings. However, the systems needed to serve a large city are very different from those that serve people in more sparsely populated areas. This section describes the following topics:

- The treatment processes used at municipal wastewater treatment plants, which receive wastewater from homes, businesses, and other institutions
- The septic systems that are typically used to handle the wastes of individual homes, or small clusters of homes, in less densely populated areas
- The composting toilet, which is gaining recognition as a sustainable solution to the age-old problem of sanitation

The section closes with a description of the US framework for the regulation of municipal wastewater treatment.

Municipal Wastewater Treatment

In most cities and towns, sewage treatment comprises a very similar set of processes, most of which are long established. After outlining the objectives of sewage treatment, this section describes those basic processes, concluding with the common but controversial step of spreading the residuals of sewage treatment on land.

As already noted, more than just sewage goes into a city's sanitary sewers, and the term *municipal wastewater* captures this reality. However, municipal wastewater's most prominent component—the component that demands prompt treatment to prevent infectious disease and for which treatment is designed—is *sewage*. In this discussion, the two terms are used interchangeably.

Objectives of Sewage Treatment

Sewage treatment has three major objectives. The first is to remove pathogens, thus preventing waterborne illness in those whose drinking water source is downstream from a sewage outfall.

The second objective is to remove organic matter, thus decreasing the ecological impact of sewage waste: a decline in dissolved oxygen in the receiving water. This is precisely the same effect seen when large quantities of animal manure are released by concentrated animal feeding operations (CAFOs). As described in Chapter 6, dissolved oxygen in the receiving water declines as oxygen is consumed by bacterial digestion of both fecal waste and the detritus of algal overgrowth. If a large quantity of sewage is released into a body of water, the bacterial decomposition can deplete oxygen in the water, causing fish and other aquatic organisms to die. This impact of sewage is measured as its **biochemical oxygen demand (BOD)**: the demand for oxygen created by the biochemical process of decomposing organic matter.*

The third objective of sewage treatment is to remove suspended solids. Sewage-laden water, even if it is free of floating solids, carries a heavy load of suspended solids, making the water cloudy. Suspended solids are assessed as **turbidity** (cloudiness), which is a measure of how much the transmission of light through water is impaired. Suspended solids not only make water cloudy but also harbor pathogens and interfere with disinfection; moreover, they contribute to BOD (because they consist partly of organic matter). Thus, removing suspended solids also serves the first two objectives of sewage treatment: removing pathogens and removing organic matter.

Basic Processes of Sewage Treatment

Basic sewage treatment consists of primary and secondary treatment, though other treatments are frequently added (see **Figure 7.5**; this diagram is an expansion of the municipal wastewater treatment step that appears in the preceding three diagrams). **Primary sewage treatment** is a mechanical process during which ever-finer materials are removed from the waste stream through a sequence of steps. Primary treatment begins with a **bar screen**—wastewater flows through a set of parallel bars that screens out relatively large objects, such as children's toys and dead rats. In most modern sewage treatment works, materials captured by the bar screen are removed mechanically; in the past, these materials were raked away by workers. Next, the waste stream passes through a grinder (sometimes called a **comminutor**), ensuring that nothing in the waste stream is large enough to clog up the works.

In the two remaining steps of primary treatment, materials are simply allowed to settle out of the waste stream. First, in the **grit chamber**, heavier particles such as sand settle out; this grit will be landfilled. Then, in the **primary clarifier**, a large uncovered vat, suspended solids containing organic matter are allowed to settle out. These solids are **sewage sludge**, which itself must be treated and disposed of. Material that floats—scum—is skimmed off for further treatment along with the sludge.

The next step, **secondary sewage treatment**, is the heart of sewage treatment. This is a biological process—an accelerated version of natural decomposition in which bacteria digest organic wastes in an aerobic environment. Different methods are used to accomplish this. In the more traditional approach, wastewater is sprayed over a **trickling filter**—a bed of rocks coated with bacteria-containing slime; as the water trickles downward, the bacteria decompose organic matter. Using newer technology, sewage is primed with bacteria and then agitated in large enclosed vats called **sludge digesters** (shown in **Figure 7.6**). Either process is followed by a resting stage in which fine matter settles out, becoming sludge, and floating scum is removed to be treated along with the sludge.

Some wastewater treatment systems, particularly in large urban areas, include **tertiary sewage treatment** tailored to specific needs. For example, very fine suspended solids might be

---

*BOD is measured (in mg/L) as the amount of dissolved oxygen consumed as microorganisms break down the waste in a given volume of water in a given time period, usually either 5 or 10 days (referred to as BOD5 and BOD10). An alternate test, which takes less time to complete, uses chemical reactions as a surrogate measure of biological decomposition, assessing chemical oxygen demand (COD) in lieu of BOD.

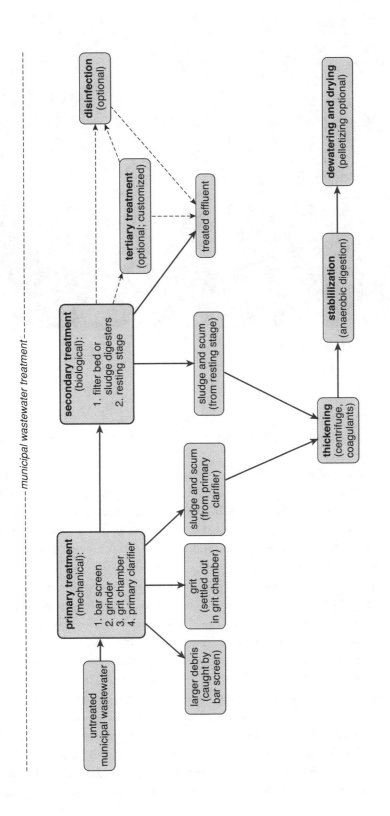

FIGURE 7.5 Steps in the treatment of municipal wastewater and sewage sludge.

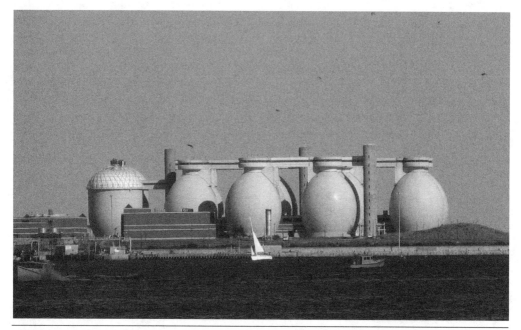

FIGURE 7.6 Pleasure boats and seabirds pass by the large egg-shaped sludge digesters of Greater Boston's Deer Island Sewage Treatment Plant.

removed, generating more sludge; or a carbon filter might be used to remove synthetic organic chemicals. Another optional step may follow tertiary or secondary treatment: **disinfection** of the waste stream, usually by chlorination.

How do these processes accomplish the basic objectives of sewage treatment? As shown in **Table 7.1**, most pathogens survive primary treatment, unless they are simply unable to survive for long outside the human body. Although secondary treatment does not specifically target pathogens, many bacteria may die simply because they run out of food; viruses are more likely than bacteria to survive secondary treatment. If disinfection is used at the end of sewage treatment, it is used with the intention of killing pathogens that remain in the waste stream. Although disinfection was used routinely in the past, it is used less commonly today because of concerns about the impact of chlorine in the aquatic environment. Also, because pathogens enter water from other sources, including farmland, the disinfection of municipal wastewater does not completely eliminate bacterial contamination of waterways.

The objective of removing organic matter from the waste stream is accomplished by removing finer and finer solids, in primary and secondary (and sometimes tertiary) treatment (Table 7.1). In contrast, primary and secondary treatment do not remove chemicals from the waste stream; this is accomplished, if at all, through optional tertiary treatment designed for this purpose. Thus, primary and secondary treatment are the core processes of treating *sewage*; it is only in tertiary treatment that other components of the waste stream may be addressed.

As described previously, some steps in the treatment of wastewater produce sludge as a by-product. Therefore, the final step in sewage treatment is to treat this sludge (see Figure 7.5).

Table 7.1 Objectives and Effects of Municipal Wastewater Treatment

| Objectives | Effects of Steps in Municipal Wastewater Treatment | | | |
| | Basic Treatment Steps | | Additional Optional Steps | |
	Primary (mechanical)	Secondary (biological)	Tertiary Treatment	Disinfection
Remove pathogens	Most survive	Many die off	—	Is effective
Remove organic waste (BOD)	Some is removed	Most is removed	Depends on treatment	—
Remove suspended solids	Some are removed	Most are removed	Depends on treatment	—
Remove chemicals	—	—	Depends on treatment	—

Although "sludge" sounds solid, the sludge that results from sewage treatment is actually mostly water, and the first step in treatment is **thickening**, for example, by centrifuging or by adding coagulants. The next step, **stabilization**, is the heart of sludge treatment. In this process, the sludge is digested by anaerobic organisms in a warm, well-circulated environment. This process reduces both the volume of sludge and its odor. Stabilization also kills many pathogens as a result of the anaerobic environment and the intense competition for food, but it is not designed specifically to rid sludge of all pathogens. Finally, the sludge is dewatered and dried; treated sludge is a soil-like material and is sometimes formed into pellets (see **Figure** 7.7). The odor of treated sludge is variable but often reflects the presence of compounds that contain sulfur or ammonia.

In the United States, some treated sludge is handled as a waste product—landfilled or incinerated—and some is applied to agricultural land as a soil additive or fertilizer. It would be feasible to landfill all sewage sludge in the United States; it would amount to about 5% of the dry weight of the solid waste that is already being landfilled.[9]

Land Application of Treated Sewage Sludge

The idea of spreading treated sewage sludge on agricultural land has great appeal.* After all, it is an organic waste, rich in nutrients, and spreading it on land solves a big disposal problem.

---

*In the early 1990s, the sewage industry coined a new term for treated sewage sludge, **biosolids**, to be used in marketing this product (Rampton S. Let them eat nutri-cake. *Harper's Magazine*, November 1998:48–49), and the term is now widely used. This term connotes a natural organic material while avoiding reference to either its sewage heritage or its nonsewage chemical constituents. Similarly, the land application of biosolids is sometimes referred to as a "beneficial reuse" of a waste product, although the benefits are accompanied by risks. This text uses the neutral descriptive terms *land application* and *treated sewage sludge* (or *treated sludge*), asking the reader to bear in mind that the sewage waste stream contains more than just sewage.

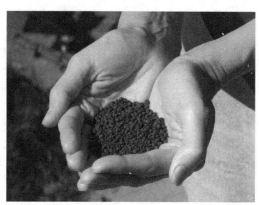

FIGURE 7.7 Treated sewage sludge, shown here in pellet form, is often used as fertilizer. *Source*: Courtesy of Keith J. Maxwell.

Unfortunately, treated sludge may be contaminated with pathogens—and also with metals, including lead, as well as organic chemicals present in the original wastewater stream and concentrated in the residue of treatment.

Although a potential exposure pathway clearly links sewage to treated sludge to crops or grazing animals consumed by people, it is difficult to quantify the human health risk of pathogens or chemicals in treated sewage sludge—and indeed, the risk is likely to be highly variable. Some computer modeling has suggested that the risk of human infection from several common fecal pathogens is low.[10] On the other hand, field studies have drawn direct links between fecal pathogens (for example, *Salmonella*) isolated from people and from treated sludge.[11] Antibiotic-resistant pathogens in treated sludge are spread in the environment (much as they are in CAFO wastes), creating the opportunity to spread resistance through bacterial gene swapping.[11] An analysis in the United Kingdom of the bovine spongiform encephalopathy (BSE) risk to cattle grazing on land to which sewage sludge had been applied (evaluated because sewage could contain prions from slaughterhouse wastes) indicated that the risk of infection was too low to sustain BSE in the UK cattle herd;[12] even so, it serves as a reminder of the multiple connections among pathogens, wastes, and food. Chemical analyses of sludge have documented the presence of dioxins,[13] flame retardants,[14] estrogenic breakdown products of alkyphenol ethoxylates found in detergents,[14] and pharmaceuticals.[15]

EPA estimates that more than 7 million dry metric tons of sewage sludge is produced annually in the United States, and that 54% of this sludge (treated sludge only) is applied to land—not only in agriculture and horticulture, but also in forests and on reclamation land.[16] Information gathered from seven states shows wide variation in the land application of treated sludge as well as some interstate commerce in this commodity. In 2000, for example, New York applied only 10% of its own treated sludge to land and exported 48% to other states. In contrast, Colorado applied 82% of its own treated sludge (a much smaller quantity than New

York's) to land and also imported treated sludge from other states, with the result that more was applied in Colorado than had been generated there.[16]

Septic Systems and Constructed Wetlands

Although about two-thirds of the US population is connected to a municipal wastewater treatment system, this arrangement is not necessary or cost-effective in areas of low population density. As a result, septic systems are widely used in exurban and rural areas.

A septic system consists of a septic tank and a leach field. The septic tank is a buried steel or concrete vault that receives wastewater from a house (see **Figure 7.8**). This holding tank allows some material to float on the surface as scum, while other material sinks and accumulates as sludge on the floor, leaving a liquid layer in the middle. Fecal bacteria are present in all these layers. The sludge that accumulates in the tank must be cleaned out periodically and disposed of. Liquid from the middle layer flows out from the septic tank as it is displaced by water entering the tank. Thus, the system is passive, driven by gravity.

The effluent leaving the septic tank is distributed over a rather large area, called a leach field or drainage field, through a buried system of branching perforated pipes, still driven by gravity. Water trickles out through the perforations and then downward through the soil to the water table. In the process, pathogens carried along with the water are adsorbed onto soil particles or become mired in bacterial slime and gradually die off because of temperature changes and lack of food.[17] These processes do not work well if the soil is wet. Thus, the leach field must be located well above the local water table so that wastewater can drain properly. In an extreme situation, if the local water table rises high enough to intrude into the leach field, ponds of untreated wastewater can form on the surface. This poses an immediate health hazard as well as impeding the biological process of the system.

In a variation on the typical septic system, an artificial wetland can be constructed between the septic tank and the leach field so that the effluent is much cleaner when it reaches the leach field. Such a constructed wetland is a man-made marsh designed to act as a wastewater

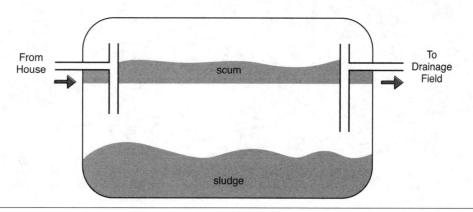

FIGURE 7.8 A septic tank.

treatment system. A constructed wetland consists of a lined basin and a layer of soil, sand, or gravel in which plants are rooted. In some constructed wetlands, the water level is above the soil surface, and water flow occurs mostly above ground; in others, the water level is below the soil surface, and water flow occurs mostly below ground.[18] In either case, the vegetation slows down the flow of water, allowing settling and filtering to occur. The plants also provide an environment in which microorganisms can thrive, and it is this microbial community that digests organic wastes. (This process is not unlike traditional secondary sewage treatment, with its bed of slime-coated rocks.) The combined septic-system-plus-constructed-wetland approach can be used not only for single homes but also for clusters of homes or apartment units.

And, in a variation on the constructed wetlands approach, an enclosed artificial ecosystem can be created for the purpose of decomposing toilet wastes. For example, the state of Vermont has installed such a system at a rest stop on the Vermont Turnpike, where poor drainage had made it difficult to construct an effective septic system.[19] A greenhouse holds a dramatic array of plants (see **Figure 7.9**). Within this carefully constructed ecosystem, microorganisms digest organic wastes; the cleaned water is recycled to the rest area's toilets.

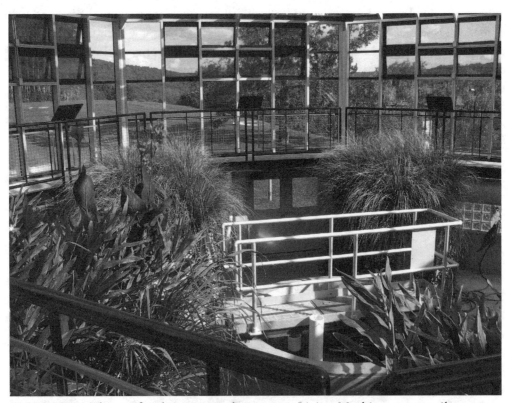

FIGURE 7.9 This artificial ecosystem, known as a Living Machine, treats toilet wastes at a rest stop on the Vermont Turnpike. *Source*: Courtesy of Keith J. Maxwell.

The Composting Toilet

In recent decades, the most fundamental sewage management decision of the 19th century—the decision to use potable water to carry sewage—has been challenged. This challenge rests on two points.[20] First, clean water is a valuable resource that should not be used to carry away urine and feces, especially in an era of increasing water scarcity. Second, human waste is itself a valuable resource, one that should not be mixed in the same waste stream with commercial and industrial discharges carrying metals and organic chemicals. Once these wastes have been mixed together in the municipal wastewater stream, the makeup of the end products—sewage sludge and treated wastewater—cannot be controlled or even predicted.

Thus, effective technologies for a sustainable approach to sanitation rest on the understanding that both clean water and human excreta are valuable resources and should be kept separate. In this spirit, **composting toilets** convert human waste into a stable compost, given adequate time and room in a ventilated composting chamber.

There are two basic variations on the composting toilet: batch systems and continuous systems.[21] Batch systems, such as the double-vault composting toilet, have two holding tanks side by side. One vault is used until it is full, and then the toilet stool is moved to the second vault. The waste in the first vault slowly dries out so that it can be removed and disposed of or used as fertilizer.[21] A batch composting toilet produces unpleasant odors as fecal waste accumulates because the composting chamber is usually vented passively, typically with a 2-inch pipe. However, the batch composting toilet is less expensive to build than the continuous composting toilet.

In a continuous (single-chamber) composting toilet, waste falls into a single tank, and coarse sawdust or wood shavings are periodically added into the composting chamber, adding carbon and helping to maintain the aerobic environment needed for decomposition.[21] The composting chamber is vented, usually with a 4- or 6-inch ventilation stack equipped with a low-voltage electric or solar exhaust fan. In the aerobic environment of the tank, bacteria digest the organic wastes, much as in garden compost. The compost is not removed for several years—and over time pathogens die off, simply losing out in the competition with composting organisms.[21] The tank has an inspection door near the top and another door at the bottom through which finished compost is removed (see **Figure 7.10**). This compost, which does not carry the chemical burden found in municipal sewage sludge, can be safely used as fertilizer.[20] Urine undergoes nitrification inside the composting tank; within a few days, it becomes an odorless, nitrogen-rich liquid fertilizer that moves through a filter at the bottom of the tank and drains into a separate storage unit below the composting tank.[21] When properly built and vented, a continuous composting toilet is virtually odorless.

In lower-income countries, the centralized sewer model is a particularly poor fit: Sewage systems are expensive to build and maintain; they create sludge that must be disposed of; and they use enormous quantities of water. In these countries, where fecal contamination of drinking water affects a large share of the population—and where most of the world's 1.8 million annual deaths from fecal disease occur[22]—the composting toilet offers the potential for dramatic im-

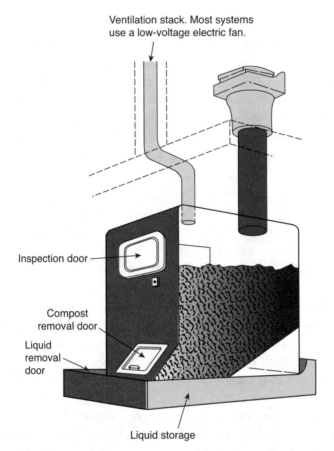

Ventilation stack. Most systems use a low-voltage electric fan.

Inspection door

Compost removal door

Liquid removal door

Liquid storage

FIGURE 7.10 The design of the continuous composting toilet features a separate holding area for liquid waste, doors to inspect and remove compost and liquid, and a ventilation stack. When properly built and vented, a continuous composting toilet is odorless. *Source*: Courtesy of the ReSource Institute for Low Entropy Systems (RILES).

provements in health and comfort at relatively low cost. Moreover, it is a *sustainable* approach to sanitation on a global scale, unlike the use of water to carry sewage to municipal treatment facilities. And, as shown in **Figures 7.11a** and **7.11b**, continuous composting toilets can be attractive, both inside and out. In the United States, continuous composting toilets such as the Clivus Multrum, though not common, are to be found in some "green" homes and office buildings, and also in some parks, camps, and other recreation areas.

Regulation of Municipal Wastewater Treatment in the United States

Under the Clean Water Act, the federal government sets standards for the quality of ambient water as well as the technological requirement to use secondary sewage treatment—primary sewage treatment is not adequate. Municipalities discharging their wastes must meet permitting requirements (under the National Pollutant Discharge Elimination System) that include both

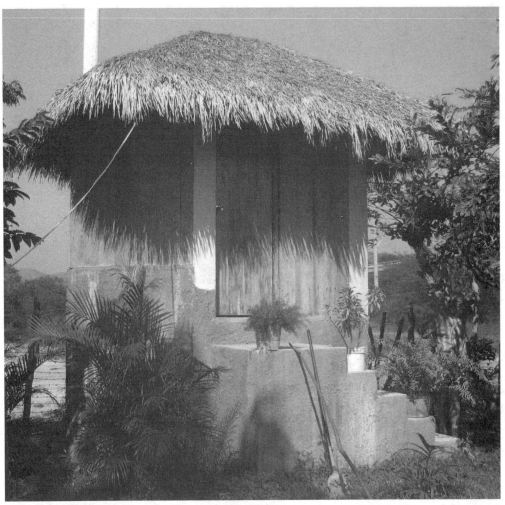

FIGURE 7.11a This continuous composting toilet in Mexico shows an exterior adapted to local conditions. *Source*: Courtesy of the ReSource Institute for Low Entropy Systems (RILES).

effluent limitations and requirements to use specific control technologies, much as for industrial wastes. Standards for a facility are designed to maintain the quality of the receiving waters. The key effluent standards for treated sewage waste are for bacteriological quality (number of fecal coliform organisms per volume of effluent) and biochemical oxygen demand, or BOD (limiting the burden of nitrogen or organic matter in the effluent). Although the federal government has ultimate enforcement authority, most of this activity is undertaken by the states.

Under federal regulations, treated sludge that is to be applied to land must meet certain standards for metals and pathogens. These regulations recognize the realities that some pathogens survive sludge treatment and that metals do not break down in the environment. At present,

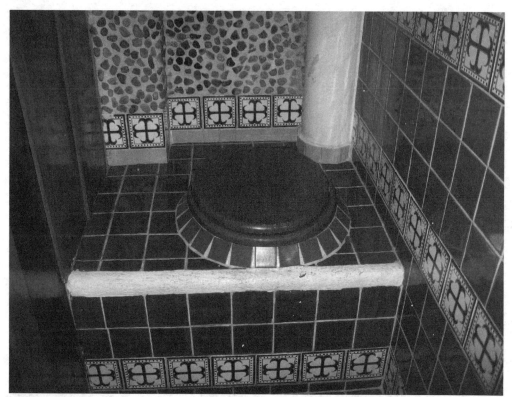

FIGURE 7.11b The interior of this continuous composting toilet in Mexico reflects local decorative traditions. *Source*: Courtesy of the ReSource Institute for Low Entropy Systems (RILES).

there are no restrictions on the various organic compounds present in sludge, though a new standard has recently been proposed to limit dioxin concentrations in sludge. There are certain restrictions on the land application of treated sludge—related to the timing of crop harvesting or animal grazing, for example—as well as requirements for recordkeeping and reporting.

Key elements of the US regulatory framework for municipal wastewater treatment appear in **Table 7.2.** This table is the seventh in a series of similar tables that place regulatory provisions within the traditional regulatory domains of environmental health.

7.3 Sources and Treatment of Drinking Water

In 2006, the US EPA estimated that almost 55,000 community water systems were serving about 264 million people[23]—about 90% of the US population. Most of those who rely on private water supplies live in rural areas and have their own wells. This section describes the following topics:

- The treatment of community drinking water, including disinfection and fluoridation
- Individual options for obtaining or treating water, including the use of private well water; use of devices to treat home water, whether from a public or private source; and

Table 7.2 Overview of US Regulatory Framework for Environmental Health Hazards (7)

Environmental Health Domain	Major Laws and Key Provisions for the Control of Environmental Health Hazards
Biological hazards	Public Health Service Act (PHSA)—development of guidelines for vaccination; use of quarantine or isolation to prevent entry of infectious diseases into the United States; conduct of surveillance and investigation of outbreaks
Air pollution	Clean Air Act (CAA)—ambient standards (NAAQS) for Criteria Air Pollutants; emissions standards for Hazardous Air Pollutants, including mercury; emission allowances for SO_2 (to control acid deposition); removal of lead from gasoline; requirement to sell reformulated gasoline in high-smog areas
Ionizing radiation	Energy Reorganization Act (ERA)—safety requirements for operating nuclear power plants, including licensing, emissions limits, storage of wastes
	Nuclear Waste Policy Act (NWPA)—requirements to build and regulate a repository for radioactive wastes, including spent reactor fuel
	Uranium Mill Tailings Radiation Control Act —standards for management of abandoned mill tailings
Alternative energy sources	Energy Policy Act (EPAct)—modest supports for alternative energy sources
Hazardous wastes	Comprehensive Environmental Response Compensation and Liability Act ("Superfund")/Superfund Amendments and Reauthorization Act (CERCLA/SARA)—identify, assess health risks of, and remediate abandoned hazardous waste sites
	Resource Conservation and Recovery Act (RCRA)—"cradle-to-grave" manifest system for hazardous wastes; standards and permits for hazardous waste storage or disposal facilities; provisions to promote hazardous waste minimization (source reduction) and recycling of hazardous wastes
Occupational health	Occupational Safety and Health Act (OSHAct)—ambient standards (Permissible Exposure Limits) for workplace air; employers must provide Materials Safety Data Sheets (MSDSs) to workers
Industrial water pollution	Clean Water Act (CWA)—ambient standards (Ambient Water Quality Criteria, or AWQC) for about 150 pollutants; technology requirements and permitting system for discharges to ambient water, from industry
Toxic chemicals	Toxic Substances Control Act (TSCA)—premanufacture notice for new chemicals; EPA can restrict manufacture, distribution, or use if new chemical poses unreasonable risk
	Emergency Planning and Community Right-to-Know Act (EPCRA)— local and state emergency response commissions; yearly chemical reporting requirements for manufacturing facilities; data available as Toxics Release Inventory; facilities must provide Materials Safety Data Sheets (MSDSs) to local commissions *(continues)*

Table 7.2   *(Continued)*

Environmental Health Domain	Major Laws and Key Provisions for the Control of Environmental Health Hazards
	Pollution Prevention Act (PPA)—support for source reduction/ waste prevention as preferable to treatment or disposal of wastes
Pesticides	Federal Insecticide, Fungicide, and Rodenticide Act (FIFRA)— registration of pesticides
Food supply	Federal Food, Drug, and Cosmetic Act (FFDCA)/Food Quality Protection Act (FQPA)—setting pesticide tolerances in food; setting food defect action levels; approval of food additives, including potential chemical by-products of irradiation; requirements for HACCP systems for food safety; BSE surveillance and controls on feed for ruminants
	Humane Methods of Slaughter Act (HMSA)—standards for humane slaughter
	Wholesome Meat Act (WMA)/Poultry Products Inspection Act (PPIA)—inspection of meat and poultry
	Magnuson-Stevens Fishery Conservation and Management Act (MSFCMA)—conservation of fisheries
	Organic Foods Production Act (OFPA)—standards for labeling food as organic
Sewage wastes and community water supply	*Clean Water Act (CWA)—ambient standards and permitting system for discharges to ambient water from municipal wastewater treatment plants; procedures for land application of treated sewage sludge*
Municipal solid waste	
Consumer products	
Environmental noise	

Note: New information appears in italics.

the substitution of commercial bottled water for drinking water from either a public or a private source

The section concludes with a snapshot of US regulatory provisions related to drinking water.

Public Water Supplies

Community drinking water is of critical importance in public health because it is a mechanism for delivering healthful water to a large number of people—or, conversely, for spreading a health hazard to the same group of people. Pathogens (protozoa, bacteria, and viruses) and chemical contaminants are of particular concern. Like wastewater treatments, technologies for the treatment of drinking water have traditionally focused on the control of pathogens. The need to remove synthetic organic chemicals is a more recent development, and communities add specialized treatment as needed.

Many large cities rely on water from surface sources because cities require a large daily supply, as well as a surplus to get through dry periods without any interruption in supply. Both Boston and the city of New York, for example, rely on large reservoirs located in less populated areas of their respective states. Quabbin Reservoir, which serves greater Boston, was built during the 1930s, submerging parts of five towns. Los Angeles draws water from rivers farther north in the state and also from the Colorado River, which forms the border between California and Arizona. The city also relies on groundwater drawn from beneath the Los Angeles basin.[24]

Smaller communities and rural areas often rely on groundwater sources. There is considerable variation in the treatment needed to ensure that the source water is safe as drinking water. In particular, some groundwater sources may require little treatment—if land uses do not compromise water quality—because groundwater undergoes natural filtering as it moves through an aquifer. As noted in Chapter 6, agricultural activities may add excess nitrates to groundwater in rural areas; specialized treatments are required to remove nitrates from water.

Before turning to the treatment of tap water in the United States—that is, to issues of water *quality*—it is useful to revisit briefly the question of water *quantity*. As described in Chapter 6, the irrigation of crops consumes enormous quantities of water, driving water use to exceed the renewable supply in parts of the US central plains, for example. Further, as noted at the start of this chapter, the typical US family of four consumes about 400 gallons of water per day—in most cases, water that has been treated to drinking water standards. Thus, as context for a description of treatment technologies for drinking water, it is appropriate to bear in mind some ways in which ordinary consumers can conserve water (**Table 7.3**).

Basic Treatment Technology for Drinking Water

Most of the common technologies to treat community drinking water are not new. A typical sequence of steps begins with allowing large particles to settle out by gravity. After this initial settling step, tiny particles of silt or clay remain suspended in the water. As in the treatment of wastewater, such turbidity is of concern because the suspended particles can harbor pathogens and interfere with disinfection. Because the particles are very fine and negatively charged, they tend to repel one another and remain suspended in the water. The second treatment step, called **coagulation and flocculation,** is designed to overcome this problem. In this step, alum (aluminum sulfate) is added to the water, which is then mixed; the alum neutralizes the particles' charge (coagulation), allowing them to stick together when they collide, forming **flocs** (flocculation). A **sedimentation** step then allows the flocs to settle out by gravity. Both the initial settling step and the later sedimentation step create sludge, which must be disposed of. Often this sludge, which is mostly water, is simply discharged into a municipal sewer system. Alternatively, it can be dried and disposed of in a landfill.

After sedimentation has cleared the water of many fine suspended particles, the water is filtered. The usual technology is a **sand filter.** The water trickles gently through a bed of sand, driven only by gravity. At regular intervals, the sand filter is cleaned by backwashing from below, using clean water under pressure. Carbon filters may also be used. These steps are very effective in reducing the turbidity of the water, and thereby removing many, though not all, pathogens.

Table 7.3   Some Simple Ways to Conserve Water at Home

Repairing or buying household items:
- insulate hot water pipes
- repair dripping faucets, running toilets, and leaky plumbing
- install low-flow showerheads
- install low-flow toilets (or if possible, reduce tank volume by putting a plastic jug filled with water into the tank)
- choose water-efficient new appliances (for example, dishwasher, washing machine)

Developing water-conscious habits indoors:
- do not flush the toilet unnecessarily (for example, to dispose of tissues)
- take shorter showers
- turn off the water while you scrub your hands, brush your teeth, or shave
- turn off the water while you wash dishes by hand—fill the sink instead
- install an instant water heater at the kitchen sink
- minimize use of garbage disposal—compost if possible
- run dishwasher only with full load
- run washing machine only with full load; or set appropriate load size

Developing water-conscious habits outdoors:
- plant grass and shrubs that do not demand a lot of water
- water using soaker hose or other drip irrigation techniques
- use mulch in gardens to keep water in the soil
- keep a shutoff nozzle on your hose
- use a broom or rake instead of the hose to sweep grass or debris from paved surfaces
- be mindful if you wash your car

Adapted from: Federal Emergency Management Agency. Are You Ready? Appendix A: Water Conservation Tips. Available at: http://www.fema.gov/areyouready/appendix_a.shtm. Accessed May 1, 2008. National Resources Conservation Service. Water Conservation. Available at: http://www.nrcs.usda.gov/feature/backyard/watercon.html. Accessed May 1, 2008.

Disinfection of Drinking Water

The final step in drinking water treatment is disinfection—that is, a treatment with the specific objective of killing pathogens. In the United States, chlorination is the most common method of drinking water disinfection. Chlorination is highly effective against bacteria but somewhat less effective against viruses and protozoa. In particular, the protozoan parasites *Giardia lamblia* and *Cryptosporidium parvum* are resistant to chlorine. These organisms can be removed by filtration or by disinfection using ozone.

When chlorination is used as the method of disinfection, residual chlorine is deliberately left in the water as it leaves the treatment plant. This is essential to maintain disinfection throughout the distribution system. Particularly in the aging infrastructures of older cities, water mains have cracks that allow soil and groundwater to enter or rough patches where microbes can collect (see **Figure 7.12**).

Unfortunately, the residual chlorine is also available to combine with organic matter present in water that comes from surface sources—for example, from the decomposition of leaves that have fallen into an open reservoir. These reactions create organic compounds known as

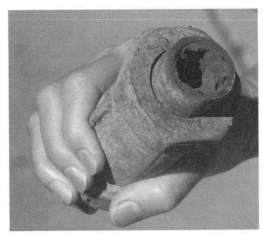

FIGURE 7.12 This 10-year-old water supply pipe has accumulated mineral deposits that make its internal surface rough. *Source*: Courtesy of Keith J. Maxwell

disinfection byproducts (DBPs). The most common disinfection byproducts belong to a group of chemicals called **trihalomethanes (THMs).** (The *halo-* in *trihalomethane* indicates that these compounds contain a halogen, such as chlorine.) Chloroform (trichloromethane) is by far the most common of the trihalomethanes found in drinking water. Exposure to trihalomethanes in drinking water does not pose an acute health risk, but epidemiologic research has documented an association between chronic exposure and increased risk of bladder cancer.[25,26] Current evidence suggests there may be an association between maternal exposure to disinfection byproducts and low birthweight,[27,28] but not spontaneous abortion.[29,30] Some municipal water systems use chloramine (created by mixing chlorine and ammonia) rather than chlorine for residual disinfection. Chloramine is more stable in the distribution system than chlorine is, thus providing longer-lasting protection and creating fewer disinfection by-products.[31]

As noted earlier, treatment with ozone is an alternative to chlorination as a method of disinfection. Ozone is effective against protozoa and viruses and does not create chlorinated byproducts, but it has no residual disinfecting effect in the distribution system.

Fluoridation of Drinking Water

Exposure to fluoride at low concentrations in drinking water is well known to prevent tooth decay, a substantial public health benefit. Community **fluoridation** programs aim to achieve fluoride concentrations in drinking water of 0.7 to 1.2 mg/liter in locations with low natural fluoride levels.[32] However, fluoride sometimes occurs naturally in water at concentrations high enough to cause a disfiguring mottling of the teeth called **fluorosis.**

In 1986, EPA set the enforceable standard (the Maximum Contaminant Level, or MCL) for fluoride in drinking water at 4 mg/liter, and the secondary, nonenforceable limit (the Secondary Maximum Contaminant Level, or SMCL) at 2 mg/liter. The secondary standard reflects concern about the cosmetic effects of fluorosis. A recent review of the fluoride standard by the National Research Council recommended that the MCL of 4 mg/liter should be lowered for two reasons[33]: First, the current standard does not protect against severe fluorosis, which is not just cosmetic but contributes to decay and infection; and second, long-term exposure to fluoride at 4 mg/liter may contribute to the risk of bone fracture. The NRC also noted that the secondary standard of 2 mg/liter may not fully protect against the cosmetic effects of fluorosis.[33]

Private Wells, Home Water Treatment, and Bottled Water

Although the great majority of Americans now get their water from public supplies, some rely on private wells, mostly in rural areas. And whatever the source of their water, increasing numbers of Americans have installed water treatment devices in their homes in recent years. Finally, bottled water, once a rarity in the United States, has become an everyday consumer item. These alternatives—or supplements—to public water supplies are described here.

Private Wells

Water from private wells is not subject to federal drinking water standards, though some state and local governments set requirements for private wells.[34] Well water is vulnerable to contamination by activities on land located upgradient of the well, as well as by surface runoff. Because most private wells are located in rural or semirural areas, upgradient land uses often include private septic systems or agriculture. As a result, private wells may be at particular risk of contamination by human fecal waste, animal wastes, pesticides, or nitrates from the use of fertilizers. As described previously, infants who consume well water contaminated with nitrates may suffer methemoglobinemia. Further, in some geologic settings, radon is a common contaminant in groundwater.

Devices for Home Water Treatment

Some people choose to install a device to treat drinking water at home—because their water supply is untreated, or because they are concerned about the quality of their water despite municipal treatment, or simply to improve the taste of their water. Most of these devices are known as **point-of-use treatment systems**—that is, they are installed at a single tap, such as the faucet at the kitchen sink. Many of these devices use carbon filters to remove contaminants; other more complex systems use reverse osmosis or distillation to remove impurities.

Bottled Water

The consumption of commercially bottled water has been increasing dramatically in recent years.[35] Compared to public drinking water, bottled water is much more expensive per gallon and is more likely to come from a groundwater source; in addition, bottled water is unlikely to be fluoridated.[36] Bottled water is not regulated by the EPA as drinking water, but rather by the FDA as a packaged food (as described later).

Some consumers prefer the taste of bottled water. Taste is, of course, a matter of personal preference, but it is not surprising that there should be differences in taste, given that the taste of any water is affected by its mineral content and by the method of disinfection used to purify the water. The mineral content of bottled water varies with its source, but because most bottled water is groundwater, it is likely to start with higher mineral content than the surface waters that are the source of most public drinking water.[36] Producers of some bottled waters also add minerals for the purpose of flavoring the water. As described earlier, chlorination is the most common method of disinfection of public drinking water in the United States. Bottled water, on the other hand, is more often disinfected using ozonation or ultraviolet light[36] because no residual disinfection effect is needed as in the distribution system of a public water supply.

Regulation of Drinking Water in the United States

The Safe Drinking Water Act (SDWA) was originally passed in 1974 and substantially amended in 1986 and 1996. It requires EPA to promulgate national standards (the National Primary Drinking Water Regulations, or NPDWR) for contaminants in public drinking water that are likely to pose a health risk and be present in waters used to supply drinking water. EPA is also required to identify, on a regular basis, contaminants that are candidates for future regulation.

EPA sets two standards: a Maximum Contaminant Level Goal (MCLG), an unenforceable goal that marks a level where no health effects are anticipated; and a **Maximum Contaminant Level (MCL)**, a standard that must be met. EPA is to set the MCL as close to the MCLG as is feasible given technological options and costs. EPA is required to conduct a health risk assessment (as described in Chapter 2) in support of a new MCL and also to estimate its benefits and costs. The EPA can impose fines on public water systems that fail to comply with the standards. MCLs have been set for some biological hazards, turbidity, and a long list of chemical contaminants. EPA may also set a nonenforceable secondary MCL (SMCL); this is a recommended guideline that individual states may choose to adopt as a standard. An SMCL addresses a contaminant's effect on the taste or odor of water, or its cosmetic effects in those who drink the water (such as discoloration of the teeth from excessive naturally occurring fluoride).

The EPA has set enforceable standards for a small number of specific pathogens, including *Cryptosporidium*, *Giardia lamblia*, and coliform bacteria.[37] In each case, the MCLG is zero, and the MCL is a requirement for a specific testing regimen and test results. The MCL for coliform bacteria, for example, requires regular sampling for total coliforms; if a threshold for positive results is exceeded, then the standard calls for testing for fecal coliform bacteria or *E. coli*. Coliform bacteria are a group of bacteria, widespread in the environment, that live in water, soil, or the intestines of warm-blooded animals; the subgroup known as fecal coliform bacteria are those that enter the environment in the feces of warm-blooded animals. *E. coli* is one type of fecal coliform bacteria.

Most fecal coliform bacteria are not pathogens; however, any substantial presence of fecal coliforms in drinking water indicates recent sewage contamination and hence the potential presence of fecal pathogens. It is impractical to monitor most fecal pathogens directly, since there are many different ones (including protozoa and viruses as well as non-coliform bacteria) and individually most are uncommon. However, since none of these pathogens occurs in the absence of fecal contamination, coliform bacteria and especially fecal coliform bacteria serve as *indicator organisms* for sewage contamination and thus for the potential presence of pathogens.

The scope of the Safe Drinking Water Act is much broader than standards for contaminants in water. As amended, it includes provisions for watershed protection at the source of the water and bans the installation of lead pipe and the use of lead solder in public water distribution systems. The law calls for regular monitoring of public drinking water for contaminants, including some not regulated under the law, and requires that information on drinking water quality be provided to the public on a regular basis.

Bottled water is regulated as a packaged food under the Federal Food, Drug and Cosmetic Act and thus falls under the purview of the US Food and Drug Administration.[35] Bottled water must be labeled as to its source (as *source* is defined legally); for example, water labeled as *spring water* may be collected at a spring, but it may also come from a well drilled into an aquifer from which water emerges as a spring at some other location.[35] Some bottled water comes from surface sources—usually a public water supply, with additional treatment.[36] FDA sets standards of quality for bottled water that are based on EPA's drinking water standards, and it also sets standards for manufacturing practices.[36] Carbonated water, soda water, seltzer water, sparkling water, and tonic water are considered soft drinks and are not regulated as bottled water.

Key elements of the US regulatory framework for municipal drinking water appear in **Table 7.4**. This table is the eighth in a series of similar tables that place regulatory provisions within the traditional regulatory domains of environmental health.

7.4 Solid Waste and Its Management

The amount of ordinary trash generated each year in the United States has increased steadily for decades; in 2005, it stood at 246 million tons, about double what it was in 1970 (121 million tons).[5] On the other hand, per capita generation appears to be leveling off, hovering around 4.5 pounds per person per day since 1990.[5] These quantities include trash from businesses—from restaurants to insurance companies—to which everyone contributes indirectly. Including these indirect contributions, the average 190-pound adult male generates his weight in trash about every six weeks.

The most common materials in the municipal solid waste stream are paper and paperboard, which together make up about one-third by weight of what we throw away (**Figure 7.13**). Yard trimmings, food scraps, and plastics together also account for more than one-third of the total. Looked at another way, by type of product, nearly one-third by weight (31%) was made up of containers and other packaging (not shown in figure).[5]

Trash, for all its homely familiarity, is not easy to manage. For one thing, trash is generated by many individual households across every city and town so that simply designing routes and schedules for trash trucks is a logistical challenge. In addition, trash contains many different items, from pencils to refrigerators. Municipal waste sometimes contains hazardous items, such as drain cleaners or mothballs. But it always includes food waste, and this means that it must be removed on a strict schedule—when trash cans overflow, odor quickly becomes a problem, as do rats and other pests. Strikes by trash collectors in New York have left vivid images of city life without this service. In the bigger picture, most trash is now disposed of in large regional facilities rather than local dumps—but most towns are not enthusiastic about hosting such a large

Table 7.4 Overview of US Regulatory Framework for Environmental Health Hazards (8)

Environmental Health Domain	Major Laws and Key Provisions for the Control of Environmental Health Hazards
Biological hazards	Public Health Service Act (PHSA)—development of guidelines for vaccination; use of quarantine or isolation to prevent entry of infectious diseases into the United States; conduct of surveillance and investigation of outbreaks
Air pollution	Clean Air Act (CAA)—ambient standards (NAAQS) for Criteria Air Pollutants; emissions standards for Hazardous Air Pollutants, including mercury; emission allowances for SO_2 (to control acid deposition); removal of lead from gasoline; requirement to sell reformulated gasoline in high-smog areas
Ionizing radiation	Energy Reorganization Act (ERA)—safety requirements for operating nuclear power plants, including licensing, emissions limits, storage of wastes
	Nuclear Waste Policy Act (NWPA)—requirements to build and regulate a repository for radioactive wastes, including spent reactor fuel
	Uranium Mill Tailings Radiation Control Act—standards for management of abandoned mill tailings
Alternative energy sources	Energy Policy Act (EPAct)—modest supports for alternative energy sources
Hazardous wastes	Comprehensive Environmental Response Compensation and Liability Act ("Superfund")/Superfund Amendments and Reauthorization Act (CERCLA/SARA)—identify, assess health risks of, and remediate abandoned hazardous waste sites
	Resource Conservation and Recovery Act (RCRA)—"cradle-to-grave" manifest system for hazardous wastes; standards and permits for hazardous waste storage or disposal facilities; provisions to promote hazardous waste minimization (source reduction) and recycling of hazardous wastes
Occupational health	Occupational Safety and Health Act (OSHAct)—ambient standards (Permissible Exposure Limits) for workplace air; employers must provide Materials Safety Data Sheets (MSDSs) to workers
Industrial water pollution	Clean Water Act (CWA)—ambient standards (Ambient Water Quality Criteria, or AWQC) for about 150 pollutants; technology requirements and permitting system for discharges to ambient water, from industry
Toxic chemicals	Toxic Substances Control Act (TSCA)—premanufacture notice for new chemicals; EPA can restrict manufacture, distribution, or use if new chemical poses unreasonable risk
	Emergency Planning and Community Right-to-Know Act (EPCRA)—local and state emergency response commissions; yearly chemical reporting requirements for manufacturing facilities; data available as Toxics Release Inventory; facilities must provide Materials Safety Data Sheets (MSDSs) to local commissions *(continues)*

Table 7.4   *(Continued)*

Environmental Health Domain	Major Laws and Key Provisions for the Control of Environmental Health Hazards
	Pollution Prevention Act (PPA)—support for source reduction/waste prevention as preferable to treatment or disposal of wastes
Pesticides	Federal Insecticide, Fungicide, and Rodenticide Act (FIFRA)—registration of pesticides
Food supply	Federal Food, Drug, and Cosmetic Act (FFDCA)/Food Quality Protection Act (FQPA)—setting pesticide tolerances in food; setting food defect action levels; approval of food additives, including potential chemical by-products of irradiation; requirements for HACCP systems for food safety; BSE surveillance and controls on feed for ruminants
	Humane Methods of Slaughter Act (HMSA)—standards for humane slaughter
	Wholesome Meat Act (WMA)/Poultry Products Inspection Act (PPIA)—inspection of meat and poultry
	Magnuson-Stevens Fishery Conservation and Management Act (MSFCMA)—conservation of fisheries
	Organic Foods Production Act (OFPA)—standards for labeling food as organic
Sewage wastes and community water supply	Clean Water Act (CWA)—ambient standards and permitting system for discharges to ambient water from municipal wastewater treatment plants; procedures for land application of treated sewage sludge
	Safe Drinking Water Act (SDWA)—standards for drinking water: Maximum Contaminant Level Goal (MCLG) and Maximum Contaminant Level (MCL), which is the standard
	Federal Food, Drug, and Cosmetic Act (FFDCA)—regulation of bottled water as packaged food
Municipal solid waste	
Consumer products	
Environmental noise	

Note: New information appears in italics.

facility. As a result of such not-in-my-backyard opposition, it is increasingly difficult to find a final resting place for trash.

There are four basic approaches to managing trash:

- Not generating it in the first place (known as source reduction or waste prevention)
- Recycling, including the composting of organic wastes

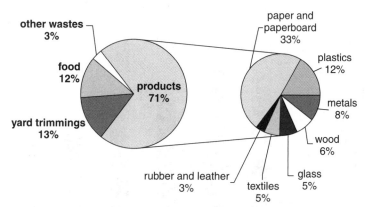

FIGURE 7.13 Makeup of municipal solid waste (by weight) in the United States, 2005. *Data from*: US Environmental Protection Agency. *Municipal Solid Waste in the United States: 2005 Facts and Figures*, 2006: Table ES-4. Available at: http://www.epa.gov/msw/pubs/mswchar05.pdf.

- Incineration
- Placement in a landfill

Clearly, it is desirable to reduce the amount of waste we produce and to recycle as much as possible of the waste that we do produce. As shown in **Figure 7.14**, only about 29% of the US municipal solid waste stream in 2005 was recycled (including composted wastes)—even though about 58% was made up of paper, plastics, metals, or glass; and about 25% was food waste or yard trimmings (Figure 7.13). About 7% of municipal solid waste in the United States in 2005 was burned in waste-to-energy incinerators, and about two-thirds was disposed of in landfills. These percentages vary substantially by geographic region.

This section first takes up the four major options for managing municipal solid waste, as listed earlier: waste prevention; recycling and composting; incineration, usually with the production of usable energy and referred to as waste-to-energy (WTE) incineration; and landfilling. Next, the section describes briefly the handling of two special types of community wastes: hazardous items in household trash, known as household hazardous wastes; and medical wastes, which may include infectious items, for example. The section concludes with a brief description of the US regulatory framework for municipal solid waste.

Preventing Waste

Waste prevention (also called source reduction), which is difficult to quantify, results from many corporate and individual decisions. Products can be designed to contain less material, or to have a longer useful life, or to be repairable rather than disposable. Packaging can be reduced, and reusable glass bottles can be substituted for plastic containers.[5]

At the consumer level, EPA encourages such practices as double-sided copying and the use of washable plates, silverware, and towels rather than disposable ones. The agency also notes the tradition of reusing both durable and nondurable goods (such as appliances, furniture, or clothing), whether by passing them on informally to friends and family or through donations to charity, as

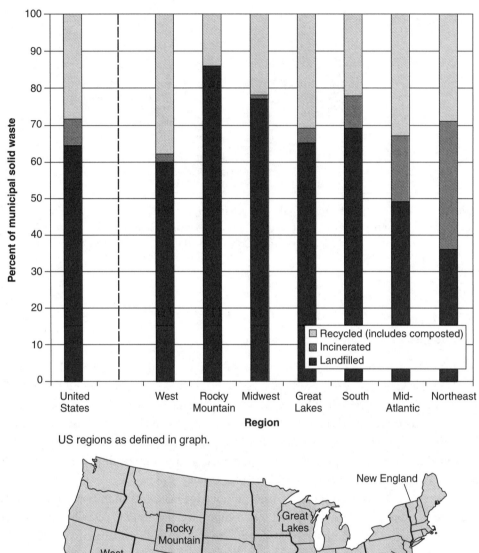

US regions as defined in graph.

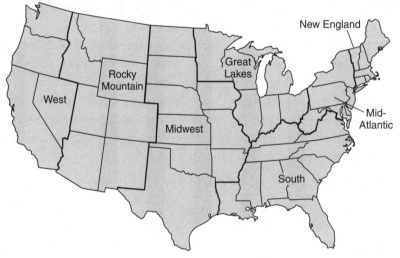

FIGURE 7.14 Fate of municipal solid waste (by weight) in the United States and by US region, 2005. *Data from*: Simmons P, Goldstein N, Kaufman S, Themelis N, Thompson J. The state of garbage in America. *BioCycle*. 2006;47(4):26.

a practice that reduces waste.[5] Thus much of what is now called source reduction at the consumer level has a commonsense ring to it, and in fact was common practice 50 or 100 years ago.

Recycling, Including Composting

Recycling of municipal solid waste removes from the waste stream items made of recyclable materials, such as glass, metal, plastics, and paper, before the wastes are disposed of. Overall, almost half of Americans (48%), about 139 million people, had access to curbside recycling in 2005.[5] Regional differences are striking, however. Curbside recycling reached a substantially higher percentage of people in the more populous Northeast and West (79% and 67%, respectively) than in the Midwest (43%) or South (23%).[5] This pattern probably partly reflects greater urbanization in the Northeast and West—although recycling can be challenging in locations of extremely high population density, it is very costly where population density is low. In the United States, symbols are commonly used to aid consumers in separating recyclable items, and in buying items made at least partly from recycled materials (see **Figure 7.15**).

In many cities and towns, residents sort recyclables (into glass, paper, and so on) before putting them out to be collected; in other communities, recyclables are not sorted by consumers. In this situation, recyclables picked up at curbside are processed at **materials recovery facilities (MRFs)**, where items are sorted using varying degrees of automation. For example, a series of tumblers perforated with larger and larger holes can be used to sort objects by size; a water bath can separate materials that float (such as wood or plastic) from those that sink (such as metals); and magnets can be used to separate out ferrous metals.

A range of organic materials can also be removed from the solid waste stream for **composting**. However, in many communities, municipal composting is limited to yard trimmings, separated by the consumer before placing trash at the curb.[5] From the municipal point of view, backyard composting by individuals is considered waste prevention, rather than recycling, because it prevents a waste from entering the municipal waste stream.

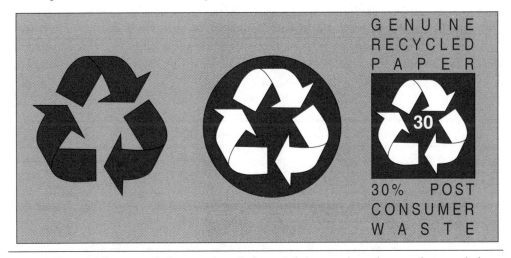

FIGURE 7.15 These symbols represent (left to right) a product that can be recycled, a product that contains at least some recycled material, and a product that contains a specified percentage of recycled material.

People with enough yard space can use a composting bin or start a composting pile out-doors. By mixing fresh materials (such as grass clippings and fruit or vegetable scraps) with dry materials (such as dead leaves or twigs), and keeping the mixture damp, the home composter creates conditions in which organic materials slowly decay into compost that can be used as fer-tilizer and soil conditioner. Even indoors, composting of plant-based food scraps can be done on a small scale using worms. This approach, called **vermicomposting**, uses a specific type of worms, known as redworms, housed in a bin. The worms consume the food scraps and produce castings (worm excrement) that can be used as potting soil.[38]

Waste-to-Energy Incineration

Waste-to-energy (WTE) incineration serves the dual purpose of disposing of municipal solid waste and generating energy, either in the form of electricity or as steam to be used in an indus-trial process. Energy produced by a municipal solid waste incinerator reduces the demand for energy from traditional sources, such as fossil or nuclear fuels. In addition, when trash is re-duced to ash by burning, its volume is decreased by 80% to 90%. Thus, trash incinerators are attractive in principle—but incineration is not a benign technology.

Certain components of trash produce hazardous emissions when burned. Thus, either some ma-terials must be removed from the waste stream before burning or the incinerator must be designed to manage these hazards. Metals—mostly as particulates but, in the case of mercury, vapors—must be captured by devices in the smokestack. And burning of plastics causes the emission of dioxins and furans unless a very high temperature is maintained in the incinerator. The incineration of trash also poses practical challenges. A trash incinerator is expensive to start up or shut down, and therefore it requires a steady flow of trash as well as a steady market for the energy it produces.

Incinerators produce two kinds of ash: **fly ash**, captured by pollution control equipment in the smokestack, and **bottom ash**, which remains on the floor of the furnace. Fly ash is produced in smaller quantities but is more toxic. Under federal law, both types of ash must be tested and then either landfilled as municipal solid waste or disposed of as hazardous waste.

According to EPA, between 1990 and 2005, incinerator emissions of dioxins were reduced by more than 99%, emissions of mercury by 93%, and emissions of lead by 95%.[39] As regula-tory controls on incinerator emissions have been tightened, many have shut down, and the ma-jority of today's incinerators are large operations (**Table 7.5**). Of the 66 large WTE facilities in

Table 7.5 Profile of US Waste-to-Energy Incinerators, 2005

Size (capacity)	Number of Units	Number of Facilities
Large (> 250 tons per day)	167 (all WTE)	66
Small (35 to 250 tons per day)	60 (58 WTE)	26
Very small (< 35 tons per day)	Not reported (mostly not WTE)	Not reported

Data from: Wayland R. Clean Air Act Section 129: Waste to Energy Overview. Presented at: Waste-to-Energy: An Integrated Waste Management Option Conference; 2007. Available at: http://www.epa.gov/Region2/cepd/pdf/2robertwaylandspresentation.pdf.

the United States in 2005, 32 were in the Northeast Corridor (from Washington, DC, through New York and New England), 9 were in Florida, and 5 were clustered in the Upper Midwest.[39]

Disposal in Landfills

Up through the 1970s, most municipal solid waste in the United States was put in a town dump. As the name suggests, this was simply a location where any type of trash could be dumped on the ground. Some dumps were located in gullies so that trash could be dumped from above, or in wet locations, which were undesirable for building. Not surprisingly, dumps were food sources that attracted various wild animals—from rats to bears—as well as insect pests. Sometimes the trash at town dumps was burned to reduce its volume and make it less attractive to pests. Many town dumps were located near a town boundary so as to offend as few local voters as possible.

However, one important environmental impact of the dump—its contamination of groundwater—was largely invisible. Rainwater seeping through waste extracts, or leaches, some constituents from the wastes. The water carrying these dissolved or suspended substances, now called *leachate*, trickles downward below the surface of the soil until it reaches the water table, and then slowly spreads in the groundwater. Over time, as domestic trash came to include more chemical products, the problem of groundwater contamination took on a new importance.

Today's **municipal solid waste landfill** is very different from the town dump. It is a licensed facility, usually operated by a corporation. It holds a very large volume of waste and is engineered specifically to prevent rainwater from leaching contaminants into groundwater. About the only feature it has in common with the town dump is that it accepts unsorted municipal solid waste.

A solid waste landfill (see **Figure 7.16**) begins as a depression dug into the earth's surface, and as the landfill fills up, it rises above the surface around it. Basic design features guard against groundwater contamination. The pit is double-lined, usually with plastic and clay liners, to prevent leachate from reaching the ground beneath the facility. Just above the liner is a network of pipes that collect leachate, which is pumped to the surface. As trash arrives at the operating landfill, heavy machinery is used to compact the waste in layers several feet deep, with a layer of soil between layers of waste. The finished landfill is capped with clay, to prevent rainwater from entering. After a landfill is closed and capped, it must be monitored and maintained. The surface area can be used for purposes that do not involve construction—for example, as a public park.

The modern landfill creates one new hazard. Open dumping allowed aerobic decomposition of waste, whereas the environment within a modern landfill is largely anaerobic—or it becomes anaerobic over time. Bacteria that decompose organic wastes in an anaerobic setting produce methane, an explosive gas. To keep methane from building up inside a landfill, pipes inserted throughout the landfill collect the gas, which can either be safely vented into the environment or collected and used as fuel in industry.

As described earlier, methane is a potent greenhouse gas. On a global scale, it has proved difficult to establish the relative importance of various sources of this gas,[40] given wide regional variation. Landfill emissions accounted for an estimated 28% of US methane emissions in 2003.[41]

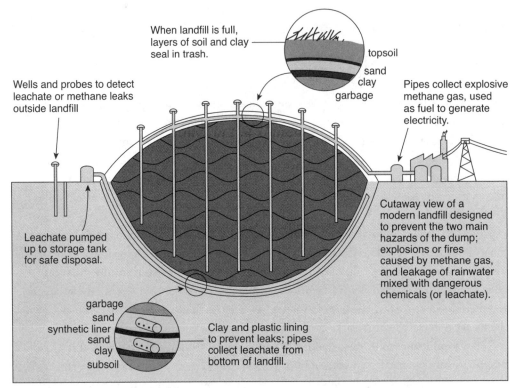

When landfill is full, layers of soil and clay seal in trash.

topsoil
sand
clay
garbage

Wells and probes to detect leachate or methane leaks outside landfill

Pipes collect explosive methane gas, used as fuel to generate electricity.

Leachate pumped up to storage tank for safe disposal.

Cutaway view of a modern landfill designed to prevent the two main hazards of the dump; explosions or fires caused by methane gas, and leakage of rainwater mixed with dangerous chemicals (or leachate).

garbage
sand
synthetic liner
sand
clay
subsoil

Clay and plastic lining to prevent leaks; pipes collect leachate from bottom of landfill.

FIGURE 7.16 A cross section of a modern municipal solid waste landfill. *Source*: Reprinted from US Environmental Protection Agency, Resource Conservation and Recovery Act (RCRA). Available at: http://www.epa.gov/superfund/students/clas_act/haz-ed/ff_06.htm. Accessed December 13, 2007.

Modern landfills that meet federal specifications are expensive to build, and because they are large they can be difficult to site in densely populated areas. However, trash is so bulky that it is not usually economical to transport it over long distances. Like waste incinerators, landfills are becoming fewer and larger—there were 6,326 municipal solid waste landfills in 1990, but only 1,654 in 2005.[5] In contrast to waste incinerators, these landfills are underrepresented in the most densely populated northeastern section of the country, which hosts only 133 such facilities.

Handling of Household Hazardous Wastes

As described in Chapter 5, industrial wastes are classified as hazardous under federal law if they are corrosive, toxic, ignitable, or reactive. Using the same criteria, some ingredients of household products are hazardous, and products containing such ingredients are classified as **household hazardous wastes**. Most are common products, such as oven cleaners, drain cleaners, and toilet cleaners; antifreeze and transmission fluid; weed killers, cockroach sprays, mothballs, and rat poison; propane tanks and lighter fluid; paint strippers and photographic chemicals; mercury thermometers or compact fluorescent light bulbs; and ordinary batteries.[42]

Discarded computers pose a special problem. Ideally, they would be reused or recycled, but the US market for outdated computers is very limited, and because computers have many parts, some of which contain toxic materials, they cannot simply be recycled like glass or plastic items. Many end up in landfills. Some communities have special programs to collect computers for recycling, but the actual work of recycling often takes place in a lower-income country, as described in Section 5.6.

Federal law does not restrict the disposal of household hazardous wastes in municipal trash—consumers are not required to separate them, and municipalities are not required to provide special handling. However, many communities do maintain sites where household hazardous wastes can be turned in, or hold special collection days for these wastes, and such opportunities make it easier for people to dispose of hazardous items properly (see **Figure 7.17**).

In the United States, 1.6 million tons of household hazardous waste is generated each year.[42] Like trash more generally, this is a waste stream that can be substantially reduced through individual decisions and actions, as more people become aware of these hazards.

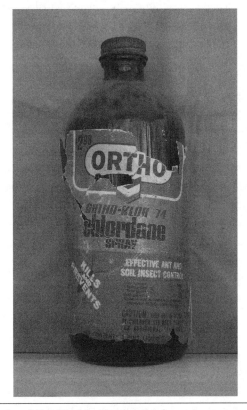

FIGURE 7.17 This bottle of liquid chlordane, which sat in a garage for 20 years after the sale of the pesticide was prohibited in the United States, was turned in at a municipal collection day for household hazardous wastes.

Medical Waste

Medical waste, produced by health care facilities, includes ordinary trash as well as items that are infectious, hazardous, or radioactive. Although some specific types of medical waste fall under various federal laws, much regulation of medical waste is at the state or local level. One particularly influential federal action was emissions requirements set for all medical waste incinerators built after 1996; these requirements are likely to push medical facilities toward other approaches to waste disposal.[43] Other and perhaps more desirable options, for example, using chemical processes or ionizing radiation in conjunction with mechanical processes, are available.[44]

Regulation of Municipal Solid Waste in the United States

The major law governing the handling of municipal solid waste is the Resource Conservation and Recovery Act. As its name suggests, its goals include not only ensuring that disposal facilities are adequate, but also encouraging source reduction, recycling, and recovering energy from wastes. Open dumping of trash is no longer legal; regulations under RCRA set requirements for landfill features including liners, leachate collection, and groundwater monitoring. Emissions from trash incinerators must meet emissions limits under the Clean Air Act.

Key elements of the US regulatory framework for municipal solid waste appear in **Table 7.6**. This table is the ninth in a series of similar tables that place regulatory provisions within the traditional regulatory domains of environmental health.

7.5 The Urban Environment

The world's population, now at more than 6 billion, is on the brink of being more than half urban, and the population of the lower-income countries is expected to cross this line by 2020 (**Figure 7.18**). The World Health Organization estimates that about 3 billion people now live in urban areas worldwide, about 1 billion of them in urban slums.[45] Thus, the challenges of managing the urban metabolism—the disposal of toilet waste and trash, and the provision of safe drinking water—are of critical importance worldwide, and especially in lower-income countries. These challenges are amplified by the fact that the world's cities are becoming ever larger—in 2005, some 20 of the world's cities were designated as **megacities**, having at least 10 million inhabitants (see **Figure 7.19**). Most of these megacities are in lower-income countries; only two are in North America.[46] Environmental health problems characteristic of urban settings in lower-income countries, and in the United States, are described in this section.

Urban Settings in Lower-Income Countries

Most urban areas are characterized by sharp socioeconomic disparities within their boundaries. In lower-income countries, rapid urbanization has overwhelmed the capacities of urban governments. Life in the urban slums of lower-income countries is characterized by extremes of poverty, overcrowding, inadequate housing, malnutrition, and lack of clean water

Table 7.6 Overview of US Regulatory Framework for Environmental Health Hazards (9)

Environmental Health Domain	Major Laws and Key Provisions for the Control of Environmental Health Hazards
Biological hazards	Public Health Service Act (PHSA)—development of guidelines for vaccination; use of quarantine or isolation to prevent entry of infectious diseases into the United States; conduct of surveillance and investigation of outbreaks
Air pollution	Clean Air Act (CAA)—ambient standards (NAAQS) for Criteria Air Pollutants; emissions standards for Hazardous Air Pollutants, including mercury; emission allowances for SO_2 (to control acid deposition); removal of lead from gasoline; requirement to sell reformulated gasoline in high-smog areas
Ionizing radiation	Energy Reorganization Act (ERA)—safety requirements for operating nuclear power plants, including licensing, emissions limits, storage of wastes
	Nuclear Waste Policy Act (NWPA)—requirements to build and regulate a repository for radioactive wastes, including spent reactor fuel
	Uranium Mill Tailings Radiation Control Act—standards for management of abandoned mill tailings
Alternative energy sources	Energy Policy Act (EPAct)—modest supports for alternative energy sources
Hazardous wastes	Comprehensive Environmental Response Compensation and Liability Act ("Superfund")/Superfund Amendments and Reauthorization Act (CERCLA/SARA)—identify, assess health risks of, and remediate abandoned hazardous waste sites
	Resource Conservation and Recovery Act (RCRA)—"cradle-to-grave" manifest system for hazardous wastes; standards and permits for hazardous waste storage or disposal facilities; provisions to promote hazardous waste minimization (source reduction) and recycling of hazardous wastes
Occupational health	Occupational Safety and Health Act (OSHAct)—ambient standards (Permissible Exposure Limits) for workplace air; employers must provide Materials Safety Data Sheets (MSDSs) to workers
Industrial water pollution	Clean Water Act (CWA)—ambient standards (Ambient Water Quality Criteria, or AWQC) for about 150 pollutants; technology requirements and permitting system for discharges to ambient water, from industry
Toxic chemicals	Toxic Substances Control Act (TSCA)—pre-manufacture notice for new chemicals; EPA can restrict manufacture, distribution, or use if new chemical poses unreasonable risk
	Emergency Planning and Community Right-to-Know Act (EPCRA)—local and state emergency response commissions; yearly chemical reporting requirements for manufacturing facilities; data available as Toxics Release Inventory; facilities must provide Materials Safety Data Sheets (MSDSs) to local commissions

(continues)

Table 7.6 *(Continued)*

Environmental Health Domain	Major Laws and Key Provisions for the Control of Environmental Health Hazards
	Pollution Prevention Act (PPA)—support for source reduction/waste prevention as preferable to treatment or disposal of wastes
Pesticides	Federal Insecticide, Fungicide, and Rodenticide Act (FIFRA)—registration of pesticides
Food supply	Federal Food, Drug, and Cosmetic Act (FFDCA) /Food Quality Protection Act (FQPA)—setting pesticide tolerances in food; setting food defect action levels; approval of food additives, including potential chemical by-products of irradiation; requirements for HACCP systems for food safety; BSE surveillance and controls on feed for ruminants
	Humane Methods of Slaughter Act (HMSA)—standards for humane slaughter
	Wholesome Meat Act (WMA)/Poultry Products Inspection Act (PPIA)—inspection of meat and poultry
	Magnuson-Stevens Fishery Conservation and Management Act (MSFCMA)—conservation of fisheries
	Organic Foods Production Act (OFPA)—standards for labeling food as organic
Sewage wastes and community water supply	Clean Water Act (CWA)—ambient standards and permitting system for discharges to ambient water from municipal wastewater treatment plants; procedures for land application of treated sewage sludge
	Safe Drinking Water Act (SDWA)—standards for drinking water: Maximum Contaminant Level Goal (MCLG) and Maximum Contaminant Level (MCL), which is the standard
	Federal Food, Drug, and Cosmetic Act (FFDCA)—regulation of bottled water as packaged food
Municipal solid waste	*Resource Conservation and Recovery Act (RCRA)—requirements for municipal solid waste landfills and waste-to-energy incinerators*
Consumer products	
Environmental noise	

Note: New information appears in italics.

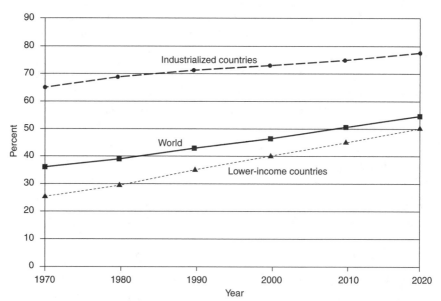

FIGURE 7.18 Percentage of the global population that is urban, 1970–2020. *Data from*: United Nations. World Urbanization Prospects: *The 2005 Revision Population Database*; Table A.2. Available at: http://www.un.org/esa/population/publications/ WUP2005/2005wup.htm. Accessed April 23, 2007.

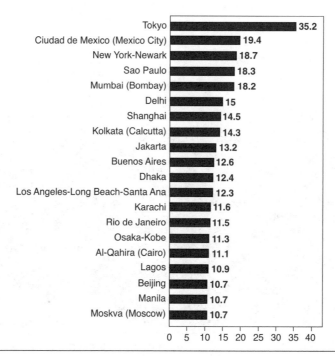

FIGURE 7.19 Populations of the world's 20 megacities, 2005. *Data from*: United Nations. World Urbanization Prospects: *The 2005 Revision Population Database*. Available at: http:// www.un.org/esa/population/publications/WUP2005/2005wup.htm. Accessed April 23, 2007.

and sanitation (see **Figure 7.20**).[45] Ambient air pollution, lead exposure from industry and from the relatively recent use of leaded gasoline, toxic wastes, traffic accidents, violence, and fires are also common hazards of these settings.[45]

Many who live in the urban slums of lower-income countries are cut off from opportunities for employment, health services, or education,[47] as well as basic municipal services. In Jakarta, for example, less than 60% of the population has access to piped water at communal taps—and water from this source must be boiled before it can be drunk safely.[48] In many cities in lower-income countries, street vendors sell water or other drinks (see **Figure 7.21**). Both sewage and trash are largely uncontrolled,[48] so many people live surrounded by wastes. All the conditions of these urban slums—crowding, trash, the lack of clean drinking water, and standing water resulting from a lack of wastewater management—are conducive to the transmission of infectious diseases, including diseases of closeness or contact, diseases of fecal origin, and vectorborne illnesses.

Urban and Suburban Settings in the United States

The cities and suburbs of the industrialized countries today, though not without infrastructure problems, have generally adequate systems for maintaining the "urban metabolism"—provision of drinking water, removal and treatment of wastewater, and removal and disposal of trash. As noted earlier, the setting that shapes daily life in urban or suburban settings is often referred to as the built environment, which includes not only buildings, but also transportation systems and public spaces.

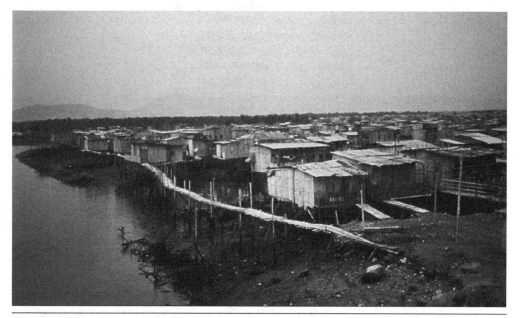

FIGURE 7.20 Slum dwellings in an Ecuadoran city perch over sewage-contaminated water. *Source*: Reprinted courtesy of CDC Public Health Image Library. ID 5323. Content Provider: CDC . Available at: http://phil.cdc.gov/phil/details.asp. Accessed September 13, 2007.

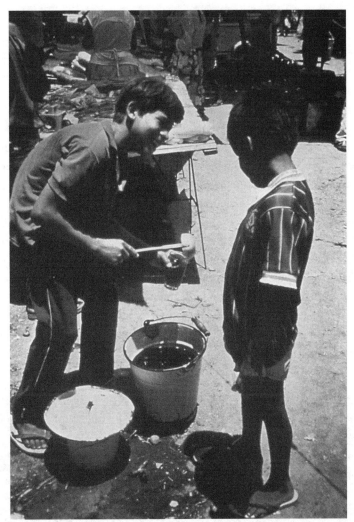

FIGURE 7.21 A young street vendor in Peru sells a homemade corn drink, using a dipper and a single glass. *Source*: Reprinted courtesy of CDC Public Health Image Library. ID 5319. Content Provider: CDC. Available at: http://phil.cdc.gov/phil/ details.asp. Accessed October 3, 2007.

As detailed in Chapter 5, in the United States, the poor and people of color bear a differential burden of industrial pollution, and such pollution is concentrated in urban areas. Zoning laws can contribute to these disparities because disenfranchised populations are more likely to live in neighborhoods zoned to allow noxious land uses, resulting in environmental burdens.[49] These burdens may include not only waste facilities themselves, but also noise, vibration, exhaust, and risk of pedestrian injuries from the associated truck traffic—and perhaps even illegal dumping.[49]

In their homes, lower-income urban residents face an elevated risk of lead poisoning, pests and the pesticides used to control them, and risk factors for asthma—including mold, cockroaches and rodents, and droppings from these pests. Urban poverty is also associated with a range of basic social risks including food insecurity[50] and the threat of violence.

Other emerging public health concerns of the built environment stem from the sprawling suburban and exurban development that has come to be known simply as **sprawl**. Suburban sprawl in the United States is marked by expansive, low-intensity construction, compared to urban settings, and by the separation of land uses in distinct locations. In these planned communities, housing (in subdivisions, as in **Figure 7.22**), stores (in malls or shopping centers), offices or industry (in office parks or industrial parks), and civic institutions such as high schools (on campuses) are built on large tracts of land designated for one use through zoning laws.[51]

Another hallmark of sprawl is the necessity for a car in daily life—simply to navigate among life's basic functions—and the resulting expansive road systems and heavy traffic.[51] All this driving, of course, contributes to air pollution on a regional scale and, along with the preponderance of single-family housing, increases per capita energy consumption in the suburbs. In contrast, traditional urban neighborhoods were not planned, but rather grew incrementally. In this setting, different land uses are interspersed, and many basic needs can be met by walking or using public transportation. A city is fundamentally a collection of such neighborhoods.

Part of the allure of the suburbs has been that they seem to offer an escape from an unhealthful urban setting characterized by crowding and pollution. But suburban life brings its own risks. Many suburban roadways carry a high volume of traffic, moving at high speed, yet

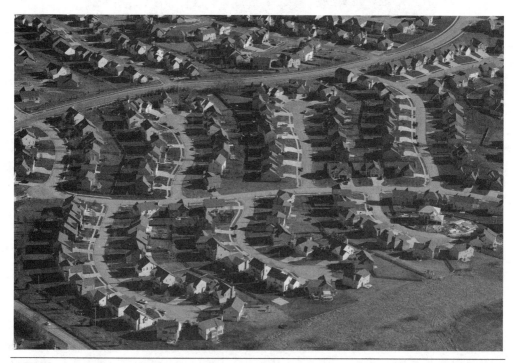

FIGURE 7.22 Suburban developments like this one, with its curving cul-de-sacs and large homes, all similar in design, are found all across the United States. © 2007 Craig L. Patterson. Used with permission.

with cars constantly entering traffic or turning off the road. In fact, traffic fatality rates are higher in higher-sprawl areas than in denser urban development—for pedestrians specifically, and also for all traffic fatalities (that is, involving private vehicles, buses, trains, taxis, bicycles, or pedestrians).[52] Finally, the inconvenience and hazards of walking in sprawled development discourage travel on foot—and this sedentary lifestyle may be associated with obesity.[53]

Risk of obesity is also associated with poverty, which is more characteristic of urban and rural settings than suburban settings. One important pathway is believed to lead through inexpensive foods, chosen as a matter of necessity when money is scarce.[54] Less expensive foods are often more energy-dense—that is, they contain refined grains, added sugars, or fats—and thus contribute to weight gain. A healthier diet, high in protein, vegetables, and fruits, is also a more expensive diet. And, as noted in Section 5.1, exposure to some synthetic organic chemicals has been linked to increased risk of obesity in animal studies.

Obesity is a serious national problem, and one that is rapidly getting worse. As shown in **Figure 7.23**, in 2005 the prevalence of obesity was at least 15% in every state and was at least 25% in 17 states. In contrast, in 1995 the prevalence of obesity in every state was between 10% and 19%.[55]

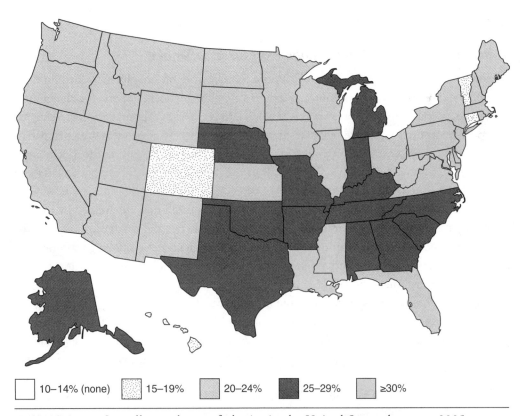

| 10–14% (none) | 15–19% | 20–24% | 25–29% | ≥30% |

FIGURE 7.23 Overall prevalence of obesity in the United States, by state, 2005. *Modified from*: US Center for Disease Control and Prevention. *US Obesity Trends 1985–2005*. Available at: http://www.cdc.gov/print.do. Accessed April 19, 2007.

7.6 Hazards of Modern Life

Although people living in the United States and other industrialized nations live in a context shaped by the community-level environmental health issues described earlier—sewage treatment, trash disposal, suburban sprawl—they spend much of their time in certain microenvironments. On average, Americans spend about 87% of their time indoors and about 69% of their time in their homes.[56] Among adults, those in the lowest income and education brackets spend the most hours indoors at home.[57] Working adults spend substantial time in their work environments, and similarly, children spend a lot of time at school.

Although most people tend to assume that indoor air is less polluted than outdoor air, the opposite is often true. As described in this section, indoor air may contain not only local ambient pollutants, but also pollutants from indoor sources—most obviously, tobacco smoke. Other indoor hazards are associated with the construction or furnishing of buildings—the use of lead paint and asbestos, the difficult-to-characterize hazards of so-called sick buildings, and the indoor accumulation of naturally occurring radon gas. The use of personal care products or other consumer products may lead to ingestion or dermal exposures as well as to inhalation of chemicals in indoor air. Finally, some products and activities result in exposure to two physical hazards—nonionizing radiation and noise. This section concludes with a description of US regulatory provisions related to these various hazards.

Tobacco Smoke and Other Indoor Exposures to Smoke

As noted in Chapter 4, in lower-income countries, smoke from burning biomass fuels for heating and cooking is the dominant source of indoor air pollution and an important cause of morbidity and mortality. In the same way, but at a much lower level of exposure, the increasing use of indoor woodstoves in the United States in recent decades has increased this source of particulates, irritant gases, and other air pollutants, including some carcinogens, in the indoor air of some homes.[58] Other activities—grilling food, for example—also contribute particulates and other pollutants to indoor air.

However, in the United States these sources of indoor air pollution are dwarfed by tobacco smoke. By the early 1900s, the large-scale production of cigarettes had emerged, along with the major companies that would continue to sell them. Although cigarette smoking was originally seen by some as a dirty habit and a sign of moral weakness (nicotine's addictive property was well known), it became increasingly popular. Cigarette rations were provided to US soldiers during World War I, and per capita consumption increased by more than 50% during World War II.[59] By 1950, cigarette smoking had been accepted as a part of American life.[59] And in that year an influential article in the *British Medical Journal* clearly linked smoking to lung cancer,[60] marking the start of what would become a massive body of scientific evidence on smoking's health effects.

In 1965, some 51% of US men and 34% of women over age 18 were smokers.[61] By this time, the US Surgeon General was issuing regular reports on smoking's health effects, and cigarette packs were required to bear a warning label about their health hazards. Through the intervening years, the tobacco corporations first denied cigarettes' health risks and then gradually admitted to some of them, all the while continuing to advertise their products. All 50 states have now signed settlement agreements (most jointly) with a group of tobacco companies.[62] Through these agreements, the companies are paying the states billions of dollars over a 25-year period to help cover costs of medical care for people with tobacco-related disease who were publicly insured; the companies have also agreed not to market tobacco products to youth.[62] In return, the states agreed not to pursue the companies' violations of state antitrust laws and consumer protection laws.

In 2004, 23% of US men and 19% of women were smokers[62]—a dramatic decline from 1965, but still a substantial share of the population. Cigarette smoke is a mix of hundreds of chemicals, of which at least 60 have been documented as carcinogens in either laboratory animals or people.[63] The mix of chemicals in cigarette smoke includes both tumor initiators and tumor promoters. The radioactive element polonium, an alpha emitter (and thus an internal radiation hazard), is also present in cigarette smoke.[64]

More than 50 years of epidemiologic study of the risks of cigarette smoking has produced a long list of ailments associated with this habit.[63] Smoking causes emphysema and other chronic lung disease, and it increases the risk of heart disease, heart attack, and stroke.[63] Cigarette smoking has been clearly linked to cancers all along its track through the body: in the oral cavity, pharynx, larynx, lung, and bladder—indeed, it accounts for most cancer at these sites.[63] It also causes cancer of the esophagus, stomach, kidney, pancreas, and cervix.[63] There is increasing evidence that active smoking, at least, causes female breast cancer—results from a recent large cohort study, for example, support this conclusion[65]—but evidence that environmental tobacco smoke causes breast cancer is lacking. Recent research from Asia, where both primary liver cancer and hepatitis B and C are more common than in the United States, suggests that smoking probably increases the risk of primary liver cancer (cancer that originates in the liver).[66,67] Some evidence suggests that smoking adversely affects hearing.[68] And finally, smoking during pregnancy increases the risk of stillbirth, low birthweight, and sudden infant death syndrome (SIDS).[63]

Exposure to **environmental tobacco smoke**, sometimes called **secondhand smoke**, is hazardous to the health of those who live or work with smokers. Like smokers, adults exposed to secondhand smoke are at increased risk of heart disease, heart attack, and lung cancer; children exposed to secondhand smoke are at increased risk of SIDS and respiratory effects, including asthma.[69]

Today, despite all our knowledge of its health effects, smoking remains a major cause of morbidity and mortality in the industrialized nations and has been exported to lower-income countries, where it is a burgeoning health problem. The World Health Organization projects that in 2025, 3 million people will die from smoking in the industrialized countries, and 7 million in lower-income countries.[70]

Lead in Paint

In the story of **lead paint**—as in the stories of leaded gasoline, asbestos, and cigarettes—corporate irresponsibility combined with regulatory failure at great cost to public health. And, like agricultural pesticides, lead paint was not released as a by-product of some process, but rather was deliberately applied widely in the environment. It was used both indoors and outdoors, by builders, homeowners, and renters in the very spaces where people spend most of their time. And unlike exposures to most environmental hazards, exposure to lead paint increases over time as it slowly wears away, shedding small particles into soil and household dust.

By 1915, the paint pigment known as white lead (which contained an inorganic lead compound) was well known to be neurotoxic to both production workers and painters.[71] Alice Hamilton, a physician and groundbreaking industrial hygienist, had published on the subject and explicitly warned major paint manufacturers on the dangers of white lead. By 1931, 11 European countries had banned or restricted the use of white lead in interior paints,[71] and scientific information on lead's effects on children continued to accumulate through the 1930s.

Yet through the coming decades, the Lead Industries Association and the National Paint Company (maker of the leading Dutch Boy brand) aggressively marketed lead paint; and the public was captivated by the new fashion for clean, bright, colorful walls, and by the paints that made them possible.[71] Adding lead to paint not only gave bright color, but also made paint more durable. Advertisements featured children and explicitly touted lead paint as clean and safe. Though a political movement to restrict lead paint in the United States had begun by the 1950s, change was slow in coming.[71]

Only in 1978, as the total quantity of lead used in gasoline was falling sharply, was lead banned from most interior and exterior paints. Each reduction of lead in gasoline meant an immediate reduction in lead entering the general environment in car exhaust. In contrast, the removal of lead from paint did not stop lead from entering the environment—in 1978, it was lead paint applied many years earlier that was crumbling to dust in rooms and in yards. In the same way, lead paint applied before the ban is still producing exposures today.

For many years, it was believed that young children were exposed to lead in paint mostly by eating chips of paint or gnawing on furniture, toys, or windowsills. This exposure indeed occurs, but later research indicated that most of children's exposure to lead paint occurs through the incidental ingestion of house dust indoors—and, to a lesser extent, contaminated soil outdoors.[72,73] Younger children, in particular, mouth objects in the environment and put their fingers into their mouths. Fortunately, relatively inexpensive landscaping techniques can substantially reduce contact with lead in the soil around a home.

Removing lead paint is expensive, and workers must be well trained to avoid spreading lead into the environment around a job site (see **Figure 7.24**). In 1998–2000, some 20 years after lead paint was restricted, about 25% of US housing units had significant lead paint hazards, whether in the form of deteriorated paint, lead in dust, or lead in exposed soil.[74] This amounts to 38 million housing units, compared to an estimated 64 million housing units with significant lead paint hazards in 1990,[74] a decline that represents the combined effects of lead abatement and the demolition or renovation of older housing. The prevalence of lead paint hazards is higher in housing units in the Northeast (40%) and Midwest (33%), reflecting the greater use of durable lead paint in harsher climates.

As shown in **Table 7.7**, much progress has been made in reducing blood lead levels in US children. As described in Chapter 4, the action level for blood lead remains at 10 µg/dL, though lead's neurotoxic effects are considered to have no threshold—that is, there is no blood lead level

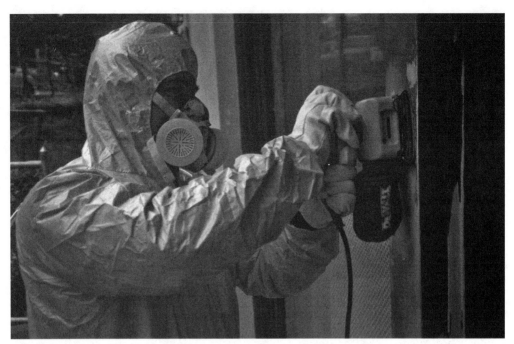

FIGURE 7.24 This worker wears protective gear as he demonstrates the use of a power sander to remove lead paint in 1999. *Source*: Reprinted courtesy of CDC Public Health Image Library. ID 7333. Content provider: CDC/Aaron L. Sussell. Available at: http://phil.cdc.gov/phil/details.asp. Accessed September 26, 2007.

that is without effect in young children. Thus, although the figures in Table 7.7 represent a success in remediation, they are also a reminder of a failure of prevention of enormous proportions. And economic and racial disparities in exposure to lead persist: In 2003–2004, when the median blood lead level for all US children ages 1 to 5 years was 1.6 µg/dL, it was 2.3 µg/dL for children in poverty, and 2.9 µg/dL for African American children in poverty. Similarly, the 90th percentile blood lead level for all US children ages 1 to 5 years was 3.9 µg/dL; but it was 5.4 µg/dL for children in poverty, and 7.7 µg/dL for African American children in poverty.[75]

Table 7.7   Decline over Time in Blood Lead Levels (µg/dL) in US Children Ages 1 Through 5 Years

Percentile	1976–1980	1988–1991	1992–1994	1999–2000	2003–2004
50th	15	3.5	2.6	2.2	1.6
90th	25	9.4	7.1	4.8	3.9

Adapted from: US Centers for Disease Control, National Center for Health Statistics. *Data from National Health and Nutrition Examination Survey (NHANES)*. Available at:
http://www.epa.gov/envirohealth/children/csv/BodyBurdens_2007.csv. Accessed December 21, 2007.

Unhealthy Construction Materials and Sick Buildings

Unlike lead paint, which mainly creates an ingestion hazard, some features of building construction or maintenance create inhalation hazards in indoor air. Asbestos, though not used in new construction in the United States, is present as insulation in many older homes and office buildings, not only in walls and ceilings, but also around furnaces and pipes. It was also installed in many schools across the country. As described earlier, people who worked with asbestos on the job are at risk of asbestosis (a fibrotic lung disease), lung cancer, and mesothelioma. And the general population continues to be exposed to asbestos fibers released from crumbling insulation in walls or around pipes or boilers—in homes, schools, and workplaces. Indeed, in the industrialized nations nearly everyone has asbestos fibers in his or her lungs.[76] People who live with asbestos building materials have exposures much lower than those experienced by workers and are very unlikely to develop asbestosis because fibrotic disease develops in response to a heavy burden of particles or fibers in the lungs. On the other hand, exposure to asbestos insulation at home or work does carry some risk of lung cancer or mesothelioma—albeit a much lower risk than that borne by workers with substantially higher exposures.

Formaldehyde—the same chemical present in some air fresheners—is widely used in the production of pressed wood products, such as particleboard and plywood, as well as creaseproof and flame-proof fabrics for curtains and furniture.[77] Formaldehyde, a gas at room temperature, is released from wood or fabric products into indoor air. In the 1970s, formaldehyde was used in the manufacture of urea-formaldehyde foam insulation, which resulted in substantial formaldehyde exposure; however, this product is rarely installed today, and insulation from the 1970s is no longer a significant source of exposure. As described previously, formaldehyde causes respiratory irritation, asthma, and cancer.

Mold and other biological contaminants, such as bacteria and pollen, may grow or accumulate in buildings, usually where water or dampness is present. These biological contaminants may cause respiratory or allergic responses in people who live or work in the building.

A so-called **sick building** is one whose occupants report a range of acute symptoms when they are in the building, and usually feel better shortly after they leave the building, but cannot pinpoint what is causing their symptoms. Occupants report such nonspecific symptoms as headache; irritation of the eyes, nose, or throat; dry cough, itchy skin, dizziness, nausea, difficulty in concentrating, and fatigue, which together are referred to as **sick building syndrome**.[78] The causes, which are usually not clearly established, may include organic chemicals in the air of the building originating from construction materials; biological agents such as mold spores, bacterial toxins, or insect feces; airborne particulates from many sources; or chemicals originating from activities in the building—all of which may be compounded by shoddy maintenance or poor ventilation. Industry standards for required ventilation rates in buildings, which were reduced in the 1970s to conserve energy, are now at least 15 cubic feet per minute of outside air per person, and are higher in many specific settings.[78] In contrast to sick building syndrome, a specific diagnosable illness that has been clearly linked to a specific feature of a building is referred to as **building-related illness**.

Radon Gas in Buildings

Another important indoor air pollutant, radon, is a natural hazard that can be enhanced by construction practices. In high-granite regions, indoor exposure to naturally occurring radon gas and radon progeny, which emit ionizing radiation, can be substantial, particularly in a building with a basement. Radon rises from the soil and seeps into the basement, from which it can circulate throughout the house. An exhaust vent in the basement—for a clothes dryer, for example—creates negative pressure, drawing more radon into the basement. In addition, if a home in a high-radon area is served by local groundwater, then radon volatilizes into the air of the home whenever tap water is used. Tight construction, though it is desirable for energy efficiency, allows radon to accumulate at higher concentrations indoors.

Because radon has no odor and is not a respiratory irritant, people can be completely unaware of a radon hazard in their home. Yet in a high-radon location, radon may be the dominant source of exposure to ionizing radiation from natural sources. Because radon is a gas, and because radon and some radon progeny are alpha emitters, lung cancer is the health risk of greatest concern. Fortunately, inexpensive radon detectors are available, and relatively simple steps, such as sealing cracks in the foundation and installing an appropriate system of vents and fans, can often mitigate radon concentrations in indoor air.

Personal Care Products

One of the hallmarks of the consumer lifestyle is the very large number of products that people deliberately apply to their bodies. Unlike cigarettes, these products aren't generally seen as unhealthful. Rather, they meet a need to maintain some combination of health, comfort, and physical appearance.

Sometimes called **personal care products**, this group includes soap, shampoo, toothpaste, moisturizers, sunblock, and feminine hygiene products—all of which are important for health or comfort—though they are often marketed, and to some extent formulated, for their cosmetic benefits. These core products are outnumbered by products that are fundamentally cosmetic: deodorants and antiperspirants; products to condition, color, curl, or straighten hair; depilatories to remove hair; nail polish and polish remover; special cleansers, moisturizers, and anti-aging products for the face; creams to lighten the skin or darken it, to screen out some of the sun's rays or enhance their tanning effect; and an array of facial make-up products. Although women use more of these products than men do, cosmetic products are being increasingly marketed to men.

It is challenging to assess the health risks of personal care products because both exposure and toxicity are hard to document. A woman may use a rather long list of products, and the list changes over time. Similarly, a single product may have many ingredients, and its composition may change often in a competitive marketplace. And, although a listing of ingredients must appear on the label of a cosmetic product, listed in order of predominance (by weight), inert ingredients need not be listed. **Inert ingredients** are those that do not serve the primary function of a particular product, but have some supporting function—for example, as solvents or spreading agents. This designation does not mean either that the ingredient is harmless or that it is chemically inert. Similarly, ingredients that are trade secrets need not be named.

The toxicity of many ingredients has not been well characterized. Phthalates, for example, have been used as plasticizers in nail polish, hair spray, and fragrances for some years, but have only recently come under scrutiny as endocrine disruptors. When the CDC did its first survey of body burdens of chemicals in the US population, which included measurements of phthalate metabolites in urine, the results were a surprise.[79] The phthalates whose metabolites were found at the highest concentrations were not breakdown products of the phthalates produced in the largest quantities and used to make plastic products (DEHP and DiNP). Rather, they were breakdown products of the phthalates used in personal care products (DBP and DEP).

Workers in hair and nail salons have elevated exposures to chemicals commonly used in cosmetic products—for example, phthalates in hair spray and nail polish, toluene in nail polish and polish remover, acetone in polish remover, and chemicals known as meth(acrylates) in artificial nails.[80] Toluene, acetone, and meth(acrylates) are all chemicals known to have neurotoxic effects.[80]

Personal care products are heavily marketed to women, sometimes naming a specific ingredient as a selling point—including some ingredients that in retrospect seem to have been poor choices. For example, during the 1950s, magazine advertisements touted estrogenic hormones in skin creams and foundation make-up, and hormones made a comeback in the advertising of hair and scalp products in the late 1970s and 1980s.[81] Yet today there is great concern about hormonally active environmental chemicals. Similarly, during the 1950s and 1960s, hexachlorophene was advertised regularly in magazines as the active ingredient in underarm deodorant, as was ammoniated mercury as the active ingredient in skin bleaching creams marketed to African American women.[81] Both of these chemicals are neurotoxic. In the early 1970s, FDA prohibited the use of mercury in most cosmetics and restricted hexachlorophene to bacteriostatic skin cleansers, with appropriate labeling.[82]

Other Consumer Products

Recent decades have also seen a proliferation of chemical products for housekeeping—detergents, fabric softeners, and stain removers for the laundry; and many products that offer protection against germs or odors, such as toilet bowl cleaners and air fresheners. Many disinfectants and other household cleaning products contain respiratory irritants, and asthma is an occupational hazard for those who work as indoor cleaners.[83] Yet it is difficult for many people to see these mundane products as potentially harmful.

Antibacterial sprays and soaps are increasingly popular. A study undertaken in 2000 showed that among national brand products at national chain stores, 26% of bar soaps and 78% of liquid soaps contained an antibacterial agent.[84] This widespread and mostly unnecessary use of antimicrobial products contributes to the emerging problem of antibiotic resistance among bacteria. In most situations, a more appropriate objective is not to kill microbes on the hands, but rather to remove microbes from the hands through careful handwashing, as described in Chapter 3.

Air fresheners range from solid blocks (from which chemicals volatilize) to aerosol sprays to electronic programmable metered mist dispensers. Many air fresheners contain formaldehyde or paradichlorobenzene.[85] Both are respiratory irritants; formaldehyde can also trigger asthma attacks.[85,86] IARC classifies formaldehyde as carcinogenic to humans (Group 1) on the basis of epidemiologic evidence on nasopharyngeal cancer.[87] Moreover, the solid air fresheners are usually fatal if eaten by children or pets.[85] Paradichlorobenzene is also a key ingredient of mothballs, along with naphthalene, which can cause damage to red blood cells.[88]

Application of pesticides in the home offers the opportunity for substantial exposure because pesticide residues may cling to surfaces, including furniture, carpet, or plush toys, for some period. Young children risk being highly exposed because of their hand-to-mouth behaviors and their tendency to mouth or chew toys. People living in urban areas, and especially those in substandard housing, are likely to have more problems with some insect pests, such as cockroaches, and may resort more often to pesticide use.

Also of concern is the accidental ingestion of illegal household pesticides, mostly by children. A series of accidental poisonings in the city of New York in the 1990s revealed that an illegal rat poison known as "Tres Pasitos" (three little steps, taken by a rat before dying) contained the carbamate insecticide aldicarb, not licensed for use as a rodenticide. Tres Pasitos continues to be sold and used around the country, mainly in Hispanic communities.[89,90] Similarly, an insecticide known as "Chinese chalk"—cockroaches are said to die if they cross a line drawn on the floor—contains deltamethrin, a potent pyrethroid pesticide.[91] Mostly illegally imported from China, it resembles ordinary blackboard chalk and thus children are likely to see it as harmless (see **Figure 7.25**).

Some items that are not themselves chemical products may nevertheless emit chemicals into the indoor environment. For example, dry-cleaned clothing releases volatile organic chemicals used in the cleaning process. As described in Chapter 5, polybrominated diphenyl ethers are

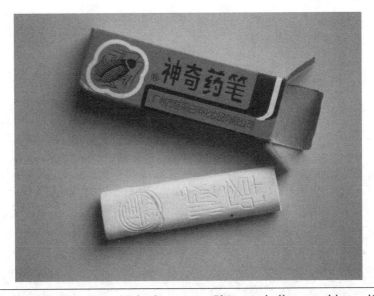

FIGURE 7.25 This illegal pesticide, known as Chinese chalk, resembles ordinary blackboard chalk. *Source*: Courtesy of Dion Lerman, Pennsylvania Integrated Pest Management Program/Pennsylvania State University.

widely used as flame retardants in many products, from mattresses to plastic television housings, and have been measured in indoor settings.

Nonionizing Radiation

Concern about exposures to nonionizing radiation has focused on three aspects of modern life (see the sidebar titled "About the Electromagnetic Spectrum" in Chapter 4). At the very long-wavelength, low-energy end of the electromagnetic spectrum is the **extremely low frequency radiation** emitted by electric power lines and electrical appliances. A large body of epidemiologic study of electromagnetic fields (EMF) associated with power lines (see **Figure 7.26**), mostly focusing on cancer, has shown mixed results, perhaps partly because it is very difficult to estimate past exposures. The most convincing evidence is for an association between exposure to electric power lines and childhood leukemia, and on the basis of this evidence IARC has classified extremely low frequency electromagnetic fields as Group 2B, possibly carcinogenic to humans.[92] Using IARC criteria, a working group of the US National Institute for Environmental Health Sciences (NIEHS) had also classified electric and magnetic fields associated with power lines into Group 2B on the basis of studies of childhood leukemia in residential studies and chronic lymphocytic leukemia in occupational studies.[93]

Cellular phones emit electromagnetic radiation in the microwave range. The potential for such **microwave radiation** to cause cancer is also an active area of research, though there is a lack of consensus on the risk of the brain malignancies and other tumors that have been studied.[94] At present, the rapid adoption of this new technology by a broad segment of the population has outpaced research on its potential health risks.

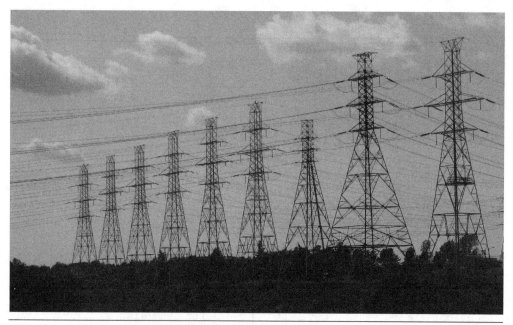

FIGURE 7.26 Electric power lines like these create very large electromagnetic fields.

A third concern is cancer risk in those who use tanning salons. Until the early 1990s, UV-A radiation was generally not considered to cause skin cancer. However, current scientific evidence makes clear that UV-A—like UV-B and UV-C—is carcinogenic. As the early public health message about the health hazards of sun exposure became prominent in the 1980s and 1990s, artificial tanning beds gained in popularity. These devices, found in special tanning salons or associated with nail and hair salons, emit mainly UV-A radiation, along with much smaller quantities of UV-B radiation. Despite new understanding on the health effects of UV-A radiation, many tanning salons continue to claim that they offer a "safe" way to tan. However, epidemiologic study has clearly linked the use of tanning beds to risk of malignant melanoma, especially with exposure before age 35, and probably also to risk of squamous cell carcinoma.[95]

Environmental Noise

Finally, exposures to noise may occur both indoors and out. For the most part, noise levels outside the occupational setting do not reach the levels found in industrial workplaces. There are exceptions: Some recreational activities, such as target shooting, are very loud and carry the risk of permanent noise-induced hearing loss.[96] Rock concerts are well known to create temporary hearing loss in those who attend and have caused permanent hearing loss in some performers. Hearing loss has recently been linked to sound exposure in musicians who play the steel pan (a percussion instrument used in Caribbean music)[97] and in adolescents who attend discos and use personal music players.[98,99] Indeed, there is concern that a whole generation of youngsters who listen regularly to music at high volume through headsets may suffer hearing loss. However, this exposure is hard to measure in an observational study because of differences in earphones among the many products on the market.

The hearing of a national sample of US children ages 6 through 19 was assessed as part of the third National Health and Nutrition Examination Survey (NHANES-III) in 1988–1994.[100] This study documented threshold shift (the standard measure of hearing loss) in 12.5% of all children tested. The prevalence of hearing loss was higher in boys (14.8%) than in girls (10.1%), and higher in children ages 12 through 19 (15.5%) than in children ages 6 through 11 (8.5%). Most of the children had a hearing loss in only one ear and were in an early stage of hearing loss—but the pattern observed is one usually associated with exposure to loud noise.[100]

The most-studied types of environmental noise are traffic noise and airport noise, and this research indicates that the health impacts of noise are not limited to hearing loss. The sounds of airports and traffic clearly cause annoyance in both adults and children, and exposure to airport noise may have cardiovascular effects, though the evidence to date is limited.[101] The best-documented nonhearing impacts of noise to date are its effects on children's cognitive performance: Exposure to airport noise at school has been associated with impairments of both reading comprehension and long-term memory.[101]

Regulation Related to Consumer Products, the Indoor Environment, and Noise

In addition to the Environmental Protection Agency, the Food and Drug Administration and the Consumer Product Safety Commission (CPSC) have roles in the regulation of consumer products and indoor air. (The CPSC's regulation of the physical safety of various consumer products, such as lawn mowers, is outside the scope of this discussion.) Key elements of the US regulatory framework related to consumer products and environmental noise appear in **Table 7.8**. This table is the tenth and last in a series of similar tables that place regulatory provisions within the traditional regulatory domains of environmental health.

The Indoor Environment

With an addition to the Toxic Substances Control Act, named the Residential Lead-Based Paint Hazard Reduction Act of 1992, the federal government directed EPA to provide technical information about managing lead hazards, as well as public education and outreach activities. EPA authorizes state programs for the surveillance and abatement of lead hazards, but it is the states that train and certify inspectors and contractors.

Similarly, the federal government provides financial support and technical assistance to states for radon programs, though states are not required to either monitor radon or control it. The Consumer Product Safety Commission regulates the safety of household products that contain chemicals, including products such as cleaning chemicals and air fresheners, but mainly as regards packaging and labeling.

Cigarettes and Cosmetics

For the most part, restrictions on smoking in specific locations are set at the state and local levels; an exception is the prohibition of smoking on domestic airline flights.[62] The major federal actions have been to require warnings on cigarette packages and to prohibit cigarette advertising on television and radio; however, agencies have passed up opportunities to regulate cigarettes as a hazardous substance, as a chemical substance, and as a consumer product.[62] As described previously, states have negotiated settlement agreements with the tobacco companies.

The Food and Drug Administration has only limited authority to regulate cosmetics. Cosmetic products and ingredients are not subject to premarket approval by FDA (except for color additives), and recall of a cosmetic product from the market is a voluntary action by the manufacturer.[102] The safety of cosmetics ingredients is reviewed by a panel of scientists, the Cosmetic Ingredient Review, established in 1976 by the Cosmetic, Toiletry, and Fragrance Association, a trade group. FDA has a nonvoting liaison member on the panel. FDA does have authority to initiate the removal of adulterated or misbranded cosmetics from the market. As of December 2006, FDA had prohibited a total of 10 ingredients for use in cosmetics, including mercury and two ingredients whose regulation originates outside the realm of cosmetics (chlorofluorocarbon propellants and prohibited cattle material). In addition, a manufacturer can ask the Food and Drug Administration to grant trade secret status for an individual ingredient with special properties that are not well known; in this case, the label need not list the ingredient, but must add the words "and other ingredients."

Noise

Regulation of noise in the United States takes place at the state or local level. Although two federal laws are on the books—the Noise Control Act of 1972 and the Quiet Communities Act of

Table 7.8   Overview of US Regulatory Framework for Environmental Health Hazards (10)

Environmental Health Domain	Major Laws and Key Provisions for the Control of Environmental Health Hazards
Biological hazards	Public Health Service Act (PHSA)—development of guidelines for vaccination; use of quarantine or isolation to prevent entry of infectious diseases into the United States; conduct of surveillance and investigation of outbreaks
Air pollution	Clean Air Act (CAA)—ambient standards (NAAQS) for Criteria Air Pollutants; emissions standards for Hazardous Air Pollutants, including mercury; emission allowances for SO_2 (to control acid deposition); removal of lead from gasoline; requirement to sell reformulated gasoline in high-smog areas
Ionizing radiation	Energy Reorganization Act (ERA)—safety requirements for operating nuclear power plants, including licensing, emissions limits, storage of wastes
	Nuclear Waste Policy Act (NWPA)—requirements to build and regulate a repository for radioactive wastes, including spent reactor fuel
	Uranium Mill Tailings Radiation Control Act—standards for management of abandoned mill tailings
Alternative energy sources	Energy Policy Act (EPAct)—modest supports for alternative energy sources
Hazardous wastes	Comprehensive Environmental Response Compensation and Liability Act ("Superfund")/Superfund Amendments and Reauthorization Act (CERCLA/SARA)—identify, assess health risks of, and remediate abandoned hazardous waste sites
	Resource Conservation and Recovery Act (RCRA)—"cradle-to-grave" manifest system for hazardous wastes; standards and permits for hazardous waste storage or disposal facilities; provisions to promote hazardous waste minimization (source reduction) and recycling of hazardous wastes
Occupational health	Occupational Safety and Health Act (OSHAct)—ambient standards (Permissible Exposure Limits) for workplace air; employers must provide Materials Safety Data Sheets (MSDSs) to workers
Industrial water pollution	Clean Water Act (CWA)—ambient standards (Ambient Water Quality Criteria, or AWQC) for about 150 pollutants; technology requirements and permitting system for discharges to ambient water, from industry
Toxic chemicals	Toxic Substances Control Act (TSCA)—pre-manufacture notice for new chemicals; EPA can restrict manufacture, distribution, or use if new chemical poses unreasonable risk
	Emergency Planning and Community Right-to-Know Act (EPCRA)—local and state emergency response commissions; yearly chemical reporting requirements for manufacturing facilities; data available as Toxics Release Inventory; facilities must provide Materials Safety Data Sheets (MSDSs) to local commissions

(continues)

Table 7.8 *(Continued)*

Environmental Health Domain	Major Laws and Key Provisions for the Control of Environmental Health Hazards
	Pollution Prevention Act (PPA)—support for source reduction/waste prevention as preferable to treatment or disposal of wastes
Pesticides	Federal Insecticide, Fungicide, and Rodenticide Act (FIFRA)—registration of pesticides
Food supply	Federal Food, Drug, and Cosmetic Act (FFDCA)/Food Quality Protection Act (FQPA)—setting pesticide tolerances in food; setting food defect action levels; approval of food additives, including potential chemical by-products of irradiation; requirements for HACCP systems for food safety; BSE surveillance and controls on feed for ruminants
	Humane Methods of Slaughter Act (HMSA)—standards for humane slaughter
	Wholesome Meat Act (WMA)/Poultry Products Inspection Act (PPIA)—inspection of meat and poultry
	Magnuson-Stevens Fishery Conservation and Management Act (MSFCMA)—conservation of fisheries
	Organic Foods Production Act (OFPA)—standards for labeling food as organic
Sewage wastes and community water supply	Clean Water Act (CWA)—ambient standards and permitting system for discharges to ambient water from municipal wastewater treatment plants; procedures for land application of treated sewage sludge
	Safe Drinking Water Act (SDWA)—standards for drinking water: Maximum Contaminant Level Goal (MCLG) and Maximum Contaminant Level (MCL), which is the standard
	Federal Food, Drug, and Cosmetic Act (FFDCA)—regulation of bottled water as packaged food
Municipal solid waste	Resource Conservation and Recovery Act (RCRA)—requirements for municipal solid waste landfills and waste-to-energy incinerators
Consumer products	*Federal Food, Drug, and Cosmetic Act (FFDCA)—limited controls on ingredients in cosmetic products*
Environmental noise	*Two federal laws on the books, the Noise Control Act of 1972 and the Quiet Communities Act of 1978, have been unfunded since the 1980s*

Note: New information appears in italics.

1978—no efforts to implement these laws have been funded since the early 1980s.[103] Thus, federal noise control is currently moribund, though a framework exists that could someday bring it back to life.

7.7 Sharing Global Impacts and Resources

Modern development, which brings many benefits in health and comfort, also drains resources and leaves its mark in wastes and chemical pollution, as described throughout this text. The products and byproducts of development may travel long distances in water or air and they may even change form, but they do not simply go away. This ecological reality highlights the importance of foresight in making the technological decisions that shape development, but in fact many such decisions have been made without much thought for their long-term implications. To date, the benefits of development have accrued mainly to the industrialized nations, whereas the negative impacts are shared more widely.

Impacts of Development

The impact of development on an ecosystem or on the global environment is often conceptualized as:

$$\text{Impact} = \text{Population} \times \text{Consumption}$$

or,

$$I = P \times C$$

a formulation known simply as the impact equation. Alternatively, with the C expanded into component factors, affluence and technology, the equation can be written as:

$$I = P \times A \times T$$

a formulation commonly referred to as the IPAT equation. This expanded version incorporates both sides of a historical difference of opinion between two leading environmentalists,[104,105] both biologists by training: Paul Ehrlich, who emphasized the importance of affluence as a driving force in environmental pollution; and Barry Commoner, who emphasized technology as the driver of pollution.

Ecosystems cannot bear unlimited impacts. Rather, an ecosystem (or the earth as a whole) has an inherent **carrying capacity**, the maximum impact that it can support for an extended period—although temporary excursions above the carrying capacity can be absorbed. Thus, if the combination of population and consumption pushes impact above the carrying capacity, this condition cannot be sustained without permanent or long-term damage to the ecosystem. In contrast, **sustainable development** can be defined as development that can be maintained over many generations, within the constraints of an ecosystem or the global environment.

In recent years, a useful measure of the impact of modern development has gained currency. The **ecological footprint** is the area on the earth's surface that is required to provide resources for, and absorb the wastes of, an individual or population with a given lifestyle. The ecological footprint was originally conceptualized as the sum of four footprints: the area required to produce food (comprising croplands and pastures), the forested area required to produce wood products, the land area covered by the built environment (called the degraded land footprint), and the forested area needed to absorb the carbon dioxide produced by burning fossil fuels (called the energy footprint or **carbon footprint**).[106] More recent analyses incorporate a fisheries footprint, and account separately for cropland and pastureland.[107]

The global average ecological footprint for 2001 was 54.1 acres per capita.[107] In the industrialized countries, the energy footprint dominates, often making up 90% or more of the total footprint. In contrast, in some of the world's poorest countries, the energy footprint makes up only one quarter to one-half of the total, and the food-related footprints (cropland, pasture, and fisheries) together account for a similar proportion of the total.[107]

A simple online calculator allows individuals to estimate their own ecological footprints, based on answers to questions about home heating, travel and transportation choices, food, recreation, and so forth.[108] Another online tool calculates carbon offsets—actions or choices that compensate for the carbon impact associated with a long airplane flight, for example.[109]

Although the ecological footprint offers important insights into human demands on ecosystems, it does not capture the health effects of toxic pollution or the depletion of fossil fuel reserves. Nor does it reflect the consumption of water—one of the most fundamental of all the resources that support human life. Most of the earth's water is salt water; the majority of its fresh water is in the form of ice and snow, and most of the remaining fresh water is found deep in the earth. Human societies rely mostly on that share of the earth's fresh water that is freely available at or near the surface. Desalination of seawater, though technically feasible, is expensive because it consumes large quantities of energy, and it is not currently a sensible option in most parts of the world.

The United Nations estimates that, as of 2000, about 20% of the people in the world lacked a natural water supply, about 15% had an abundant natural supply, and the remaining two-thirds had a low-to-moderate natural supply.[110] Behind these global figures, of course, is a collection of local and regional issues, given that conserving water in one location does not ease shortages in another part of the world. Shortages of potable water are looming in locations around the world as water is degraded by sewage or industrial pollution, or is lost to evaporation through irrigating crops, or is withdrawn from aquifers and not returned to them. The World Health Organization lists 15 countries, mostly in the Middle East, northern Africa, or Central Asia, whose yearly water use in 2005 exceeds even a theoretical maximum renewable supply.[110]

The Global Future

From the vantage point of the early 21st century, three global environmental realities stand out starkly. First, Western-style development patterns are not sustainable at the global scale: In 2001, the global average ecological footprint, at 54.1 acres per capita, exceeded the global carrying capacity of 38.8 acres per capita. In other words, the global impact was 39% greater than the global capacity to sustain human populations.[107] The global ecosystem can absorb these excesses temporarily—but the world's population is now taking out an ecological loan that will have to be repaid in reduced ecological impact by future generations.

Second, enormous disparities persist between the world's richer and poorer countries. Expressed in terms of ecological impact, in 2001 the United States had one of the highest na-

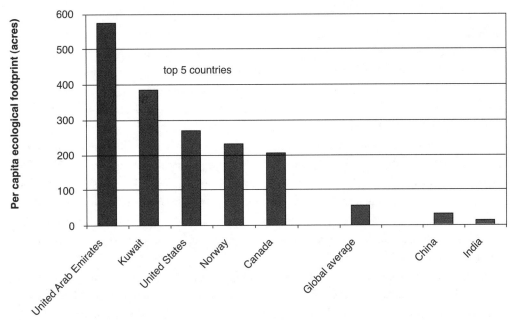

FIGURE 7.27 Per capita ecological footprints of selected countries, 2004. *Data from*: Venetoulis J, Talberth J. *Ecological Footprint of Nations: 2005 Update: Redefining Progress*; 2006:Appendix 1. Available at: http://www.rprogress.org/publications/ 2006/Footprint%20of%20Nations%202005.pdf. Accessed May 3, 2008.

tional ecological footprints at 269 acres per capita, about 5 times the global average (see **Figure 7.27**). Two oil-rich Middle Eastern nations had much higher per capita footprints, though smaller populations. China and India had footprints of 31 and 12 acres per capita, respectively. Most countries in sub-Saharan Africa had per capita ecological footprints lower than that of India, as did Bangladesh, Cambodia, Burma (Myanmar), Nepal, and Haiti.[107]

These disparities in per capita ecological footprint are reflected in other statistics. For example, of the more than 8 million lives claimed each year by ongoing hunger (as opposed to famine emergencies), most are in sub-Saharan Africa and South Asia.[111] Disparities between richer and poorer countries are also reflected in their overall **burden of disease**, a metric developed by the World Health Organization. The burden of disease is quantified using **disability-adjusted life years (DALYs)**—for a population, the years of healthy life *lost* to premature mortality or to disability, compared to a standard life expectancy. This approach uses disability weights for persons living in various health states, thus counting years lived in poor health as partial years of life lost.[112,113] Using this metric, the total burden of disease in countries classified by WHO as high-mortality developing countries is more than twice that in developed countries (358 vs 156 DALYs per 1000 population).[114] Further, in high-mortality developing countries, infectious diseases accounted for 58%, and non-infectious diseases for 31% of the total burden of disease. (The remainder is attributable to injuries.) In the developed countries, this picture was reversed: Infectious diseases accounted for 8%, and non-infectious diseases for 79%, of the total burden of disease.[114]

And finally, despite the very high *per capita* ecological footprints of the United States and some other industrialized nations, the strain on the earth's *total* carrying capacity in the future is likely to be driven mostly by increasing footprints in regions with much larger populations. In particular, China and India, with populations of about 1.3 billion and 1.1 billion, respectively, in 2007[115]—more than one-third of the world's people—have relatively low per capita footprints today, but are rapidly embracing many aspects of Western-style development, with its industry, consumption of fuels, and consumerism.

In light of these ecological and demographic realities, the world faces a difficult challenge in devising a global future that is both more sustainable and more equitable than the present. The IPAT equation, although it frames the limits of environmental sustainability, also offers some hope of a more positive role for technology. As the framework was originally conceived, technological development was seen as a contributor to pollution. But as technology is re-oriented toward the "green"—reflecting a broader social shift toward environmentally conscious decision-making—it can become a part of the solution.[104]

For those living in the industrialized nations, and especially in the United States with its generous natural endowments, the earth's physical limits have not always been apparent. They were not of concern when we elected to use clean water to carry sewage, or when we began to draw down the Ogallala Aquifer, or when we subsidized meat with grain subsidized in turn by oil. But today both foresight and fairness call for a more sustainable way of living in a world linked not only by the global transport of pollutants and pathogens, but by the very climate that will frame our future.

Study Questions

1. Explain how the major objectives of sewage treatment are met through the major processes of sewage treatment.

2. Make a list of some specific situations that you are familiar with in an industrialized country in which a modern continuous composting toilet could be a reasonable option.

3. In your current residence, can you identify ways to reduce the quantity of your household trash or to better separate out hazardous or recyclable components?

4. Describe the health risks associated with urban settings in industrialized and lower-income countries.

5. Using an online calculator, estimate your carbon footprint and test out the effects of some variations. Are there changes you could readily make that would reduce your footprint?

References

1. Tarr J. *The Search for the Ultimate Sink: Urban Pollution in Historical Perspective.* Akron, Ohio: University of Akron Press; 1996.

2. Strasser S. *Waste and Want.* New York, NY: Henry Holt; 1999.

3. US Environmental Protection Agency. *Indoor Water Use in the United States.* 2007. Available at: http://www.epa.gov/watersense/docs/indoor508.pdf. Accessed April 29, 2007.

4. US Environmental Protection Agency. *Outdoor Water Use in the United States.* 2007. Available at: http://www.epa.gov/watersense/docs/outdoor508.pdf. Accessed April 29, 2007.

5. US Environmental Protection Agency. *Municipal Solid Waste in the United States: 2005 Facts and Figures.* 2006. Available at: http://www.epa.gov/msw/pubs/mswchar05.pdf. Accessed April 29, 2008.

6. US Environmental Protection Agency. *Your Community and the CSO Universe.* Available at: http://www.epa.gov/reg3wapd/cso/YourCommunity.htm. Accessed March 31, 2007.

7. Massachusetts Water Resources Authority. *About MWRA.* Available at: http://www.mwra.state.ma.us/02org/html/whatis.htm. Accessed March 31, 2007.

8. Massachusetts Water Resources Authority. *Combined Sewer Overflows.* Available at: http://www.mwra.state.ma.us/03sewer/html/sewcso.htm. Accessed March 31, 2007.

9. Hale R, La Guardia M. Have risks associated with the presence of synthetic organic contaminants in land-applied sewage sludge been adequately assessed? *New Solutions.* 2002;12(4):371–386.

10. Gale P. Land application of treated sewage sludge: quantifying pathogen risks from consumption of crops. *J Appl Microbiol.* 2005;98:380–396.

11. Sahlstrom L, de Jong B, Aspan A. Salmonella isolated in sewage sludge tracked back to human cases of salmonellosis. *Letters Appl Microbiol.* 2006;43:46–52.

12. Gale P, Stanfield G. Towards a quantitative risk assessment for BSE in sewage sludge. *J Appl Microbiol.* 2001;91:563–569.

13. Rideout K, Teschke K. Potential for increased human foodborne exposure to PCDD/F when recycling sewage sludge on agricultural land. *Environ Health Perspect.* 2004; 112(9):959–969.

14. Hale R, La Guardia M, Harvey E, Gaylor M, Mainor T, Duff W. Persistent pollutants in land-applied sludges. *Nature.* July 2001;412:140–141.

15. Golet E, Strehler A, Alder A, Giger W. Determination of fluoroquinolone antibacterial agents in sewage sludge and sludge-treated soil using accelerated solvent extraction followed by solid-phase extraction. *Anal Chem.* 2002;74(21):5455–5462.

16. US Environmental Protection Agency. *Land Application of Biosolids.* 2002. Available at: http://www.epa.gov/oigearth/reports/2002/BIOSOLIDS_FINAL_REPORT.pdf. Accessed April 29, 2008.

17. Minnesota Pollution Control Agency. *Sewage Treatment in a Soil System.* 2001. Available at: http://proteus.pca.state.mn.us/publications/wq-wwists1-11.pdf. Accessed April 29, 2008.

18. US Environmental Protection Agency and US Department of Agriculture. *A Handbook of Constructed Wetlands.* Available at: http://www.ci.austin.tx.us/wri/treat8.htm. Accessed April 29, 2008.

19. Zezima K. Vermont blends "green" flush toilets and a greenhouse. *New York Times,* August 31, 2005.

20. Rockefeller A, Goodland R. What is environmental sustainability in sanitation? In: Goodland R, Orlando L, Anhang J, eds. *Toward Sustainable Sanitation.* Fargo, ND: International Association of Impact Assessment; 2001:7–16.

21. Orlando, L. Personal communication. January 7, 2008.

22. World Health Organisation. Statistical Annexe, World Health Report 2000—Changing History; Table 2. Available at: http://www.who.int/whr/2004/en/. Accessed February 7, 2008.

23. US Environmental Protection Agency. *Public Drinking Water Systems: Facts and Figures.* Available at: http://www.epa.gov/ogwdw/pws/index.html. Accessed December 27, 2007.

24. US Geological Survey. *Probing the Los Angeles Basin—Insights into Ground-Water Resources and Earthquake Hazards* 2002. Available at: http://geopubs.wr.usgs.gov/fact-sheet/fs086-02/. Accessed April 29, 2008.

25. Villanueva C, Cantor K, Grimalt J, Malats N, Silverman D, Tardon A, et al. Bladder cancer and exposure to water disinfection by-products through ingestion, bathing, showering, and swimming in pools. *Am J Epidemiol.* 2007;165(2):148–156.

26. Chang C-C, Ho S-C, Wang L-Y, Yang C-Y. Bladder cancer in Taiwan: relationship to trihalomethane concentrations present in drinking-water supplies. *J Toxicol Environ Health.* 2007;70(Part A):1752–1757.

27. Nieuwenhuijsen M, Toledano M, Eaton N, Fawell J, Elliott P. Chlorination disinfection byproducts in water and their association with adverse reproductive outcomes: a review. *Occup Environ Med.* 2000;57(2):73–85.

28. Wright J, Schwartz J, Dockery D. Effect of trihalomethane exposure on fetal development. *Occup Environ Med.* 2003;60:173–180.

29. Howards P, Hertz-Picciotto I. Invited commentary: disinfection by-products and pregnancy loss—lessons. *Am J Epidemiol.* 2006;164(11):1052–1055.

30. Savitz D, Singer P, Herring A, Hartmann K, Weinberg H, Makarushka C. Exposure to drinking water disinfection by-products and pregnancy loss. *Am J Epidemiol.* 2006;164(11):1043–1051.

31. US Environmental Protection Agency. *Information About Chloramine in Drinking Water.* Available at: http://www.epa.gov/safewater/disinfection/chloramine/. Accessed December 27, 2007.

32. US Centers for Disease Control and Prevention. *Community Water Fluoridation.* Available at: http://www.cdc.gov/fluoridation/. Accessed December 27, 2007.

33. National Academy of Sciences. *Fluoride in Drinking Water: A Scientific Review of EPA's Standards (Report in Brief).* 2006. Available at: http://dels.nas.edu/dels/rpt_briefs/fluoride_brief_final.pdf. Accessed April 29, 2008.

34. US Environmental Protection Agency. *Private Drinking Water Wells.* Available at: http://www.epa.gov/safewater/privatewells/index2.html. Accessed December 27, 2007.

35. US Food and Drug Administration, Center for Food Safety and Applied Nutrition. *Bottled Water Regulation and the FDA.* August/September 2002. Available at: http://www.cfsan.fda.gov/~dms/botwatr.html. Accessed December 27, 2007.

36. US Environmental Protection Agency. *Bottled Water Basics.* 2005. Available at: http://www.epa.gov/OGWDW/faq/pdfs/fs_healthseries_bottlewater.pdf. Accessed April 29, 2008.

37. US Environmental Protection Agency. *Drinking Water Contaminants.* Available at: http://www.epa.gov/safewater/contaminants/index.html. Accessed: April 30, 1008.

38. US Environmental Protection Agency. *Vermicomposting.* Available at: http://www.epa.gov/compost/vermi.htm. Accessed December 12, 2007.

39. Wayland R. Clean Air Act Section 129: Waste to Energy Overview. Presented at: Presentation for the Waste-to-Energy: An Integrated Waste Management Option Conference; 2007. Available at: http://www.epa.gov/Region2/cepd/pdf/2robert waylandspresentation.pdf. Accessed April 29, 2008.

40. Intergovernmental Panel on Climate Change. IPPC, 2007: *Summary for Policymakers.* In: *Climate Change 2007: The Physical Science Basis.* Contribution of Working Group I to the Fourth Assessment Report of the Intergovernmental Panel on Climate Change. Cambridge, England, and New York, NY: Cambridge University Press; 2007.

41. US Energy Information Administration. *Emissions of Greenhouse Gases in the United States 2004.* 2005. Available at: http://www.eia.doe.gov/oiaf/1605/archive/gg05rpt/pdf/executive_summary.pdf . Accessed April 19, 2008.

42. US Environmental Protection Agency. *List of Common HHW Products.* Available at: http://www.epa.gov/msw/hhw-list.htm. Accessed March 30, 2007.

43. US Environmental Protection Agency. *Medical Waste.* Available at: http://www.epa.gov/epaoswer/other/medical/. Accessed March 31, 2007.

44. Health Care Without Harm. *Non-Incineration Medical Waste Treatment Technologies.* Washington, DC; 2001. Available at: www.noharm.org/us/medicalwaste/issue. Accessed April 29, 2008.

45. World Health Organization. *A Billion Voices: Listening and Responding to the Health Needs of Slum Dwellers and Informal Settlers in New Urban Settings.* 2005. Available at: http://www.who.int/social_determinants/resources/urban_settings.pdf. Accessed April 29, 2008.

46. United Nations. *World Urbanization Prospects: The 2005 Revision Population Database.* Available at: http://www.un.org/esa/population/publications/WUP2005/2005wup.htm. Accessed April 23, 2007.

47. Vlahov D, Galea S, Gibble E, Freudenberg N. Perspectives on urban conditions and population health. *Cadernos de Saude Publica.* 2005;21(3):949–957.

48. Marshall J. Megacity, mega mess. *Nature.* 2005;437:312–314.

49. Maantay J. Zoning, equity, and public health. *Am J Public Health.* 2001;91(7):1033–1041.

50. Evenson K, Laraia B, Welch V, Perry A. Statewide prevalences of concern about enough food, 1996–1999. *Public Health Rep.* July–August 2002;117:358–365.

51. Duany A, Plater-Zyberk E, Speck J. *Suburban Nation: The Rise of Sprawl and the Decline of the American Dream.* New York, NY: North Point Press; 2000.

52. Ewing R, Schieber R, Zegeer C. Urban sprawl as a risk factor in motor vehicle occupant and pedestrian fatalities. *Am J Public Health.* 2003;93(9):1541–1545.

53. Frumkin H. Urban sprawl and public health. *Public Health Rep.* May–June 2002;117:201–212.

54. Drewnowski A, Specter S. Poverty and obesity: the role of energy density and energy costs. *Am J Clin Nutr.* 2004;79:6–16.

55. US Centers for Disease Control and Prevention. *US Obesity Trends 1985–2005.* Available at: http://www.cdc.gov/print.do. Accessed April 19, 2007.

56. Klepeis N, et al. The National Human Activity Pattern Survey (NHAPS): a resource for assessing exposure to environmental pollutants. *J Expo Anal Environ Epidemiol.* 2001;11(3):231–252.

57. Echols SL, Macintosh DL, Hammerstrom KA, Ryan B. Temporal variability of microenvironmental time budgets in Maryland. *J Expo Anal Environ Epidemiol.* 1999; 9:502–512.

58. Naeher L, Brauer M, Lipsett M, Zelikoff J, Simpson C, Koenig C, et al. Woodsmoke health effects: a review. *Inhalation Toxicol.* 2007;19(1):67–106.

59. US Centers for Disease Control and Prevention. *Reducing Tobacco Use: A Report of the Surgeon General.* 2000. Available at: http://www.cdc.gov/tobacco/data_statistics/sgr/sgr_2000/sgr_tobacco_chap.htm. Accessed April 29, 2008.

60. Doll R, Hill A. Smoking and carcinoma of the lung; preliminary report. *Br Med J.* 1950;2(4682):739–748.

61. National Center for Health Statistics. *Health, United States, 2006.* 2006. Available at: http://www.cdc.gov/nchs/hus.htm. Accessed April 29, 2008.

62. US Centers for Disease Control and Prevention. *Smoking and Tobacco Use.* Available at: http://www.cdc.gov/tobacco/data_statistics/by_topic/policy/legislation.htm. Accessed April 9, 2007.

63. National Cancer Institute. *Cigarette Smoking and Cancer: Questions and Answers.* Available at: http://www.cancer.gov/cancertopics/factsheet/Tobacco/cancer. Accessed April 5, 2007.

64. US Environmental Protection Agency. *Radiation Protection: Tobacco Smoke.* Available at: http://www.epa.gov/rpdweb00/sources/tobacco.html. Accessed December 16, 2007.

65. Reynolds P, Hurley S, Goldberg D, Anton-Culver H, Bernstein L, Deapen D, et al. Active smoking, household passive smoking, and breast cancer: evidence from the California Teachers Study. *J Natl Cancer Inst.* 2004;96(1):29–37.

66. Jee S, Ohrr H, Sull J, Samet J. Cigarette smoking, alcohol drinking, hepatitis B, and risk for hepatocellular carcinoma in Korea. *J Natl Cancer Inst.* 2004;96(24):1851–1856.

67. Tanaka K, Tsuji I, Wakai K, Nagata C, Mizoue T, Inoue M, et al. Cigarette smoking and liver cancer risk: an evaluation based on a systematic review of epidemiologic evidence among Japanese. *Jpn J Clin Oncol.* 2006;36(7):445–456.

68. Palmer K, Griffin M, Syddall H, Coggon D. Cigarette smoking, occupational exposure to noise, and self reported hearing difficulties. *Occup Environ Med.* 2004;61:340–344.

69. US Centers for Disease Control and Prevention. *Fact Sheet: Secondhand Smoke.* 2006. Available at: http://www.cdc.gov/tobacco/data_statistics/Factsheets/SecondhandSmoke.htm#. Accessed April 5, 2007.

70. World Health Organization. *The Tobacco Atlas*; 2002. Report No. ISBN 92 4156 209 9. Available at: http://www.who.int/tobacco/statistics/tobacco_atlas/en/. Accessed April 29, 2008.

71. Markowitz G, Rosner D. *Deceit and Denial: The Deadly Politics of Industrial Pollution.* Berkeley: University of California Press; 2002.

72. Lanphear BP, Burgoon DA, Rust SW, Eberly S, Galke W. Environmental exposures to lead and urban children's blood lead levels. *Environ Res.* 1998;76(Section A):120–130.

73. Lanphear BP, Matte TD, Rogers J, Clickner RP, Dietz B, Bornschein RL, et al. The contribution of lead-contaminated house dust and residential soil to children's blood lead levels: a pooled analysis of 12 epidemiologic studies. *Environ Res.* 1998;79(Section A):51–68.

74. Jacobs DE, Clickner RP, Zhou JY, Viet SM, Marker DA, Rogers JW, et al. The prevalence of lead-based paint hazards in U.S. housing. *Environ Health Perspect.* 2002; 110(10):A599–A606.

75. US Environmental Protection Agency. *America's Children and the Environment (ACE) / See the Data.* Available at: http://www.epa.gov/envirohealth/children/seedata.htm. Accessed December 21, 2007.

76. Robinson BS, Musk AW, Lake RA. Malignant mesothelioma. *Lancet.* 2005;366:397–408.

77. Miller EW, Miller RM. *Indoor Pollution.* Santa Barbara, Calif: ABC-CLIO; 1998.

78. US Environmental Protection Agency. *Indoor Air Facts No. 4 (revised): Sick Building Syndrome.* Available at: http://www.epa.gov/iaq/pubs/sbs.html. Accessed April 7, 2007.

79. US Centers for Disease Control and Prevention. *National Report on Human Exposure to Environmental Chemicals.* 2001. Available at: http://www.cdc.gov/exposurereport/. Accessed January 20, 2002.

80. LoSasso GL, Rapport LJ, Axelrod BN. Neuropsychological symptoms associated with low-level exposure to solvents and (meth)acrylates among nail technicians. *Neuropsychiatry Neuropsychol Behav Neurol.* 2001;14(3):183–189.

81. Maxwell NI. Social differences in women's use of personal care products: a study of magazine advertisements, 1950–1994. Silent Spring Institute; 2000. Available at: http://library.silentspring.org/publications/pdfs/magazinestudy.pdf. Accessed April 29, 2008.

82. US Food and Drug Administration. *Ingredients Prohibited and Restricted by FDA Regulations*, 2006. Available at: http://www.cfsan.fda.gov/~dms/cos-210.html. Accessed April 5, 2007.

83. Zock J-P, Kogevinas M, Sunyer J, Almar E, Muniozguren N, Payo F, et al. Asthma risk, cleaning activities and use of specific cleaning products among Spanish indoor cleaners. *Scand J Work Environ Health.* 2001;27(1):76–81.

84. Perencevich EN, Wong MT, Harris AD. National and regional assessment of the antibacterial soap market: a step toward determining the impact of prevalent antibacterial soaps. *Am J Infect Control.* 2001;29:281–283.

85. US Environmental Protection Agency. *Learn About Chemicals Around Your House: Air Fresheners.* Available at: http://www.epa.gov/kidshometour/products/airf.htm. Accessed April 4, 2007.

86. US Environmental Protection Agency. *An Introduction to Indoor Air Quality: Formaldehyde.* Available at: http://www.epa.gov/iaq/formalde.html. Accessed April 7, 2007.

87. International Agency for Research on Cancer. *Agents Reviewed by the IARC Monographs.* Available at: http://monographs.iarc.fr/ENG/Classification/Listagents alphorder.pdf. Accessed February 4, 2007.

88. US Agency for Toxic Substances and Disease Registry. *ToxFAQs: Naphthalene.* 2005.

89. Anonymous. Poisonings associated with illegal use of aldicarb as a rodenticide—New York City, 1994–1997. *MMWR Weekly.* 1997;46(41):961–963.

90. City of New York, Department of Health and Mental Hygiene. *Poisonings Associated with the Use of an Illegal Pesticide, Tres Pasitos, in New York City.* 2006. Available at: http://www.nyc.gov/html/doh/downloads/pdf/cd/06md38.pdf. Accessed April 29, 2008.

91. US Environmental Protection Agency. *Insecticide Chalk.* Available at: http://www.epa.gov/pesticides/health/illegalproducts/chalk.htm. Accessed April 5, 2007.

92. International Agency for Research on Cancer. *IARC Monographs on the Evaluation of Carcinogenic Risks to Humans: Volume 80: Non-Ionizing Radiation, Part 1: Static and Extremely Low-Frequency (ELF) Electric and Magnetic Fields.* World Health Organization; 2002. Available at: http://monographs.iarc.fr/ENG/Monographs/vol80/volume80.pdf. Accessed April 29, 2008.

93. National Institute of Environmental Health Sciences Working Group. *Assessment of Health Effects from Exposure to Power-Line Frequency Electric and Magnetic Fields.* 1998. Available at: http://www.niehs.nih.gov/health/topics/agents/emf/docs/niehs-report.pdf. Accessed April 9, 2007.

94. Kundi M. Mobile phone use and cancer. *Occup Environ Med.* 2004;61:560–570.

95. International Agency for Research on Cancer Working Group on Artificial Ultraviolet (UV) Light and Skin Cancer. The association of use of sunbeds with cutaneous malignant melanoma and other skin cancers: a systematic review. *Int J Cancer.* 2006;120:1116–1122.

96. Nondahl DM, Cruickshanks KJ, Wiley TL, Klein R, Klein BE, Tweed TS. Recreational firearm use and hearing loss. *Arch Family Med.* April 2000;9:352–357.

97. Juman S, Karmody CS, Simeon D. Hearing loss in steelband musicians. *Otolaryngol Head Neck Surg.* 2004;131:461–465.

98. Biassoni EC, Serra MR, Richtert U, Joekes S, Yacci MR, Carignani R, et al. Recreational noise exposure and its effects on the hearing of adolescents. Part II: development of hearing disorders. *Int J Audiol.* 2005;44(2):74–85.

99. Serra MR, Biassoni EC, Richter U, Minoldo G, Franco G, Abraham S, et al. Recreational noise exposure and its effects on the hearing of adolescents. Part I: an interdisciplinary long-term study. *Int J Audiol.* 2005;44(2):65–73.

100. Niskar AS, Kieszak SM, Holmes AE, Esteban E, Rubin C, Brody DJ. Estimated prevalence of noise-induced hearing threshold shifts among children 6 to 19 years of age: the Third National Health and Nutrition Examination Survey, 1988–1994, United States. *Pediatrics.* 2001;108(1):40–43.

101. Stansfeld SA, Matheson MP, Mark P. Noise pollution: non-auditory effects on health. *Br Med Bull.* 2003;68:243–257.

102. US Food and Drug Administration. *FDA Authority over Cosmetics.* Available at: http://www.cfsan.fda.gov/~dms/cos-206.html. Accessed April 5, 2007.

103. US Environmental Protection Agency. *Noise.* Available at: http://www.epa.gov/history/topics/noise/index.htm. Accessed April 9, 2007.

104. Chertow, MR. The IPAT equation and its variants: changing views of technology and environmental impact. *Journal of Industrial Ecology.* 2001;4(4):13–29.

105. Chertow, M. *IPAT Equation.* In: Encyclopedia of Earth (Washington, DC: Environmental Information Coalition, National Council for Science and the Environment); topic editors C. Cleveland and J. Felleman. Available at: http://www.eoearth.org/article/IPAT_equation. Accessed May 1, 2008.

106. Palmer, AR. Ecological footprints: evaluating sustainability. *Environmental Geosciences.* 2004; 6(4):200–204.

107. Venetoulis J, Talberth J. *Ecological Footprint of Nations: 2005 Update: Redefining Progress.* 2006. Available at: http://www.rprogress.org/publications/2006/Footprint%20of%20Nations%202005.pdf. Accessed April 23, 2007.

108. Redefining Progress. *Ecological Footprint Quiz.* Available at: http://www.myfootprint.org/. Accessed January 25, 2008.

109. Carbon Footprint Ltd. *Reducing Your Impact.* Available at: http://www.carbonfootprint.com/. Accessed January 25, 2008.

110. United Nations. *Water: A Shared Responsibility.* Paris: UNESCO; 2006. Report No. 92-3-104006-5. Available at: http://unesdoc.unesco.org/images/0014/001444/144409E.pdf. Accessed May 20, 2007.

111. United Nations Secretariat. *Bulletin on the Eradication of Poverty* (2003 annual edition). 2004. Available at: http://www.un.org/esa/socdev/poverty/documents/boep_10_2003_EN.pdf. Accessed April 29, 2008.

112. World Health Organisation. *About the Global Burden of Disease Project.* Available at: http://222.who.int/healthinfo/bodabout/en/index.html. Accessed May 1, 2008.

113. World Health Organisation. *Disability adjusted life years (DALY).* Available at: http://www.who.int/healthinfo/boddaly/en/index.html. Accessed May 1, 2008.

114. World Health Organisation. Revised Global Burden of Disease (GBD) 2002 Estimates. Available at: http://www.who.int/healthinfo/bodgbd2002revised/en/. Accessed May 1, 2008.

115. The World Bank. *Data Factoids: China and India.* Available at: http://go.worldbank.org/7ACCTX3730. Accessed April 23, 2007.

Appendix Location of Traditional Environmental Health Topics within This Textbook's Chapter Organization

Topics	Chapters in this textbook					
	Chapter 2 Science and Methods	Chapter 3 Living with Other Species	Chapter 4 Producing Energy	Chapter 5 Producing Manufactured Goods	Chapter 6 Producing Food	Chapter 7 Living in the World We've Made
Environmental health science and methods	✓					
Environmental health policy and regulation		✓	✓	✓	✓	✓
Sustainability and alternatives			✓	✓	✓	✓
Biological hazards (infectious disease, foodborne illness)		✓			✓	
Air quality and climate change			✓	✓	✓	
Ionizing radiation			✓			
Non-ionizing radiation			✓			✓
Alternative energy sources			✓			
Manufacture and use of toxic chemicals				✓		

(continues)

Appendix (Continued)

Topics	Chapters in this textbook					
	Chapter 2 Science and Methods	Chapter 3 Living with Other Species	Chapter 4 Producing Energy	Chapter 5 Producing Manufactured Goods	Chapter 6 Producing Food	Chapter 7 Living in the World We've Made
Hazardous wastes of industry				✔		
Industrial water pollution				✔		
Occupational health			✔	✔		
Pesticides					✔	
Food supply					✔	
Sewage wastes and community water supply						✔
Municipal solid and hazardous wastes						✔
Consumer products						✔
Environmental noise						✔

✔ = primary treatment of topic   ✔ = secondary treatment of topic

Glossary

A

absorbed dose
the quantity of a toxicant that passes through the human envelope, thereby entering the body

absorption
passage of a toxicant (or toxin) through the human envelope into the body

acid deposition (or *acid rain*)
precipitation made acidic by the atmospheric conversion of nitric oxide and nitrogen dioxide to nitrates and nitric acid, and of sulfur dioxide to sulfates and sulfuric acid

acid mine drainage
water, originating as rainwater, that has been made acidic by passing through mine shafts or the waste rock from a coal mine

acid rain
see *acid deposition*

active immunity
the immunity, usually permanent, that results after the immune system has mounted a counterattack against a foreign substance

active ingredient
in a pesticide, the chemical ingredient that is intended to kill the pest

acute exposure
a brief exposure

aerosol
very fine airborne solid or liquid particles

aflatoxin
a mycotoxin produced by a mold, *Aspergillus flavus*, that grows most commonly on peanuts and corn in storage; a potent liver carcinogen

air pollution
pollution of the troposphere

Air Quality Index
EPA's daily rating of local air quality, and associated health concern, for five major air pollutants

allergen
a foreign but harmless substance to which a person's immune system mounts an unnecessary response

allergic rhinitis (hay fever)
an allergic reaction in the upper airway, with symptoms of sneezing, runny nose, and watery eyes

allergy
a disease in which the immune system mounts an unnecessary response to a foreign but harmless substance

alpha particle
a particle consisting of two protons plus two neutrons that is ejected from the nucleus of an atom during radioactive decay

alveolar ducts
the smallest airways of the lungs, whose walls have many clusters of tiny sacs

alveoli
tiny sacs, occurring in clusters as outpocketings of the alveolar ducts, where gas exchange occurs in the lungs

analytic epidemiology
epidemiology using a study design intended to test a hypothesized association between risk factor and health outcome

animal epidemiology
the use of epidemiologic methods to conduct health studies in animals

antagonism
the occurrence of a joint effect of two exposures that is less than the sum of their individual effects

anthropogenic
originating from human activities as opposed to natural sources; man-made

antibiotic resistance
bacterial resistance to an antibiotic

antibiotics
pharmaceuticals that kill or inhibit bacteria

antibodies
special proteins produced as part of the immune system's response to an antigen

antigen
a foreign substance, such as bacteria or viruses, that elicits a response from the body's immune system

aqueous solubility
the tendency of a chemical to dissolve in water

aquifer
geologic material that is porous enough to hold and transmit water

arbovirus (*ar*thropod-*bo*rne *virus*)
a virus transmitted by an arthropod

area monitoring
measurement of the concentration of a toxicant in a microenvironment (for example, in the soil of a yard or the air of a room)

artesian well
a well drilled into a confined aquifer in which water under pressure rises without pumping to a level above the top of the aquifer or sometimes above ground level

arthropod
any of a group of animals that includes insects (for example, mosquitoes, flies, lice, and fleas) and arachnids (for example, ticks, mites, and spiders)

asbestos
a durable and noncombustible mineral fiber used as insulation in many products and settings

asbestosis
fibrotic lung disease caused by exposure to asbestos

asthma
an immune illness in which the bronchi are chronically inflamed and prone to bronchoconstriction

asthma attack
an acute flare-up of the chronic condition, with inflammation, bronchoconstriction, and overproduction of thick mucus; and coughing, wheezing, and shortness of breath

averaged over time
refers to a dose; adjusted by dividing by time (for chronic exposures, usually in days)

B

back end (of the nuclear fuel cycle)
the disposal of radioactive wastes from nuclear power plants

bacteria
single-celled microorganisms, smaller than protozoa and containing DNA but no true nucleus; some are pathogenic

bar screen
a set of parallel bars through which municipal wastewater flows at the start of primary treatment

basal cell carcinoma
a type of skin cancer that originates in the deeper cells of the epidermis

Becquerel (Bq)
unit of radioactivity of a source of radiation (disintegrations per second); replaces *Curies* of earlier terminology

beta particle
an electron ejected from the nucleus of an atom during radioactive decay

bias
in epidemiology, a systematic error in the way subjects were selected or information was gathered

bioaccumulation
the building up of a chemical in an individual organism's tissues over its lifetime, as the organism continually takes in more than it excretes

bioassay
toxicity test in rodents or other laboratory animals

biochemical oxygen demand (BOD)
the demand for oxygen created by the biochemical process of decomposition of organic matter in surface waters receiving sewage wastes

bioconcentration
the movement of a chemical from water into the fatty tissues of animals; a biological consequence of a chemical's lipophilic tendency

biological hazards
hazards that stem from living things, most prominently agents of infectious disease

biological vector
an organism that is a host species of an infectious disease and also transmits the disease to one or more other host species (for example, a mosquito that transmits malaria to humans by biting)

biologically effective dose
the quantity of a toxicant (or toxin) or its breakdown product that is available to interact with some vulnerable tissue in the body (*not* the quantity of a toxicant or its breakdown product that is required to induce a biological effect)

biomagnification
the process by which a chemical becomes more concentrated in the tissues of organisms at each higher level of the food chain within an ecosystem

biomarker
a biological marker of exposure within the body; a measure of the absorbed dose, the biologically effective dose, or a change in tissue structure or function

biomass
any plant material or animal dung

biomass energy
energy stored in plant material or animal dung

biomass fuel
any fuel that either consists of biomass or is derived from biomass

biomonitoring (biological monitoring)
the measurement of a biological marker of exposure inside the body

biosolids
a term used to refer to treated sewage sludge

biotech gene
see *transgene*

biotechnology
often used synonymously with *genetic engineering*, but may refer more broadly to applied biological science

bioterrorism
the use of pathogens as weapons

bioweapons
pathogens that are deliberately transmitted by human action as weapons; or the means for such transmission

bisphenol A
a synthetic organic chemical widely used in the production of plastics

black lung
see *pneumoconiosis*

blood lead action level
the blood lead level at which action should be taken to reduce a child's exposure to lead

blood lead level (BLL)
the concentration of lead in blood measured in micrograms of lead per deciliter of blood (µg/dL) and used as a biomarker of children's exposure to lead

blue baby syndrome
see *methemoglobinemia*

body burden
the total quantity of a chemical present in the body at a given point in time

bottom ash
ash that is produced by a waste-to-energy incinerator and that settles to the floor of the furnace

bovine growth hormone (or *bovine somatotropin*)
a natural hormone in cows that, among other things, regulates milk production

bovine somatotropin
see *bovine growth hormone*

bovine spongiform encephalopathy (BSE) (or *mad cow disease*)
a prion disease of cattle

broiler
a chicken raised for its meat

bronchi (singular *bronchus*)
the two cartilaginous airways, one serving each lung, into which the trachea divides

bronchioles
small airways formed by the branching of the bronchi

bronchoconstriction
a reduction in the diameter of the bronchi caused by muscle constriction

brown lung
see *byssinosis*

brownfields
contaminated industrial sites

building-related illness
a specific diagnosable illness that has been clearly linked to a specific feature of a building

built environment
the man-made structures that shape life in urban and suburban settings, including buildings, transportation systems, and public spaces

burden of disease
the combined loss of life and loss of quality of life sustained by a population due to death and disability; quantified as disability-adjusted life years

byssinosis (or *brown lung*)
fibrotic lung disease caused by exposure to cotton dust

C

Campylobacter species
common bacterial contaminants of raw poultry

cancer
a disease of cells in which cells divide without restraint, operating outside of the body's normal controls

cancer latency
the period between the exposure that initiates a malignant tumor and the recognition of the cancer

cancer slope factor (CSF)
the slope of the dose–response curve for the carcinogenicity of a chemical in humans; specifically, the slope in the low-dose range where human exposures may actually occur; the cancer slope factor has units of incremental risk per unit increase in dose

carbamate insecticides
a class of synthetic organic insecticides

carbon footprint
the forested area of the earth's surface that is required to absorb the carbon dioxide produced through burning of fossil fuels by an individual or a population with a given lifestyle

carcinogen
a substance that increases the risk of cancer

carcinogenesis
the process by which cancer occurs in the body

carrying capacity
the maximum impact that an ecosystem, or the global environment as a whole, can support for an extended period

case-control study
an observational epidemiologic study in which subjects are selected according to their disease status (for example, lung cancer [cases], no lung cancer [controls]), and then compared on their past exposures to some factor of interest (for example, cigarette smoking)

case series
a description of a set of cases, often noticed by a clinician, that have some noteworthy characteristic in common; a type of descriptive epidemiology

chelation
a treatment for lead poisoning that increases the excretion of circulating lead

chemical hazards
environmental hazards that are chemical in nature; many, but not all, are synthetic (man-made) organic chemicals

chloracne
a painful and disfiguring skin condition caused by acute exposure to PCBs or dioxins, and which can last for months or years

chlorinated hydrocarbon insecticides
see *organochlorine insecticides*

chlorofluorocarbons (CFCs)
a subgroup of halocarbons that contain chlorine, fluorine, and carbon in different combinations; the major cause of stratospheric ozone depletion

chronic exposure
a long-term exposure, typically at a low level

chronic obstructive pulmonary disease (COPD)
a condition in which breathing is impaired by changes to the airway or alveoli, as in emphysema or chronic bronchitis

chronic rodent bioassay
a rodent bioassay lasting about 2 years, approximately the lifetime of the test animals, which provides information on both cancer and noncancer effects

ciguatera poisoning
an illness with a range of symptoms caused by eating food, usually warm-water reef fish, contaminated with toxins produced by marine algae

cilia
tiny finger-like protrusions of the cells that line the trachea and bronchi

circadian
referring to the cycles of roughly 24 hours that occur in various physiological processes

Clostridium botulinum
a foodborne pathogen that produces a neurotoxin that can be denatured by heat but is potentially fatal

coagulation and flocculation
a step in the treatment of municipal drinking water, in which the negative charge of very fine suspended particles is neutralized, allowing the particles to form flocs that settle out

cohort study
an observational epidemiologic study in which subjects are selected according to exposure status (for example, smoker, nonsmoker) and then compared on disease status (for example, lung cancer, no lung cancer)

combined sewer overflow (CSO)
an overflow valve in a combined sewer system that releases some wastewater untreated when the combined flow of municipal wastewater and storm runoff exceeds the capacity of the wastewater treatment plant

comminutor
a grinder through which municipal wastewater flows after passing through a bar screen

community-based participatory research
an approach to environmental health research that features genuine participation by those affected by the research, equitable power sharing between community and researchers, and an emphasis on practical solutions

composting
a type of recycling in which organic materials slowly decay into compost that can be used as fertilizer

composting toilet
a toilet that stabilizes human waste in a composter that is part of the unit, avoiding the use of water to carry sewage

concentrated animal feeding operation (CAFO)
open feedlot (for cattle) or building (for swine and poultry) in which animals are held while being brought to market weight

confined aquifer
an aquifer that is sandwiched between layers of impermeable or nearly impermeable rock

confounding
in epidemiology, the mixing of effects that occurs when a factor that is associated with the risk factor of interest is itself a risk factor for the health outcome of concern

consensus conference (specifically, the Danish-style consensus conference)
a 3-day conference in which a diverse group of citizens deliberates a complex issue and offers its collective judgment to government and scientists

constructed wetland
a man-made marsh designed to act as a wastewater treatment system

control rods
in the core of a nuclear reactor, rods of a neutron-absorbing material used to slow down the nuclear chain reaction

cosmic radiation
the shortest-wavelength electromagnetic radiation, originating in outer space; a type of ionizing radiation

Creutzfeldt-Jakob disease (CJD)
a transmissible spongiform encephalopathy that occurs sporadically in humans

Criteria Air Pollutants
six widespread air pollutants regulated under the Clean Air Act: carbon monoxide, nitrogen dioxide, sulfur dioxide, particulate matter, lead, and ground-level ozone

critical control point
a point in the production of food at which food safety hazards can be controlled or eliminated in the context of a Hazard Analysis and Critical Control Point (HACCP) system

cross-contamination
in food safety, the contamination of food after cooking by an implement or a surface previously in contact with the raw food

cross-sectional study
an observational epidemiologic study in which the subjects are cross-classified on exposure and health outcome; in this study design it may not be clear that exposure preceded outcome

crude incidence rate
calculated as the number of new cases that arise in a given population divided by the person-years of observation

Curie
see *Becquerel*

D

danger zone
in food safety, the temperature range from 40°F to 140°F at which human pathogens can survive and multiply

DDT (dichloro-diphenyl-trichloroethane)
an early organochlorine pesticide, still in use in some parts of the world

decibel (dB)
unit of intensity (wave amplitude) of sound; a logarithmic, composite, weighted scale

deoxyribonucleic acid (DNA)
the hereditary material in the cells of human beings and other organisms

depleted uranium
the excess uranium-238 removed from yellowcake through enrichment

dermal contact
a major route of exposure to environmental contaminants, through the skin

descriptive epidemiology
epidemiology using a study design intended to describe patterns of disease rather than link risk factors to health outcomes

developmental toxicity
the occurrence of an adverse effect on the developing organism in utero, during infancy, or during childhood (that is, before puberty)

dioxins and furans
a large group of structurally related chlorinated compounds that often co-occur; never manufactured, but rather created as by-products of various chemical processes

direct discharge
a discharge of industrial waste to some body of water, separate from the municipal wastewater system

disability
a substantial and/or long-term physical or mental limitation on a major age-appropriate life activity related to work, school, or caring for oneself

disability-adjusted life years (DALYs)
at the population level, the years of healthy life lost to premature mortality or to disability, compared to a standard life expectancy

disease of fecal origin
see *infectious diarrheal disease*

disinfection
a treatment with the specific objective of killing pathogens

disinfection byproducts (DBPs)
organic compounds formed when residual chlorine from the disinfection of drinking water combines with organic matter present in the water

distribution
movement of a toxicant (or toxin) around the body via the bloodstream or lymph system

dose
the quantification of an exposure

dose–response assessment
in a risk assessment for a chemical, a quantitative estimate of the relationship between dose and effect (a reference dose for a noncancer effect; and a cancer slope factor and weight-of-the-evidence classification for carcinogenicity); in a risk assessment for a site, gathering published toxicity values (reference dose, cancer slope factor, and weight-of-the-evidence classification) for chemicals found on the site; and deriving missing toxicity values as needed

dose–response curve
the graphical representation of a dose–response relationship, plotting dose on the *x*-axis and response on the *y*-axis, and typically having the shape of a flattened *S*

dose–response relationship
the quantitative relationship between a dose and a toxic effect ("response"), often summarized in a graph

downgradient
in the direction of groundwater flow within an aquifer; analogous to *downstream* in surface water

drainage basin
the area drained by a river and the streams that feed it (see also *watershed*)

drainage field
see *leach field*

E

ecologic study
an observational epidemiologic study in which all information on health outcomes, exposures, or other characteristics is at the level of the community rather than at the level of the individual

ecological footprint
the area on the earth's surface that is required to provide resources for, and absorb the wastes of, an individual or a population with a given lifestyle

ecosystem
a local or regional community of living things (including animals, plants, and microorganisms) and the physical setting in which they live

effect modification
in epidemiology, a joint effect of two risk factors that is either greater than or less than the sum of their individual effects

electromagnetic radiation
energy traveling through space in the form of waves that have electric and magnetic components

electromagnetic spectrum
the set of distinct types of electromagnetic radiation, arranged in order of wavelength

emerging (or reemerging) infectious diseases
infectious diseases that have only recently been identified or are making an unexpected comeback

endemic (adjective, referring to a disease)
normally present at a low to moderate level in a given population or location

endocrine disrupting compound
see *endocrine disruptor*

endocrine disruptor (or *endocrine disrupting compound*)
a chemical that interferes in some way with the body's endocrine system (hormone system)

energy conservation
reducing the amount of energy consumed

energy efficiency
getting more out of energy that is consumed

enrichment (of yellowcake)
a process that increases the ratio of uranium-235 to uranium-238 in yellowcake, achieved by removing uranium-238

environment
the complex natural system comprising all living things on the earth as well as the elements of the physical setting (air, water, soil, rock) in which they live

environmental epidemiology
the use of epidemiologic methods to study environmental hazards to human health

environmental half-life
the period of time after which one-half of the original quantity of a chemical in a given environmental medium is expected to have been chemically or biologically transformed

environmental hormone
an endocrine disruptor in the environment

environmental impact statement (EIS)
a report, required of federal agencies in the executive branch of government under the National Environmental Policy Act, that discloses and evaluates the environmental impacts of a proposed action

environmental justice
narrowly defined, equal protection from
environmental health hazards and equal access
to governmental decision-making processes for
people of all incomes and racial or ethnic
groups; more broadly, includes redress of social
inequities in the burden of environmental
pollution and industrial facilities, especially
unjust burdens on people of color

environmental modeling
mathematical estimation of the
concentration of a toxicant at or near the
location of exposure, using information
 from further back along the exposure
pathway

environmental monitoring
measurement of the concentration of a
toxicant in air, water, or soil

environmental sustainability
see *sustainable*

environmental tobacco smoke (or
secondhand smoke)
cigarette smoke, mostly in indoor air, from
smoking by other people

epidemic
the occurrence of a disease at an unusually
high rate in a population; now sometimes
used for chronic as well as infectious diseases;
also used as an adjective

epidemiology
a quantitative research method for the study
of the distribution and determinants of
health outcomes in human populations

epigenetic effect
a heritable change in how a gene is expressed,
without a change to the DNA itself

ergotism
poisoning caused by eating a toxin produced
by the mold ergot

Escherichia coli O157:H7 (*E. coli* O157:H7)
a strain of *E. coli* bacteria that may
contaminate raw beef, causing bloody
diarrhea and potentially fatal complications

eutrophication
an overgrowth of algae and other plant life in
surface water, caused by overloading of the
nutrients phosphorus and nitrogen

evaporation
the change from a liquid to a gaseous state,
occurring at a temperature below the boiling
point

excretion
removal of a toxicant (or toxin) or its
metabolites outside the human envelope by
way of exhaled air, urine, feces, or other
routes

experimental study
a type of epidemiologic study, used to
evaluate associations between risk factors and
health outcomes, in which the researcher
assigns study subjects to different exposure or
treatment groups and then gathers
information on health outcomes

exposure
contact of an environmental toxicant with
the human envelope

exposure assessment
an applied science comprising methods to
measure or estimate human contact with
environmental contaminants; in a risk
assessment for a chemical or site, an
estimation of the exposure of the
population(s) of concern to the chemical(s)
of concern

exposure modeling
the mathematical estimation of exposure,
using information or assumptions about
contact by ingestion, by inhalation, or
through the skin

exposure pathway

the pathway linking the environmental source of a contaminant to the point of exposure

extremely low frequency radiation

a type of nonionizing electromagnetic radiation emitted by electric power lines and electrical appliances

F

fate and transport

the behavior of contaminants in the environment, including their chemical or physical transformations (fate) and their movements with or between environmental media (transport)

fecal–oral pathway

any exposure pathway by which pathogens that cause infectious diarrheal disease are transmitted from feces to the mouth

fibrosis (or *fibrotic lung disease*)

excessive fibrous tissue (scar tissue) in the lungs, formed as a reaction to a physical irritant such as particulates and causing a loss of flexibility that impairs breathing

fibrotic lung disease

see *fibrosis*

fine particulates

generally, particulates 2.5 microns or less in diameter

floc

a loose mass of fine particles

fluoridation

the addition of fluoride to community drinking water at low concentrations to prevent tooth decay

fluorosis

a disfiguring mottling of the teeth caused by an excess of fluoride in drinking water

fly ash

ash that is produced by a waste-to-energy incinerator and that is captured by pollution control equipment in the smokestack

fomite

an inanimate object that passively transmits pathogens in the environment

food additive

the US regulatory term for a substance deliberately added to a food during processing to achieve a specific purpose (for example, a preservative or a sweetener)

food defect

the US regulatory term for a foreign substance in food (for example, insect fragments or rodent hairs)

foodborne illness

any infectious illness transmitted in food

foodborne transmission (of pathogens)

transmission in food of pathogens from fecal or other sources

formaldehyde

a chemical used in many applications and products; a gas at room temperature and a respiratory irritant

fossil fuels (or *hydrocarbon fuels*)

fuels formed from decayed plants and animals laid down millions of years ago and then subjected to heat and pressure underground (for example, coal, petroleum, and natural gas); also refers to fuels derived from fossil fuels (for example, gasoline)

front end (of the nuclear fuel cycle)

the mining and milling of uranium and the fabrication of reactor fuel

fuel

a substance that releases energy when it is changed, mostly through burning or nuclear fission

fuel fabrication
the production of fuel rods (metal tubes containing pellets of enriched uranium) to be used in nuclear reactors

fungicide
a pesticide used against fungi

furans
see *dioxins and furans*

G

gamma radiation
a high-frequency, ionizing type of electromagnetic radiation emitted from the nucleus of an atom undergoing radioactive decay

genetic engineering
the use of technology to create *genetically modified* organisms

genetic traits
inherited characteristics, encoded in an individual's DNA

genetically engineered
see *transgenic*

genetically modified (GM)
see *transgenic*

geographic information system (GIS)
a computerized system that combines a database of spatially linked information with application software for spatial analyses and mapping

geothermal energy
the earth's internal heat energy

global carbon cycle
the set of natural processes by which carbon moves from the physical environment

through living things and back into the physical environment

global climate change
the enhancement of the natural greenhouse effect by the production of anthropogenic greenhouse gases, resulting in overall warming and other impacts on climate

global warming
the enhancement of the natural greenhouse effect by the production of anthropogenic greenhouse gases; this term has been supplanted in the scientific literature by *global climate change*

Gray (Gy)
unit of dose of ionizing radiation (energy delivered per gram of tissue); replaces *rads* of earlier terminology

greenhouse gases
gases in the troposphere that absorb some of the heat energy radiated outward from the earth and then reradiate this energy back toward the earth's surface

grit chamber
a step in primary wastewater treatment in which heavier particles such as sand settle out

groundwater
water in the saturated zone of an aquifer

H

half-life
the time it takes for half the atoms in a sample of a radioactive element to undergo radioactive decay

halogens
a group of highly reactive chemicals that includes chlorine, fluorine, bromine, and iodine

hand-to-mouth exposure
exposure to a contaminant in soil or dust that is carried to the lips by the hands (for example, in eating or smoking)

hand-to-mouth transmission (of pathogens, especially fecal pathogens)
transmission of pathogens from feces or soil to the mouth via the hands while eating, smoking, or gesturing

hazard
a factor that causes harm or may cause harm

Hazard Analysis and Critical Control Point (HACCP) system
an approach to food safety that rests on identifying critical control points in the production of food, and then establishing preventive, monitoring, and corrective procedures around these control points

hazard identification
in a risk assessment for a chemical, a qualitative evaluation of the toxic effect(s) of a chemical, focused either on carcinogenicity or on noncancer effects; in a risk assessment for a site, identification of the chemicals contaminating the various environmental media on the site, and characterization of the degree of contamination

hazard quotient
the ratio of an actual or estimated dose to a reference dose

hazardous waste
under US law, any waste that is corrosive, toxic, ignitable, or reactive; the definition also lists specific commercial chemical products (for example, pesticides) when they are discarded, and some specific wastes from named industries or industrial processes

hazardous waste landfill
under current US regulations, a landfill designed and managed specifically to hold hazardous wastes safely; formerly, any landfill in which hazardous wastes had been placed

health impact assessment
the assessment of the likely health impacts of a proposed policy or action in a population, made before the policy or action is implemented

heavy metal
a metal with a high atomic weight; lead, mercury, arsenic, cadmium, and chromium are heavy metals

herbicide
a pesticide used against plant pests

herd immunity
the practical protection from an infectious disease experienced by a community when enough of its members have immunity against a disease that it becomes difficult to maintain a chain of infection

host (in infectious disease)
an organism in which a pathogen becomes established

household hazardous waste
any item in household waste that meets the legal definition of hazardous waste

human envelope
the envelope that separates the interior of the human body from the exterior environment; in environmental health, refers mostly to the skin, the lining of the gastrointestinal tract, and the lining of the respiratory tract

hybrid car
a car that uses both a gasoline-powered combustion engine and electric power

hydrocarbon fuels
see *fossil fuels*

hydrocarbons
organic compounds composed of only hydrogen and carbon; methane, propane, and benzene are hydrocarbons

hydrogen fuel cell
a device in which a simple chemical reaction converts hydrogen fuel and oxygen into electricity, producing water as a by-product

hydrologic cycle
the complex web of processes through which the earth's water moves through the environment

hydropower
the energy of moving water, captured by a turbine or a water wheel

I

in situ leaching
the use of an acidic or alkaline solution to dissolve uranium from the ore in which it is embedded; an alternative to mining

incidence
the occurrence of new (incident) cases of a disease in a given population during a given period of time

incidental ingestion
inadvertent swallowing of small amounts of water or dust

incremental lifetime cancer risk
the additional cancer risk, over a 70-year lifetime, that would result from a particular exposure

indirect discharge
a discharge of industrial wastes into the municipal wastewater treatment system

inert ingredient
a regulatory term referring to an ingredient that does not serve the primary function of a particular product but rather has some supporting function

infection (foodborne)
foodborne illness in which pathogens cause symptoms in the host simply through infection

infectious diarrheal disease (or *disease of fecal origin*)
an infectious disease with diarrhea as a major symptom; most often transmitted by the fecal-oral pathway

infectious disease
illness caused by microorganisms that become established in a host organism and that can be transmitted to other hosts by various means

ingestion
a major route of exposure to environmental contaminants, through eating or drinking

inhalation
a major route of exposure to environmental contaminants, through ordinary continuous breathing

insecticide
a pesticide used against insect or arachnid pests

integrated pest management (IPM)
an approach using multiple tactics (for example, biological and chemical) to manage multiple pests in a manner consistent with ecological principles

intervention study
an experimental epidemiologic study in which subjects are randomly assigned to groups receiving different health interventions, and the effectiveness of the interventions is compared across groups

intoxication (foodborne)
foodborne illness in which pathogens produce toxins that cause the symptoms of foodborne illness

ionizing radiation
radiation that has enough energy to knock an electron out of orbit, creating an ion

isolation
the separation of persons who have an infectious illness

isotope
a variant of a chemical element; different isotopes of an element have the same number of protons, but different numbers of neutrons in their nuclei

K

kuru
a transmissible spongiform encephalopathy of humans documented in New Guinea and linked to the ritual eating of body parts of corpses of people also afflicted with the disease

L

lag phase
in the growth of a population of bacteria, the first few hours in a new environment, during which time the bacteria multiply only slowly

latency
see *cancer latency*

LD_{50}
the dose of a test chemical that is acutely lethal to 50% of test animals exposed to it

leach field (or *drainage field*)
as part of a septic system, the area over which wastewater is distributed through a system of perforated pipes

leachate
the liquid substance, containing dissolved or suspended materials, that results from leaching

leaching
the dissolving or suspension of some components of a substance (for example, soil or wastes) in water as the water percolates through it

lead
a neurotoxic heavy metal

lead paint
paint containing the pigment known as white lead, which contains an inorganic lead compound

lipophilic
fat-soluble; tending to move from water to an oily medium

liquefied natural gas (LNG)
natural gas that has been cooled to a very low temperature, transforming it into liquid form

Listeria monocytogenes
a highly fatal foodborne pathogen common in mammals, birds, and soil

log phase
a period of logarithmic growth in a population of bacteria, following the lag phase

low-level radioactive wastes
radioactive wastes originating from nuclear power production or from other sources (for example, research, medicine), and which have much lower levels of radioactivity than spent reactor fuel

lowest observed adverse effect level (LOAEL)
the lowest dose at which an effect is observed in a chronic rodent bioassay

M

mad cow disease
see *bovine spongiform encephalopathy*

malignant melanoma
a cancer of melanocytes, cells in the skin that produce pigment (melanin)

mammalian feed ban
a ban on feeding any mammalian protein (that is, meat and bone meal from rendered mammals) to ruminants

materials recovery facility (MRF)
a facility where recyclable materials are separated from municipal solid waste (if not separated at curbside) and are sorted by type (for example, glass, metal, plastic, paper)

Materials Safety Data Sheet (MSDS)
a summary of an individual chemical's health effects, which employers must provide to workers under US law; also available to the public

Maximum Contaminant Level (MCL)
under US law, the maximum allowable concentration of a specific contaminant in drinking water

meat and bone meal
a high-protein meal produced from rendered animal remains from which the fat has been separated out

mechanical vector
an organism that is not a host species of an infectious disease but transmits the disease in mechanical fashion (for example, a housefly that transfers fecal pathogens that cling to its feet)

medical waste
waste produced by health care facilities; includes some ordinary trash but also items that are infectious, hazardous, or radioactive

megacity
an urban conglomeration with at least 10 million inhabitants

mercury
a neurotoxic heavy metal that is liquid at room temperature

mesothelioma
a cancer of the pleura (the membranes that coat the outsides of the chest organs and the inside of the chest cavity) or the peritoneum (a similar membrane in the abdominal cavity)

metabolism
chemical transformation of a toxicant (or toxin) by enzymes in the body

metabolite
a product of the body's metabolism of a chemical; a breakdown product

metal
an element that is shiny, is solid at room temperature (mercury is an exception), can be melted or formed using heat, and conducts electricity and heat

methemoglobinemia (or *blue baby syndrome* when it occurs in infants)
a medical condition in which hemoglobin in the bloodstream is converted into a form that cannot carry oxygen; most common in infants and young children

methicillin-resistant *Staphylococcus aureus* (MRSA)
a virulent strain of *Staphylococcus aureus*, widespread in hospitals, that is resistant not only to methicillin, but also to related antibiotics, including penicillin and amoxicillin

methylmercury
a neurotoxic organic mercury compound formed by the action of bacteria on elemental mercury

miasma
in early theories of infectious disease causation, an atmospheric emanation that rose from the earth or from rotting organic matter and that caused disease

microenvironment
the immediate environment of an exposure (for example, a room, yard, or workstation)

microwave radiation
a nonionizing type of electromagnetic radiation emitted by devices including cellular phones; also used to heat food in microwave ovens

mine tailings
crushed rock wastes of mining (for example, of uranium)

morbidity
a diseased (morbid) state; often quantified as prevalence

mortality
the number of deaths in a given population during a given period of time; the incidence of death

mucociliary escalator
the slow movement of mucus upward in the trachea and bronchi, propelled by cilia beating in unison

multilevel study
in epidemiology, a study whose design and analysis include both individual-level and community-level variables

municipal solid waste (or *trash*)
a community waste stream consisting mainly of paper, plastics, metals, glass, and organic wastes

municipal solid waste landfill
under current US regulations, a waste disposal facility in which waste is buried, usually in layers, and with features intended to isolate the wastes from the surrounding environment; formerly, any site where waste was buried

municipal wastewater (see also *sewage*)
a community waste stream consisting mainly of urine and feces but including everything that goes down the drain in homes or offices

mutagen
an agent that binds chemically to DNA, causing a change in its structure

mutation
a change to the DNA of a cell

mycotoxins
toxins produced by molds or other fungi

N

nanomaterials
see *nanoparticles*

nanoparticles (or *nanomaterials*)
engineered particles less than 100 nanometers (0.1 microns) in diameter

nanotechnology
technology for designing and producing nanoparticles

National Ambient Air Quality Standards (NAAQS)
maximum allowable concentrations for the six Criteria Air Pollutants as regulated under the Clean Air Act

National Priorities List
a national register of abandoned hazardous waste sites, created under the Comprehensive Environmental Response, Compensation, and Liability Act (Superfund)

no observed adverse effect level (NOAEL)
the highest nonzero dose at which no effect is observed in a chronic rodent bioassay

noise
unwanted sound; sound that can damage hearing or otherwise harm health

nonionizing radiation
radiation that does not have enough energy to knock an electron out of orbit

nonpoint source
a US regulatory term referring to a source of water pollution that releases contaminants over a large area

nonrenewable energy resources
energy resources that cannot be renewed (that is, produced in nature) on the human time scale

nonselective herbicide
an herbicide that kills all types of plants

normalized to (averaged over) body weight
refers to a dose; adjusted by dividing by the body weight of the person exposed

nuclear fission
the splitting of the nucleus of an atom, with the release of energy

nuclear fuel cycle
the full sequence of activities related to the production of nuclear power

nuclear power
the production of energy through the use of controlled nuclear fission

O

observational study
a type of epidemiologic study, used to evaluate associations between risk factors and health outcomes in which the researcher does not manipulate exposures but rather observes and documents exposures and outcomes

occupational asthma
asthma caused by an exposure at work

organic chemical
any of a large group of chemicals that includes most carbon-containing chemicals

organic farming
agriculture that uses sustainable practices and does not use synthetic pesticides or commercial fertilizers

organic solvent (or *solvent*)
an organic chemical that dissolves other substances

organochlorine insecticides (or *chlorinated hydrocarbon insecticides*)
the first generation of synthetic organic insecticides; includes DDT

organophosphate insecticides
a class of synthetic organic insecticides

ozone
the triatomic form of oxygen (O_3)

P

pandemic
an infectious disease epidemic of global proportions; also used as an adjective

paralytic shellfish poisoning
an illness with neurologic symptoms caused by eating food, usually mollusks, contaminated with toxins produced by marine algae

parasite
an organism that must spend a part of its life cycle inside an animal host on which it depends for certain benefits

particulates or **particulate matter (PM)**
a complex mixture that may consist of both small solid particles and fine liquid droplets, and composed of soil particles (dust), sulfates, metals, and organic chemicals

passive immunity
the temporary immunity gained from a vaccine that contains antibodies or from antibodies transported across the placenta to an infant in utero

pathogen
an agent that causes a specific infectious disease in a host

perfluorochemicals (PFCs)
a group of synthetic fluorine-containing chemicals, used in producing nonstick coatings

Permissible Exposure Limit (PEL)
under US regulations, the allowable concentration of a specific chemical in workplace air; as an 8-hour time-weighted average, a 15-minute time-weighted average, and a ceiling

persistence
the tendency of a chemical to remain in the environment without being transformed into another chemical or chemicals

persistent toxic substances
chemicals that are persistent in the environment and known to be toxic to human beings (see text for a discussion of related terms: *persistent organic pollutants*; *persistent, bioaccumulative, and toxic chemicals*; and *ubiquitous bioaccumulative toxins*)

personal care product
a product that people apply to their bodies for the sake of physical comfort and/or physical appearance

personal environment
the immediate vicinity of a person's body, wherever he or she goes

personal monitoring
measurement of the concentration of a toxicant in an individual's personal environment

personal protective equipment
equipment worn by a worker to reduce exposure to workplace hazards; for example, goggles, ear protectors, and respirators

pest
any animal or plant judged to interfere with people's well-being or interests (not a biological category)

pesticide
any chemical used to kill pests

pesticide resistance
the capacity of a pest to survive exposure to a pesticide as a result of its genetic makeup

pesticide tolerance
in the US regulatory framework, the maximum pesticide residue allowed in human food

photochemical smog
smog created through a complex series of chemical reactions among nitrogen oxides, volatile organic compounds, and other chemicals in the presence of sunlight

photovoltaic cell (or *solar cell*)
a device that converts sunlight directly into electrical energy

phthalates
a group of semivolatile synthetic organic chemicals used as plasticizers

physical hazards
hazards that stem from contact with some form of energy; for example, radiation and noise

plasticizers
chemicals used in manufacturing plastics to make them flexible (ie, plastic)

plastics
a large group of materials made with high-molecular-weight synthetic organic chemicals that have at least some flexibility (plasticity) and can be formed into items of almost any shape (for example, three-dimensional objects, thin sheets, filaments)

plume
a trail of smoke in air, or of a chemical in groundwater, which becomes broader and less concentrated with increasing distance from the source

PM$_{10}$
particulate matter 10 microns or less in diameter

PM$_{2.5}$
particulate matter 2.5 microns or less in diameter

pneumoconiosis (or *black lung*)
fibrosis associated with exposure to coal dust

point mutation
a mutation that causes only local damage within a gene

point-of-use treatment system
a treatment device for drinking water (for example, a carbon filter) installed at a single tap, such as the faucet at the kitchen sink

point source
a US regulatory term referring to a source of water pollution that releases contaminants at a specific location

polluter-pays principle
the idea that the party responsible for pollution should pay the costs of remediation

pollution
any output of human activity that is considered harmful or unpleasant; historically referred mostly to chemical wastes, smoke, and dust; but by extension used to refer to, for example, radiation, unwanted sights or sounds, or genetically modified plant species

polybrominated diphenyl ethers (PBDEs)
a large group of structurally related synthetic brominated compounds, used mainly as flame retardants

polychlorinated biphenyls (PCBs)
a group of high-molecular-weight synthetic organic chemicals, used mainly to insulate electrical devices

polycyclic aromatic hydrocarbons (PAHs)
a group of related organic compounds that are products of incomplete combustion and are ubiquitous in the environment

potable water
water deemed suitable for drinking

precautionary principle
the concept that early indications that a substance or activity causes serious harm should trigger precautionary measures before harm is proven

pretreatment (of industrial wastes) treatment of industrial wastes before they enter a municipal wastewater system

prevalence
the proportion of a population that has a disease at a given point in time

primary clarifier
a step in primary wastewater treatment in which suspended solids containing organic matter settle out

primary prevention
in public health, steps taken to prevent a health outcome from occurring (for example, through the elimination of an exposure)

primary sewage treatment
a mechanical process during which ever-finer materials are removed from municipal wastewater through a sequence of steps

prion
a type of protein found on the surface of normal nerve cells of some mammalian species; abnormal prions cause a set of degenerative brain diseases called transmissible spongiform encephalopathies

protozoa
single-celled microorganisms with a true nucleus containing DNA; some are pathogenic and parasitic

pufferfish
a fish in which some organs may contain potentially fatal neurotoxins

pyrethroid insecticides
a class of synthetic organic insecticides

pyrethrum
a pesticide extracted from chrysanthemums

Q

quarantine
the separation of persons who have been exposed to an infectious agent and may become ill

R

rad
see *Gray*

radiation
energy that is radiated from a source as particles or as waves

radiation sickness
the set of symptoms caused by high-level exposure to radiation, characterized by effects on the central nervous system, the gastrointestinal tract, and the bone marrow

radioactive
exhibiting radioactive decay

radioactive decay
the spontaneous ejection of a part of the nucleus of an atom

radiolytic chemical
a chemical created by the action of radiation

radionuclide
a radioactive isotope

radon
a gaseous radioactive element in the decay chain of uranium-238

radura
the symbol used to signify that food has been irradiated

recharge
the replenishing of water in an aquifer by water trickling downward through the zone of aeration

recharge area
the area on the ground surface through which rainfall feeds an aquifer

recombinant bovine growth hormone (rBGH)
a genetically engineered version of bovine growth hormone

recycling
separating and processing of waste materials so that they can be used again

reference dose (RfD)
a dose expected to have no adverse effects in people who are particularly sensitive to the chemical's effects and who are exposed over a 70-year lifetime; the reference dose has units mg/(kg*day)

regulatory toxicology
toxicity testing done in support of regulatory decision making

relative biological effectiveness (RBE)
a factor used in radiation dosimetry to adjust for the fact that some types of radiation do more damage to tissue than others, per unit of energy delivered

rem
see *Sievert*

rendering
the heating of animal remains in batches for the purpose of separating fat from other material

renewable energy source
an energy source that is either continually renewed in nature or can readily be renewed through human effort

reprocessing (of spent nuclear fuel)
extracting remaining uranium-238 from nuclear power plant wastes and fabricating it again into fuel pellets to be used in a reactor

reproductive toxicity
the occurrence of an adverse effect on the reproductive system or reproductive capacity of an organism

respirable particulates
generally, particulates 10 microns or less in diameter

respiratory bronchioles
very small conducting airways formed by the branching of the bronchioles

ricin
a potent toxin produced by the castor bean plant

risk
the probability of harm from some hazard

risk assessment
an applied science consisting of formal procedures for evaluating and integrating scientific information on exposure and toxicity to estimate the real-world public health risk of a hazard

risk characterization
in a risk assessment for a chemical, bringing together information on exposure and information on toxicity at different exposures, allowing the risk assessor to estimate the risk to human health; in a risk assessment for a site, summary of the cancer risk and noncancer hazard associated with exposure to chemicals on the site, under the exposure scenarios considered

risk communication
the provision or exchange of information about environmental health hazards; more broadly, public participation in research or policy making

risk factor
a factor that has been shown to pose a risk of a specific harm

risk management
actions taken to prevent or mitigate environmental health hazards; the process balances risks, benefits, and costs, and also considers social context

rodenticide
a pesticide used against rodents

routes of exposure
routes by which people contact and absorb environmental contaminants (mainly inhalation, ingestion, and dermal contact)

ruminant
an animal that has a multichambered stomach and regurgitates and rechews previously swallowed food

ruminant feed ban
a ban on feeding ruminant protein (that is, meat and bone meal from rendered ruminants) to ruminants

S

Salmonella (nontyphoid species)
common bacterial contaminants of raw poultry

sand filter
a filter in which water trickles gently through a bed of sand, driven by gravity; used in drinking water treatment

sanitation
the control of environmental factors, especially human waste and food waste, to prevent disease and promote health

saturated zone
the underground zone below the zone of aeration in which all pore spaces are filled with water, and in which water can move in any direction

scombroid poisoning
foodborne poisoning by a toxin produced by certain types of bacteria, usually associated with the spoilage of tuna and related fish

scrapie
a transmissible spongiform encephalopathy that affects sheep

secondary pest outbreak
a rapid increase in the population of a pest that was the prey of a target pest following the application of a pesticide to kill the target pest

secondary pollutant
a pollutant formed in the environment through the chemical transformation of the original pollutant

secondary prevention
in public health, steps taken to prevent a health problem from progressing (for example, through early detection of disease)

secondary sewage treatment
a biological process in which bacteria digest organic wastes in an aerobic environment

secondhand smoke
see *environmental tobacco smoke*

sedimentation
a step in the treatment of municipal drinking water in which flocs are allowed to settle out by gravity

selective herbicide
an herbicide that kills broad-leaved plant species but not plants in the grass family

sensitization
an immune response on first exposure to a specific allergen after which any future exposure to this allergen will produce an allergic response

sentinel illness
an illness caused solely (or almost solely) by exposure to a single substance and which is therefore considered a marker of exposure to that substance

septic system
a system, consisting of a septic tank and a leach field, used for the on-site treatment of household wastewater

septic tank
a buried steel or concrete holding tank that receives wastewater from a building or buildings

sewage
urine and fecal waste; but often used interchangeably with *municipal wastewater*

sewage sludge
material that originates as sludge and scum removed from the municipal wastewater stream during primary and sometimes secondary treatment

shipbreaking
the dismantling of oceangoing vessels to obtain scrap metal

sick building
a building whose occupants report a range of nonspecific symptoms when they are in the building

sick building syndrome
the set of nonspecific symptoms reported by occupants of a so-called sick building

Sievert (Sv)
unit of dose of ionizing radiation (energy delivered per gram of tissue), weighted by the relative biological effectiveness of the radiation; replaces *rems* of earlier terminology

silicosis
fibrosis associated with exposure to silica

slope (of a dose–response curve)
the increase in toxic response for a given increase in dose

sludge digester
large vat, used in secondary sewage treatment, in which sewage is primed with bacteria and then agitated to facilitate bacterial digestion of organic wastes

smog (a contraction of *smoke* and *fog*)
visible air pollution; or photochemical smog specifically

social epidemiology
the use of epidemiologic methods to study the social determinants of health

social or behavioral hazards
hazards that originate in a person's social circumstances or from the person's own behaviors

solar cell
see *photovoltaic cell*

solar power
the energy in sunlight, captured using various technologies

solvent
see *organic solvent*

source reduction (or *waste prevention*)
an approach to managing pollution by reducing the amount of waste produced

spore (bacterial spore)
dormant bacterial cell with a hard coating, able to survive inhospitable conditions

sprawl
the style of development typical of modern US suburbs, which is of relatively low density overall and in which major land uses are generally separated rather than intermixed

squamous cell carcinoma
type of skin cancer that originates in the most superficial cells of the epidermis

stabilization (of sewage sludge)
the second step in the treatment of sewage sludge; digestion of sludge by anaerobic organisms in a warm, well-circulated environment

standardized incidence ratio (SIR)
a ratio whose numerator is the *observed* (actual) number of cases of a disease in a population of interest during a given time period, and whose denominator is the number of cases that would be *expected* in the population if the age-specific rates of some reference population were applied to the local population; often abbreviated as "observed over expected"

standardized mortality ratio (SMR)
the ratio of observed deaths to expected deaths, calculated in the same manner as the SIR

standardized rate (SR)
the rate of disease that would occur in a given location if it had the age distribution of some reference population, but its age-specific rates were unchanged

standardized rate ratio (SRR)
the ratio of two standardized rates, both of which are standardized to the same reference population

Staphylococcus aureus
a common foodborne pathogen that is a normal inhabitant of human skin

statistically significant
of a statistical association; unlikely to be due to chance alone (according to an agreed criterion)

storage
removal of a toxicant (or toxin) or its metabolites from circulation to be stored in, for example, fat or bone

stratosphere
the layer of the earth's atmosphere above the troposphere, reaching to an altitude of about 30 miles (48 kilometers)

stratospheric ozone layer
a layer within the stratosphere in which the concentration of ozone is much higher than at other altitudes within the stratosphere

strip mining
see *surface mining*

subchronic rodent bioassay
a 90-day rodent bioassay, conducted as a preliminary to a chronic bioassay

Superfund
colloquial name for the Comprehensive Environmental Response, Compensation, and Liability Act; also refers to the fund for the cleanup of abandoned hazardous waste sites created by this law

surface mining (or *strip mining*)
a coal-mining technique in which the earth overlying a seam of coal is removed

surveillance
the tracking of disease or injury rates and the comparison of rates over time or across places or diseases; a type of descriptive epidemiology

surveillance biomonitoring
biomonitoring undertaken at the population level as a means of surveillance

sustainable; also **sustainable development**
(development) capable of being maintained indefinitely within the constraints of an ecosystem or the global environment

synergism
the occurrence of a joint effect of two exposures that is greater than the sum of their individual effects

synthetic organic chemical
any manufactured organic chemical

T

tallow
the animal fat product of the rendering process

target organ
in toxicity testing, the organ that is affected first as the dose of a test chemical is increased from zero (*not* an organ that a toxic chemical seeks out in the body)

target pest
the specific pest that is the target of a pesticide application

target pest resurgence
the rebounding of the target pest population after the population of a natural predator is reduced through the use of a pesticide

temperature inversion
a local weather condition in which a mass of cooler, heavier air becomes trapped at ground level beneath a layer of warmer, less dense air

teratogen
a substance that causes teratogenesis

teratogenesis
the occurrence of a structural defect in the developing organism as a result of an exposure that occurs between conception and birth

tertiary sewage treatment
specialized treatment technologies, used after primary and secondary sewage treatment, and tailored to local needs

thermohaline circulation
the global circulation of deep ocean waters along predictable paths, driven mainly by differences in the density of the water related to temperature (*thermo*) and salinity (*haline*)

thickening (of sewage sludge)
the first step in the treatment of sewage sludge, usually accomplished by centrifuging or adding coagulants

threshold (of a dose–response curve)
the highest dose at which no toxic effect occurs

Threshold Limit Value
concentration of a specific chemical in workplace air that is expected to be without material adverse health effect; published by the American Council of Governmental Industrial Hygienists

threshold shift
an upward shift in an individual's hearing threshold; a marker of hearing loss

tinnitus
a ringing in the ears that occurs after a short-term exposure to a very loud noise

Toxics Release Inventory (TRI)
a publicly available online database of the quantities of chemicals released to air or water, placed on land, or transferred offsite by industrial facilities

toxicant
a toxic substance that results from human activities; also, naturally occurring agents that are not produced by a plant or animal

toxicity
poisonous effect; harm to the body

toxicity testing
the practical work of assessing chemicals' toxicity to living things

toxicodynamics
the processes that constitute the effects of a toxicant in the body; changes in tissue structure or function, and resulting adverse effects on health

toxicokinetic modeling
estimation of the ultimate disposition of a chemical from what is known about its absorption, distribution, metabolism, storage, and excretion

toxicokinetics
the combined processes of absorption, distribution, metabolism, storage, and excretion

toxicology
the science of the disposition and effects in the body of toxic substances, including man-made chemicals, natural toxins, and physical hazards such as asbestos fibers and radiation

toxin
a naturally produced toxic substance, especially one produced by a plant or animal

trachea
the cartilaginous windpipe below the larynx, considered a part of the lower respiratory system.

transgene (or *biotech gene*)
a gene that codes for a desired characteristic and that is transferred from the DNA of one species into the DNA of the species being modified (for example, corn)

transgenic (or *genetically engineered* or *genetically modified*)
modified by the insertion of a transgene

transmissible spongiform encephalopathy (TSE)
a degenerative brain disease caused by abnormal prion proteins that can be transmitted between hosts

transpiration
a process through which water taken up by the roots of plants is released to the atmosphere through their leaves

trash
see *municipal solid waste*

trickling filter
in secondary sewage treatment, a bed of rocks coated with bacteria-containing slime over which municipal wastewater is sprayed and allowed to trickle downward to facilitate bacterial digestion of organic wastes

trihalomethanes (THMs)
a family of chemicals that are common disinfection by-products

troposphere
the innermost layer of the earth's atmosphere, extending to an altitude of approximately 8 miles (13 kilometers)

turbidity
the cloudiness of water; specifically, a measure of how much the transmission of light through water is impaired

U

ultrafine particulates
generally, particulates 0.1 microns or less in diameter

ultraviolet radiation
a form of electromagnetic radiation that includes both ionizing wavelengths (UV-C radiation) and nonionizing wavelengths (UV-A and UV-B)

uncertainty factor
a multiplier used in deriving a reference dose to set the reference dose lower (ie, to make it more protective) to account for a specific limitation in the available toxicity data

unconfined aquifer
see *water table aquifer*

upgradient
in the direction opposite to the direction of groundwater flow within an aquifer; analogous to *upstream* in surface water

uranium
a radioactive metallic element used as fuel in nuclear power reactors

uranium mill tailings
depleted uranium ore in the form of sandy sludge, a waste of the production of yellowcake

V

vaccine
an antigen preparation administered to a person to produce an immune response without causing illness

vaccine-preventable diseases
the set of diseases for which a vaccine is presently available

variant Creutzfeldt-Jakob disease (vCJD)
a transmissible spongiform encephalopathy of humans, linked to eating beef from cattle afflicted with bovine spongiform encephalopathy

vector (of infectious disease)
any living transmitter of pathogens

vectorborne disease
an infectious disease that is transmitted by biological vector

vermicomposting
indoor composting of plant-based food scraps by worms housed in a bin

virus
a parasite consisting of a strand of DNA or RNA with a coat of protein; cannot reproduce without a host organism

volatile organic compound (VOC)
a naturally occurring or man-made organic compound that volatilizes significantly at ordinary environmental temperatures

volatility
the tendency of a liquid chemical to change into gaseous form (that is, to volatilize)

volume threshold
the lowest volume at which sound at a given frequency can be heard

W

waste prevention
see *source reduction*

waste-to-energy (WTE) incineration
burning of municipal solid waste in an incinerator that also generates energy

water table
the boundary between the zone of aeration and the saturated zone

water table aquifer (or *unconfined aquifer*)
an aquifer in which the recharge area is directly above the aquifer, with no intervening impermeable layer

waterborne illness
any infectious disease transmitted in drinking water; often fecal in origin

waterborne transmission (of infectious disease)
the transmission of pathogens, often pathogens of fecal origin, in water used for drinking

watershed
in environmental health, the area drained by a river and the streams that feed it (synonymous with *drainage basin*); in common speech, also refers to the divide between two drainage basins

weed
a plant pest

weight-of-the-evidence categories
a set of categories describing the likely human carcinogenicity of a chemical, based on the total body of scientific evidence

wind farm
a group of wind turbines installed together

wind power
the energy of moving air, captured by a wind turbine

worms
multicellular organisms ranging widely in size, but all visible to the naked eye; some are parasitic and pathogenic

X

xenoestrogen
an environmental chemical that mimics the effect of estrogen in the human body

X-rays
an ionizing form of electromagnetic radiation, widely used for medical imaging

Y

yellowcake
the uranium concentrate that is extracted from uranium ore through milling

Z

zone of aeration
a subsurface zone within which the pore spaces are partly filled by water, and water moves only downward

zoonosis
an infectious disease that can be transmitted to humans from nonhuman animals, either domestic or wild

Index

A